Speech and Language Therapy
A Primer

Providing a comprehensive introduction to speech and language therapy, this book introduces students to the linguistic, medical, scientific and psychological disciplines that lie at the foundation of this health profession. As well as examining foundational disciplines, the volume also addresses professional issues in speech and language therapy and examines how therapists assess and treat clients with communication and swallowing disorders. The book makes extensive use of group exercises that allow SLT students opportunity for practice-based learning. It also includes multiple case studies to encourage discussion of assessment and intervention practices, and end-of-chapter questions with answers to test knowledge and understanding. In addition to providing a solid theoretical grounding in communication disorders, this volume will equip students with a range of professional skills, such as how to treat patients, how to diagnose and assess clients, how to help parents support children with communication disabilities, and how to assess the effectiveness of the various practices and methods used in intervention.

LOUISE CUMMINGS is Professor in the Department of English at The Hong Kong Polytechnic University. She teaches and conducts research in pragmatics and clinical linguistics. She is the author of several books, including *Case Studies in Communication Disorders* (2016), *Pragmatic and Discourse Disorders: A Workbook* (2015) and *The Communication Disorders Workbook* (2014). She has also edited a number of books including *Research in Clinical Pragmatics* (2017) and *The Cambridge Handbook of Communication Disorders* (2014).

Speech and Language Therapy

A Primer

LOUISE CUMMINGS
The Hong Kong Polytechnic University

CAMBRIDGE UNIVERSITY PRESS

CAMBRIDGE
UNIVERSITY PRESS

University Printing House, Cambridge CB2 8BS, United Kingdom

One Liberty Plaza, 20th Floor, New York, NY 10006, USA

477 Williamstown Road, Port Melbourne, VIC 3207, Australia

314–321, 3rd Floor, Plot 3, Splendor Forum, Jasola District Centre, New Delhi – 110025, India

79 Anson Road, #06–04/06, Singapore 079906

Cambridge University Press is part of the University of Cambridge.

It furthers the University's mission by disseminating knowledge in the pursuit of education, learning, and research at the highest international levels of excellence.

www.cambridge.org
Information on this title: www.cambridge.org/cummingsSLT
DOI: 10.1017/9781316796061

© Louise Cummings 2018

This publication is in copyright. Subject to statutory exception and to the provisions of relevant collective licensing agreements, no reproduction of any part may take place without the written permission of Cambridge University Press.

First published 2018

Printed in the United Kingdom by TJ International Ltd. Padstow Cornwall

A catalogue record for this publication is available from the British Library.

Library of Congress Cataloging-in-Publication Data
Names: Cummings, Louise, author.
Title: Speech and language therapy : a primer / Louise Cummings.
Description: Cambridge, United Kingdom ; New York, NY : Cambridge University Press, 2019. | Includes bibliographical references and index.
Identifiers: LCCN 2017034628 | ISBN 9781107174665 (hardback : alk. paper) | ISBN 9781316626719 (paperback)
Subjects: | MESH: Speech Therapy | Language Therapy | Communication Disorders–therapy | Communication Disorders–diagnosis | Professionalism
Classification: LCC RC423 | NLM WL 340.2 | DDC 616.85/5–dc23
LC record available at https://lccn.loc.gov/2017034628

ISBN 978-1-107-17466-5 Hardback
ISBN 978-1-316-62671-9 Paperback

Cambridge University Press has no responsibility for the persistence or accuracy of URLs for external or third-party internet websites referred to in this publication and does not guarantee that any content on such websites is, or will remain, accurate or appropriate.

Contents

List of Figures	*page* ix
List of Tables	xi
Acknowledgements	xiii
Preface	xv

1	Introduction to Speech and Language Therapy	1
	1.1 What Is Speech and Language Therapy?	1
	1.2 Why Study Speech and Language Therapy?	11
	1.3 What Do SLT Students Need to Learn?	15
	1.4 SLT and Clients with Communication and Swallowing Disorders	18
	1.5 SLT and Families and Carers	22
	1.6 SLT and Public Health	27
	Suggestions for Further Reading	30
	Questions	31
2	Linguistic Disciplines	34
	2.1 Introduction	34
	2.2 Phonetics	35
	2.3 Phonology	41
	2.4 Morphology	45
	2.5 Syntax	48
	2.6 Semantics	51
	2.7 Pragmatics	55
	2.8 Discourse	61
	2.9 Sociolinguistics	65
	2.10 Psycholinguistics	69
	2.11 Neurolinguistics	76
	2.12 Child Language Acquisition	78
	Suggestions for Further Reading	82
	Questions	83
3	Medical and Scientific Disciplines	87
	3.1 Introduction	87
	3.2 Epidemiology and Aetiology	89
	3.3 Anatomy and Physiology	92
	3.4 Neurology	96

	3.5 ENT Medicine	100
	3.6 Audiology	107
	3.7 Psychiatry	117
	3.8 Other Medical Disciplines	120
	Suggestions for Further Reading	124
	Questions	125
4	**Psychological Disciplines**	**129**
	4.1 SLT and Psychology	129
	4.2 Developmental Psychology	134
	4.3 Educational Psychology	140
	4.4 Cognitive Psychology	146
	4.5 Neuropsychology	151
	4.6 Clinical Psychology	157
	Suggestions for Further Reading	162
	Questions	163
5	**Assessment and Diagnosis**	**166**
	5.1 Introduction	166
	5.2 Formal and Informal Assessment	170
	5.3 Clinical Assessments: Speech	176
	5.4 Clinical Assessments: Language	183
	5.5 Clinical Assessments: Fluency	195
	5.6 Clinical Assessments: Voice	201
	5.7 Clinical Assessments: Swallowing	206
	5.8 Diagnostic and Classification Systems	210
	Suggestions for Further Reading	216
	Questions	217
6	**Intervention and Outcomes**	**220**
	6.1 Introduction	220
	6.2 Direct and Indirect Approaches to Intervention	223
	6.3 Clinical Interventions: Speech	227
	6.4 Clinical Interventions: Language	237
	6.5 Clinical Interventions: Fluency	245
	6.6 Clinical Interventions: Voice	249
	6.7 Clinical Interventions: Swallowing	254
	6.8 Evidence-Based Practice	260
	Suggestions for Further Reading	265
	Questions	265
7	**The Profession of Speech and Language Therapy**	**268**
	7.1 Introduction	268
	7.2 SLT in Multidisciplinary Teams	269
	7.3 SLT across Contexts and Countries	275

7.4 SLT Professional Bodies and Associations	284
7.5 SLT and Charitable Organizations	290
Suggestions for Further Reading	299
Questions	300
Notes	302
Answers	304
Appendix	317
Glossary	318
Bibliography	377
Index	411

Colour plate section can be found between pages 204 and 205

Figures

2.1a	Diagram of sound wave showing amplitude, frequency and wavelength	*page* 38
2.1b	Spectrogram and waveform of a sentence read aloud	38
2.2	Structure of the ear	39
2.3	A simplified model of the stages of language production	73
2.4	A simplified model of the stages of language comprehension	75
3.1	External auditory canal atresia	101
3.2	Grades of microtia	102
3.3	Audiogram in noise-induced hearing loss	104
3.4	Audiogram in sensory presbycusis	108
3.5	Audiogram in conductive hearing loss	109
3.6	Pure tone audiometry typical of Ménière's disease	110
3.7	Normal type A tympanogram and type B tympanogram in otitis media with effusion	112
3.8	An MRI of a right-sided acoustic neuroma	113
3.9	Diagram showing the components of a cochlear implant	115
4.1	The scales of the *Wechsler Intelligence Scale for Children – Fifth Edition* (WISC-V)	142
4.2	Model of language processing in *Psycholinguistic Assessments of Language Processing in Aphasia (PALPA)*	148
4.3	Stimulus pictures from the *Pyramids and Palm Trees Test*	150
4.4	Trail-Making Test, Part B	155
5.1	(a) A cuffed tracheostomy tube. (b) Tracheostomy tube in situ with cuff inflated	169
5.2	Pictures from the *Goldman-Fristoe Test of Articulation – Third Edition* (GFTA-3) for younger and older examinees	181
5.3	The *Predictive Cluttering Inventory* (PCI)	199
5.4	Flexible fibreoptic nasolaryngoscopy	203
5.5	The components of the WHO's *International Classification of Functioning, Disability and Health* (ICF) framework	215
6.1	SLT interventions arranged along a direct-indirect intervention continuum	224

6.2	Submucosal haemorrhage of the right vocal fold	252
6.3	Three methods of alaryngeal communication	255
6.4	A PEG tube – the MiniONE® Balloon Button	258
7.1	*The King's Speech* has been used in awareness-raising campaigns by a range of charitable and non-profit organizations	297

Tables

1.1	Roles of the speech and language therapist	*page* 4
1.2	Number of students by intervention area served by speech-language pathologists in ASHA's (2014) Schools Survey	9
5.1	Advantages and disadvantages of formal and informal assessments	175
5.2	Core and supplemental phonological processes in the *Khan-Lewis Phonological Analysis – Third Edition* (KLPA-3)	182
5.3	The *Clinical Evaluation of Language Fundamentals – Fifth Edition* (CELF-5) tests and their objectives	186
5.4	The domains and subtests in the standard version of the *Boston Diagnostic Aphasia Examination – Third Edition* (BDAE-3)	190
5.5	Diagnostic criteria for social communication disorder in *Diagnostic and Statistical Manual of Mental Disorders – Fifth Edition* (DSM-5)	212
6.1	Speech interventions in children	229
6.2	Language interventions in children	238
7.1	Data from ASHA's 2015 SLP Health Care Survey showing SLT services in a range of facilities	276
7.2	Data from ASHA's 2016 Schools Survey showing SLT services in a range of facilities	277
7.3	ASHA membership categories for year-end 2015	284
7.4	Clinical guidelines of Speech Pathology Australia	287
7.5	Charities that support people with communication and swallowing disorders	291
7.6	Titles of research studies funded by the Stroke Association in the UK	295

Acknowledgements

There are a number of people whose assistance I wish to acknowledge. I particularly want to thank Helen Barton, Commissioning Editor in Language and Linguistics at Cambridge University Press, for responding positively to the proposal for this book. I am grateful to a number of individuals and organizations for permission to use images throughout this book: Jenny Loehr; Mark Liberman; Laughlin Dawes; Sheryl Lewin; Joe Hinz; Leah Garaas; Maurice H. Miller; John Rutka; Valeria Abusamra; Daniel Low; David A. Daly; James P. Thomas; Bechara Y. Ghorayeb; Woods Hole Oceanographic Institution; MED-EL; International Hearing Society; Occupational Safety and Health Administration, USA; GN Otometrics; Pearson; Taylor & Francis Ltd; US Department of Transportation; World Health Organization; Cook Medical; Otolaryngology Houston; InHealth Technologies; Applied Medical Technology, Inc.; The Stuttering Foundation of America. I also wish to acknowledge the assistance of Judith Heaney who collated the manuscript. Finally, I have been supported by family members and friends who are too numerous to mention individually. I am grateful to them for their kind words of encouragement during my many months of work on this volume.

Preface

I have very clear recollection of my time as a student of speech and language therapy. When I began my course, my initial thoughts could be summarized in a single question: How would I ever get to grips with the large range of subjects that this course was demanding of me and my peers? I was continually moving between lectures in phonetics and syntax, anatomy and physiology, developmental and cognitive psychology, and the physics of speech, sound and hearing. Evenings and weekends were also devoted to many hours of study in different linguistic, medical and scientific disciplines. I felt that much more was demanded of a student of speech and language therapy in terms of disciplinary breadth and scope than of students in other subject areas. And so it continued for four years, with classes in neurology and cognitive neuropsychology occurring alongside lectures in pragmatics, psychiatry and audiology. Clinical practice brought additional challenges, with all manner of knowledge relating to assessment and intervention demanded during our assigned placements. My classmates and I knew what it was like to have to find our feet quickly in diverse subject areas and juggle different disciplinary terminology and frameworks.

We did, of course, find our feet. But it occurred to me any number of times that we could have done so more easily if we had had access to a single, self-contained resource that served as a comprehensive introduction to each of the disciplines that we were studying for the first time. This book is intended to be that resource. The student who reads this volume and works through its questions and exercises will receive the best possible grounding in all the linguistic, medical, scientific and psychological disciplines that a degree course in speech and language therapy (or speech-language pathology) has to offer. The same student will also be well versed in techniques of assessment and intervention in all six areas of concern to SLTs: speech; language; fluency; hearing; voice; and swallowing. Ultimately, students of speech and language therapy enter a profession that must respond to agendas in healthcare, such as evidence-based practice, and deal with the challenges of a growing elderly population with complex health needs. Professional issues ranging from continuing professional development to models of service delivery are ever present for SLTs. This volume will also introduce students to the profession that they will join upon graduating from their studies at university.

To convey all of the above in a clear and accessible manner, this volume includes a wide range of pedagogical features. These features are listed below.

Most of these features are designed to facilitate student learning by providing opportunities to rehearse knowledge and to explore clients and their communication disorders in more detail. Other features are designed to ensure easy navigation around the volume and to reduce the need to consult other sources for definitions of terms and background information. The combination of these features provides a complete learning package for students who are approaching a course of study in speech and language therapy for the first time:

- Key points boxes at the end of each section, which summarize main points
- Special topics boxes for further exploration of SLT and communication disorders
- Case studies that encourage discussion of assessment and intervention practices
- Group exercises that permit reflection and problem-solving among students
- End-of-chapter questions with answers to test knowledge
- A glossary with over 600 entries
- Bold terms throughout the text that relate to entries in the glossary
- Annotated suggestions for further reading
- www.cambridge.org/9781107174665 with 140 self-test questions and answers and other resources
- A detailed index

Every author wants his or her book to make a significant and original contribution to the literature in a certain field. The contribution that I would like this volume to make can best be described in terms of the perceptions of its student readers. I would like the readers of this book to have a 'one-stop shop' that they can use to obtain a thorough grounding in all the disciplines that they will encounter in an SLT course. If this volume accomplishes this task well, it will go a substantial way towards reducing the feelings of disciplinary overload that are experienced by many new students of speech and language therapy.

1 Introduction to Speech and Language Therapy

1.1 What Is Speech and Language Therapy?

Speech and language therapy (SLT) is an important health discipline that is responsible for the management of children and adults with communication and swallowing disorders. The individuals who practise this discipline – speech and language therapists (SLTs) – assess, diagnose and treat these disorders as well as perform a number of other key roles. SLT is a large and growing profession. The Royal College of Speech and Language Therapists (RCSLT), the professional body for SLTs in the United Kingdom, has more than 16,000 members. Its counterpart association in the United States, the American Speech-Language-Hearing Association (ASHA), reports that at the end of 2014 it had 150,468 **speech-language pathologists** (SLPs) as certified members and non-members. In this chapter, you will be introduced to the work of this rewarding health profession. In the rest of this section, the roles that are performed by SLTs will be examined. In addition to assessment, diagnosis and treatment, these roles include education of clients and families as well as advocacy for people with communication disorders. This section will also address the many misconceptions about SLT that exist among the general public. These misconceptions can be troublesome in that they can dissuade people both from entering the profession and from availing of the services that SLT can offer.

Later sections in the chapter will expand your understanding of the professional remit of SLT. In section 1.2, the question 'Why study speech and language therapy?' is posed. The answer to this question involves several dimensions, the most important of which is that communication and swallowing disorders cause distress to, and limit the life chances of, a large number of individuals. A society that rightly values these individuals will seek to mitigate the negative effects of these disorders by providing appropriate clinical services. In section 1.3, the question 'What do SLT students need to learn?' invites examination of the knowledge base that informs SLT. This knowledge base is very large indeed and includes academic learning of linguistic and medical-scientific disciplines, on the one hand, and a range of clinical skills on the other hand. In section 1.4, the children and adults who are the primary concern of SLT are examined. These individuals have developmental and acquired communication and swallowing disorders. Some of these disorders will be examined in this section. SLT is almost never conducted in isolation from the families and carers of people with communication disorders. The important roles that these individuals play in SLT intervention with clients will be addressed in section 1.5. Finally, in section 1.6, the growing calls for SLT to make a contribution to public health are examined.

As a window onto the work of SLT, let us consider the following scenario. Mary is a 50-year-old primary school teacher. She is married and has three teenage children. She has enjoyed good physical and mental health as an adult. Mary drives the 10 miles to her work each day. On her way to work one day, she is involved in a serious road traffic accident. She sustains a severe head injury as well as chest and abdominal injuries. Upon arrival at hospital, she undergoes a **CAT scan** which reveals a **subdural haematoma** in her brain. Emergency surgery is undertaken to relieve pressure on her brain. Her condition after surgery is monitored in the hospital's intensive care unit. When the neurologist in charge of Mary is satisfied that she is out of immediate danger, a referral is made to the hospital's speech and language therapy department. An SLT visits Mary, who has now been moved to the high-dependency unit. She is alert and appears to be oriented to time and place. However, she is completely mute and cannot make use of gestures. A bedside assessment reveals comprehension of simple four- and five-word utterances. Mary indicates her understanding of these utterances through eye movements. Longer, more complex utterances do not receive a response. Mary is receiving non-oral feeding. The SLT continues to work with Mary while she is an inpatient in the head trauma rehabilitation unit in the hospital. Mary is discharged from hospital six months after admission. After discharge, the SLT continues to work with her as an outpatient, both on a one-to-one basis and during weekly group therapy with other head trauma clients.

The above scenario does not describe an actual case. However, it serves to illustrate the types of circumstances that may cause clients to access SLT services. Among other difficulties, Mary's head injury has resulted in impairments of communication and swallowing. The information presented above is limited. Yet, it is nonetheless clear that Mary has a **language disorder**, as she is unable to understand utterances beyond a certain level of linguistic complexity. She is also unable to produce or express utterances. Her difficulties with the expression of language are compounded by the presence of a **motor speech disorder** that prevents her from producing intelligible speech sounds. As well as a language and speech disorder, Mary has a disorder of swallowing, or **dysphagia**. It is her inability to swallow safely that necessitates non-oral feeding. It is the responsibility of the SLT to assess and diagnose each of these disorders and to undertake an appropriate course of intervention. However, the SLT's duty of care towards Mary does not end there. Mary has a husband and three teenage children who are distressed by their inability to communicate effectively with her. The SLT has an important role to play in educating Mary's family members about her communication and swallowing problems. This educational role should include advice about the adjustments that they can make to facilitate communication with

Mary, including specific techniques that may make it easier for Mary to understand them.

So far, four roles of the SLT in the management of Mary's case have been identified: it is the role of the SLT to *assess*, *diagnose* and *treat* Mary's communication and swallowing disorders and to *educate* her family members about these disorders and what adjustments they can undertake in order to lessen their impact on communication. But the SLT is also performing three further roles that may not be so evident in the above scenario. The reason Mary has received SLT services during her stay as an inpatient in the hospital's head trauma rehabilitation unit is because of the SLT's role as an *advocate* of clients with communication disorders. It is through the role of advocate that the SLT has pressed the case for continued funding of SLT services against a backdrop of reduced healthcare spending. This role may bring the SLT into contact with health service managers and private medical insurers who need to be persuaded of the long-term benefits of SLT services to clients who sustain head trauma. As part of Mary's rehabilitation, she also participates in weekly group therapy with other head trauma clients. The intervention that is offered to these clients is the focus of a research study in which the SLT is the principal clinical investigator. In the role of *researcher*, the SLT aims to establish if group therapy can achieve significant improvements in the social communication skills of clients with head trauma. Finally, two junior therapists in the SLT department also participate in Mary's group therapy. It is the SLT's role to act as a *mentor* to these colleagues in order that they may acquire the clinical skills that are needed to work with this complex client group. All seven roles of the SLT are summarized in Table 1.1.

Having established the roles of the SLT, it is now necessary to consider certain misconceptions about speech and language therapy. For the most part, these misconceptions exist among members of the public. However, somewhat surprisingly, they are also often found among other medical and health professionals. The three misconceptions that will be addressed in the rest of this section are: (1) SLT is a career for women only; (2) SLTs work only with children who have speech disorders; and (3) SLT is concerned with accent improvement and elocution. Although other 'myths' about SLT do exist, these misconceptions are the most commonly encountered mistaken beliefs about the profession. They are also some of the most harmful beliefs in that they can deter individuals from considering SLT as a career or clients from seeking a range of SLT services. It is hoped that the exposure of these misconceptions will go some way towards reducing their influence or even eliminating them altogether.

The misconception that SLT is a career for women only is explicable to some extent. Notwithstanding the growing participation of both genders in a range of occupations, it remains the case today that considerably more women than men pursue a career in SLT. Data from the Office of National Statistics in the UK show that between April to June 2015, 21,000 people were employed as SLTs. Women accounted for 19,000 of these employees. By year end 2014, men comprised only 3.7% of the SLPs certified by ASHA. Speech Pathology

Table 1.1 *Roles of the speech and language therapist*

SLT role	Description	Examples
Assessment	SLTs use a range of clinical tools to assess the speech, language, voice, fluency and swallowing abilities of clients. Assessment establishes if there is a need for intervention and creates a baseline against which progress in therapy can be charted.	The SLT can use **standardized tests** to assess the language skills of children (e.g. Clinical Evaluation of Language Fundamentals; Semel et al., 2003). Some forms of assessment must use specialist equipment (e.g. the use of **videofluoroscopy** to evaluate swallowing).
Diagnosis	SLTs use the results of assessment to arrive at a diagnosis of a client's communication or swallowing disorder. Internationally recognized diagnostic systems can be used to guide diagnosis (e.g. ***Diagnostic and Statistical Manual of Mental Disorders – Fifth Edition*** (DSM-5); American Psychiatric Association, 2013).	The SLT can use results from the Boston Diagnostic Aphasia Examination (Goodglass et al., 2001) to diagnose an adult with a specific **aphasia** syndrome following a **cerebrovascular accident** (CVA or stroke). The SLT can use criteria in DSM-5 to diagnose a child with social (pragmatic) communication disorder.
Treatment	SLTs use a range of interventions to treat communication and swallowing disorders. Most interventions aim to achieve measurable gains in speech and language skills. Where improvements in these skills are not possible (e.g. in clients with severe neurological impairment), use may be made of **augmentative and alternative communication** (AAC).	SLTs use different approaches, techniques and equipment to treat communication and swallowing disorders. Some interventions are indirect in nature and involve advice to parents and carers (e.g. environmental modifications proposed to the parents of a dysfluent child). Other interventions involve direct work with clients (e.g. phonological therapy in children with unintelligibility).
Education	SLTs undertake important educational work with clients, families, carers, other medical and health professionals and the general public. This	Clients with **voice disorders** may need to be educated about the lifestyle factors that contribute to **dysphonia**. Spouses of clients with

Table 1.1 (*cont.*)

SLT role	Description	Examples
	educational work often occurs alongside intervention or it may be a stand-alone activity (e.g. an awareness-raising campaign among the general public about communication disorders).	aphasia must receive education about this language disorder and its implications for communication. Carers and support workers of adults with **intellectual disability** require education and training in AAC (e.g. **Makaton**).
Advocacy	Owing to their communication disability, children and adults with communication disorders require others to be advocates for them. The SLT performs an important advocacy role for these clients at local, regional and national levels.	The SLT may act as an advocate for the teenager with speech, language and communication needs in the criminal justice system. The SLT can act as an advocate for clients with progressive, neurological disorders who have limited communication at the end of their lives.
Research	SLTs also contribute to the knowledge base of their discipline by undertaking clinical research. This research role can be pursued through a programme of study (e.g. masters or doctoral studies) or as part of a therapist's routine clinical practice.	The SLT's research role can take many forms including the selection of clients according to study criteria, the implementation of a particular intervention, the recording and analysis of linguistic data, and the preparation of a journal article or book for publication.
Mentoring	The SLT also has a duty to mentor less experienced therapists and to act as a mentor to SLT students who are on clinical placements.	The SLT's mentoring role might involve regular meetings to discuss progress and concerns of junior colleagues, or observation of and feedback on clinical sessions in the case of SLT students on placements.

Australia has approximately 6,000 practising members. Of this number, 98% are women and only 2% are men. The predominance of women in the profession is in stark contrast to the predominance of men in the client groups that are assessed and treated by SLTs. Significantly more boys and men than girls and women have communication disorders such as **speech sound disorders**, **specific language impairment** (SLI) and developmental **stuttering**, and males account for the majority of individuals with conditions such as **autism spectrum disorder** (ASD) and **attention deficit hyperactivity disorder** (ADHD). If for no other reason than that SLTs are not representative of the clients they serve, efforts should be taken to correct this gender imbalance.

Central to these efforts will be a better understanding of why men are not inclined to pursue a career in SLT. A study by Litosseliti and Leadbeater (2013) gives us some insight into widely held perceptions and beliefs that may discourage men from entering the profession. One influential factor is the perceived prestige, status and salary of the profession. A careers adviser and SLT teacher in this study remarked:

> A lot of my boys to be honest, they want to be engineers or they want to earn lots of money in the city. (careers adviser)
>
> I think, you know, that one of the contributing factors when men look at this as a profession could be the erm ... although it's much better, is the career progress, the career structure and the pay-scales. (SLT teacher)

Other influential factors identified by Litosseliti and Leadbeater included the perception that SLT is 'women's work'. Women are perceived to be carers and nurturers, and these are attributes associated with all the healthcare professions, including SLT. There is also a general perception that women are better communicators than men, and so women are more suited to an occupation that assesses and treats people with communication disorders:

> I think there's the perception that women are more communicative than men whether it turns out to be more realistic ... communication and talking is always just thought of as a female thing. (female SLT)

Many of these perceptions were challenged by the careers advisers, SLT teachers and SLTs in Litosseliti and Leadbeater's study. Nevertheless, their presence is still sufficiently widespread to act as a significant disincentive to men to enter the profession. Until these perceptions can be more effectively challenged than it has been possible to achieve to date, it seems almost certain that SLT will continue to be viewed as a career for women only. This will represent a loss not only for men who would find SLT a challenging and rewarding career, but also for certain male clients with communication disorders (e.g. in the criminal justice system) who might respond more favourably to the presence of male therapists.

SPECIAL TOPIC: The SLT Workforce

SLT is widely perceived to be a 'white female' profession. This perception is borne out by the demographics of the SLT workforce. Figures from Health Workforce Australia (2014) confirm that SLT is a predominantly female profession. Between 1996 and 2011, females accounted for well over 90% of the workforce:

> 1996 (96.7% female)   2001 (97.1% female)
> 2006 (97.2% female)   2011 (97.5% female)
>
> The workforce in the UK and USA is also predominantly female. In September 2013, the SLT workforce in England was 2.5% male and 97.5% female (Health and Social Care Information Centre, 2014). By the end of 2015, males accounted for 3.7% of speech-language pathologists who were members of the American Speech-Language-Hearing Association. This pattern is replicated in the number of males enrolled in communication sciences and disorders courses at university. In the academic year 2014–2015, some 36,498 undergraduate students were enrolled in these courses in the USA (Council of Academic Programs in Communication Sciences and Disorders & ASHA, 2016). Only 4.8% of these students were male. To the extent that most SLT training places are also occupied by women, it appears unlikely that the gender imbalance of the profession will change any time soon.
>
> There is little ethnic diversity in SLT. Most members of the profession are white. By year-end 2015, 7.8% of ASHA members belonged to a racial minority. This compared with 27.6% of the US population, according to data from the 2010 Census. In 2011, only 11 of 5,296 speech pathologists in Australia had Aboriginal and Torres Strait Islander status (Health Workforce Australia, 2014). Reasons for the under-representation of ethnic minorities in the SLT workforce were examined by Greenwood et al. (2006). These investigators examined attitudes towards, and awareness of, SLT in 651 school and college students who were close to selecting degree courses. Among ethnic minority students, there was a lack of awareness that SLT is a degree course. These students also placed greater importance on studying for a degree, a profession and a scientific career, and were more influenced by a career's prestige and a high salary.
>
> Age is another important demographic feature of the SLT workforce. Knowledge of the age profile of the profession is vital to workforce planning. For example, if a large proportion of the workforce is close to retirement age, it may be necessary to increase the number of SLT training places. In 2011, 6.8% of speech pathologists in Australia were aged 55 years and older (Health Workforce Australia, 2014). Currently, the age profile of speech-language pathologists in the USA is evenly distributed, as demonstrated by the following data from ASHA for year-end 2015:
>
> 34 and younger   35 to 44   45 to 54   55 and older
> (27%)   (29%)   (21%)   (24%)
>
> The SLT workforce in the UK is relatively young. A large proportion of SLTs who work in the National Health Service are in their early 30s. Only 1.9% of the workforce is 60 or older. This indicates either an early retirement age or older SLTs choosing to work outside the National Health Service (Centre for Workforce Intelligence, 2014).

The second misconception about SLT – that SLTs work only with children who have speech disorders – is related to the first misconception in that a perceived child-caring role acts as a disincentive to men to pursue a career in SLT. The roots of this second misconception are to a large extent historical in nature. According to Duchan (2011), most histories of speech pathology in the

USA place the origins of the profession around 1925. At the same time, Duchan remarks, a number of influential US books were published. These books included Edward Wheeler Scripture's book *Stuttering and Lisping* (Scripture, 1912), which was published again 11 years later under the title *Stuttering, Lisping, and Correction of the Speech of the Deaf* (Scripture, 1923), and a book by Margaret Gray Blanton and Smiley Blanton entitled *Speech Training for Children* (1920). The focus of both volumes is on children with speech disorders, as these comments from the preface of Scripture's text indicate: 'This book has been prepared to meet the needs of physicians and teachers; both are constantly confronted with the problem of what is to be done with a lisping or a stuttering child' (1912: vi). (Lisping is Scripture's term for an **articulation disorder**.) Its historical origins aside, the misconception that SLTs work only with children with speech disorders still persists to the present day.

In section 1.4, the diverse clients who are assessed and treated by SLTs will be examined in more detail. But in order to demonstrate just how limited a view of the work of SLT this second misconception is, it will serve us to give some thought to the different conditions that are assessed and treated even just by paediatric SLTs. Speech disorders are only one of the ways in which communication can be impaired in children. Children may have language disorders such as specific language impairment. They may have voice disorders such as **puberphonia**. **Fluency disorders** such as stuttering and **cluttering** are managed by paediatric SLTs. **Conductive hearing loss** and **sensorineural hearing loss** also come under the purview of SLT. Aside from communication disorders, paediatric SLTs also assess and treat children with swallowing disorders. In the 2014 Schools Survey conducted by the American Speech-Language-Hearing Association (2014), SLPs were asked to respond to the following question: Indicate how many students you serve in each of the following areas. Across all facility types, the mean number of students served in each intervention area is indicated in Table 1.2. Table 1.2 shows that, taken together, speech disorders account for only a minority of the clients who are served by school SLPs in the USA. There is, therefore, no basis to the claim that SLTs work only or even mainly with children who have speech disorders.

It is also not true to characterize the work of SLTs as only or even mainly undertaken with children. SLTs work with clients of all ages. This can include babies with swallowing problems, preschool children with speech sound disorder, school-age children with specific language impairment, teenagers with stuttering, young adults with motor speech disorders, older adults with aphasia and elderly people with **cognitive-communication disorders** related to **dementia**. SLTs assess and treat communication and swallowing disorders across the entire life span. Figures from the 2015 SLP Health Care Survey Summary Report (ASHA, 2015a) reveal that, if anything, speech-language pathologists in the USA spend more clinical time working with adult clients. In this survey, respondents were asked: Of the time that you spend providing clinical services, approximately what percentage is spent with the following age groups? Across

Table 1.2 *Number of students (mean) by intervention area served by speech-language pathologists in ASHA's (2014) Schools Survey*

Intervention area	Number of students
Articulation/phonological disorders	20.5
Auditory processing disorder	6.9
Autism spectrum disorders	8.5
Childhood apraxia of speech	2.9
Cognitive-communication disorders	9.9
Dysphagia (swallowing/feeding)	2.6
Fluency disorders	2.5
Hearing loss	2.9
Language disorders: pragmatics/social communication	11.0
Language disorders: semantics, morphology, syntax	22.1
Nonverbal, AAC	4.7
Reading and writing (literacy)	14.6
Selective mutism	1.3
Traumatic brain injury	1.0
Voice or resonance disorders	1.5

all facility types, the mean percentages were 16.1% for infants and toddlers, 15.8% for preschool children, 14.5% for school-age clients and 53.6% for adult clients. The idea that SLTs treat children for the most part is not supported by the findings of this ASHA survey.

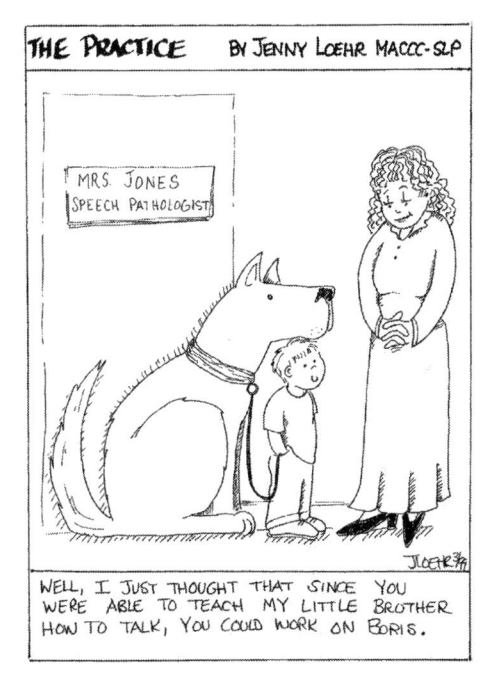

The third and final misconception that we will consider is that SLT is concerned with accent improvement and elocution.[1] As with the second misconception, this view of SLT has a historical basis. Duchan (2011) describes how a number of elocutionists who practised in the early nineteenth century saw communication disorders as within their scope of interest and practice. In his book *Analysis of the Principles of Rhetorical Delivery as Applied in Reading and Speaking*, the elocutionist Ebenezer Porter remarked of **stammering** as follows:

> As directly connected with articulation, a few remarks on impediments seem to be necessary. Stammering may doubtless exist from such causes, and to such a degree as to be insurmountable; though in most cases, a complete remedy is attainable by the early use of proper means. (1831: 32)

The elocutionist movement in the UK, which began around 1750, also had an interest in communication disorders. Duchan (2011) describes how one British elocutionist, James Hunt (1833–1869), worked to cure stammering and established his own practice in speech and voice disorders. Elocution is still widely practised today. But while regulatory bodies such as the Health & Care Professions Council in the UK prevent its practitioners from claiming to offer speech and language therapy, there has been no way of preventing the perception in people's minds that SLT is practising elocution. This perception of the work of SLTs is well entrenched and still persists today. It is not unusual for SLTs to be asked to work with clients for no other reason than that they have a socially undesirable accent. The following scenario is, unfortunately, not uncommon:

> Lee Dein, a speech and language therapist from north London, refuses to treat accents. 'Six months ago, a very posh chief executive telephoned and asked me to take on one of his employees who had a Birmingham accent. It was the first and last time I dealt with accents. During the fourth session, the woman broke down. She didn't see why she should be treated as if she had a speech problem and I agreed. The more people who treat accents in this way, the more it will be considered OK to discriminate against them.'
> ('Oi, You! Read This', *The Guardian*, 29 September 1999)

In the UK, the Shropshire paediatric speech and language therapy service has attempted to address this misconception directly by listing 'elocution and working on accents' as one of the services it does *not* offer to clients on its website. Another manifestation of this misconception is that individuals who are interested in pursuing a career in SLT must speak with a certain accent in order to be considered suitable candidates for the profession. The following comment from an online discussion forum reflects this view:

> I am interested in learning more about speech pathology as a career, and I have a question. This may be kind of weird to ask, but do all speech pathologists need to have perfect 'standard' accents and no speech problems themselves? For instance, if someone from the US had a very strong

southern accent, would this be a major problem if he or she chose to study speech pathology and pursue it as a career?

(Comment posted on *The Student Doctor Network*, 21 December 2012)

As with the other misconceptions examined in this section, the view that SLT is concerned with elocution and accent improvement not only is a misrepresentation of the work of SLTs but is also detrimental to recruitment to the profession

---

KEY POINTS: What Is Speech and Language Therapy?

- The most widely recognized roles of the SLT are the *assessment*, *diagnosis* and *treatment* of clients with communication and swallowing disorders.
- Other roles of the SLT include the contribution of knowledge to the discipline as a *researcher*, an *advocate* for those with communication disorders who cannot represent their own needs and views, an *educator* of clients and their families as well as the public about communication disorders, and a *mentor* of less experienced clinicians and student therapists.
- Misconceptions about SLT are commonplace in the general public and among other health professionals. They need to be exposed and resisted as they can deter individuals from pursuing a career in SLT, and clients from seeking SLT services.
- Three common misconceptions are that SLT is a career for women only, SLTs work only with children who have speech disorders and SLT is concerned with accent improvement and elocution.

1.2 Why Study Speech and Language Therapy?

Beyond leading to a rewarding career, the study of SLT is important for other reasons. Chief among them is that individuals with communication and swallowing disorders can experience considerable personal distress, social devaluation and occupational disadvantage. The interventions that SLT is able to offer these clients can mitigate many of these adverse consequences. These interventions can only be competently and effectively delivered by clinicians who have pursued a course of study in SLT at university or college. In addition to reducing the different impacts of communication and swallowing disorders, there is another reason why SLT should be considered a priority for academic and clinical study. The costs to society of communication and swallowing disorders are very large and growing. For the most part, these costs are measured in reduced economic productivity when individuals with these disorders are unable to work. But in addition to the costs of a lack of workplace activity, further costs are incurred when unemployed adults with communication and swallowing disorders receive state support for them and their families. Accordingly, there is a significant economic imperative for countries to invest in programmes of study that produce clinicians who can offer SLT services. In this section, we examine the impact of communication and swallowing disorders on the individuals who have these disorders. We also consider the economic case for prioritizing SLT as an area of academic and clinical study.

The impact of communication and swallowing disorders can be characterized in six different, but interrelated ways. The **psychological impact** of these disorders can include depression, anxiety, low self-esteem or even suicidal ideation related to a communication disorder. This type of impact may not arise immediately after the injury, illness or disease that causes a communication disorder, but it can persist for many months and years after the onset of a disorder (e.g. depression in adults with aphasia). The **social impact** of communication and swallowing disorders may be measured in various ways. It can include reduced friendship networks in adults who sustain a **traumatic brain injury** (TBI), victimization and bullying of children with specific language impairment, avoidance of certain social situations in teenagers who stutter and social withdrawal in adults with a cognitive-communication disorder. For the purposes of clinical study, the psychological and social impacts of communication and swallowing disorders are often examined alongside each other in investigations of the psychosocial impact of these disorders. This impact has been extensively investigated in a range of clients with communication disorders (see chapter 5 in Cummings, 2014a, for discussion).

The **behavioural impact** of communication and swallowing disorders is most often addressed in children who may display challenging behaviours in the classroom or at home as a result of a speech or language disorder. However, adults with communication disorders may also display hostile or aggressive behaviours that are related to their inability to communicate effectively. When problematic behaviours escalate into antisocial behaviour in the form of damage to property and harm to individuals, clinicians talk about the **forensic impact** of communication disorders. It is through this type of impact that children and adults with communication disorders are brought into contact with the criminal justice system (RCSLT, 2017). Many communication disorders can compromise learning and academic performance. The **academic impact** of a communication disorder may be measured in the number of qualifications achieved at different stages of formal education. Clearly, this particular impact is related to the **vocational impact** of communication disorders, especially in children, as poor academic qualifications directly limit the types of occupations that an individual can pursue. However, the adult who sustains a **stroke** may also experience the vocational impact of a communication disorder when he or she is unable to return to work on account of aphasia.

To illustrate these different impacts of communication disorders, consider the following scenario. Paul is a 7-year-old boy who has been diagnosed with significant expressive and receptive language delay. He attends a mainstream school where he receives SLT three times a week. Paul's teacher has observed a number of social and behavioural difficulties. His poor expressive language skills have created problems for him in his ability to initiate and maintain social interactions with other children in his class. When these interactions are unsuccessful, he responds with frustration and sometimes aggressive behaviour towards other children. His academic attainment is a cause of concern, as he is performing well below the class average in spelling and reading skills. At secondary school, Paul continues to experience academic difficulties. The school psychologist reports that he displays low self-esteem and has limited friendship networks in comparison to the other pupils. He has also been disciplined for smoking on school premises and can display temper outbursts in class when he is struggling with academic tasks. At 16 years of age, Paul achieves only three passes in his GCSE[2] subjects. He decides to undertake a vocational qualification in construction at his local college. While at college, he begins to engage in antisocial behaviour in the company of other boys on his course. This involves the use of illicit drugs, which brings him into contact with a juvenile court in the criminal justice system. His convictions for drug use make it difficult for him to secure employment in construction.

Although this is not an actual case, it resembles very closely the experiences of many children, and particularly boys, who have speech, language and communication needs. It is possible to identify all six of the impacts that were described above. These impacts arise directly and indirectly from Paul's expressive and receptive language delay. Paul's communication disorder appears to have a psychological impact in that the school psychologist has identified that he exhibits low self-esteem. The social impact of his communication disorder is manifested both in Paul's difficulty engaging in social interactions with other children and in his limited friendship networks when he attends secondary school. There is also a clear behavioural impact of Paul's language difficulties. When he is unable to initiate social interaction with other children, he can sometimes display aggressive behaviour. He is also prone to temper outbursts in class when he is confronted with challenging academic tasks. As Paul passes through secondary school and into college education, there are the first signs of a forensic impact of his communication disorder in the form of rule transgressions and other antisocial behaviour. He is disciplined for smoking on school premises and, when he attends college, he has contact with a juvenile court on account of illicit drug use. There is a considerable academic impact of his language difficulties in that he is well below the class average in spelling and reading and emerges with passes in only three GCSE subjects. Finally, Paul's limited academic attainment finds him pursuing a non-professional vocational role, with even that placed in jeopardy by his convictions for drug use.

To recap, a key reason for studying SLT is that the interventions it provides can go some way towards mitigating these different impacts of communication disorders. But this is not the only reason why individuals and societies should place emphasis on the study of SLT. There is also a strong economic imperative. Communication and swallowing disorders can cause reduced economic productivity. This is not just the case for the individuals who have these disorders but also for family members, many of whom leave employment to care for these individuals. In 2000, the economic cost of communication disorders in the USA was estimated to be between $154 billion and $186 billion per year, which is equal to 2.5% to 3% of Gross National Product (Ruben, 2000). The estimated lifetime costs in 2003 dollars are expected to total $2.1 billion for persons born in 2000 with hearing loss (RTI International and CDC, 2004). Most of these costs will come from lost wages due to inability or limited ability to work. SLT makes a significant contribution towards tackling these massive costs of communication disorders to the economies of countries. A report commissioned by the Royal College of Speech and Language Therapists in the UK and published in 2010 found that SLT across aphasia, specific language impairment and autism delivers an estimated net benefit of £765 million to the British economy each year (Marsh et al., 2010). If the impact of communication disorders alone does not persuade the reader of the need to study SLT, then surely this economic argument succeeds in making the case.

KEY POINTS: Why Study Speech and Language Therapy?

- Communication and swallowing disorders have adverse consequences for all aspects of an individual's life and functioning.
- These consequences are characterized in terms of a number of impacts which SLT interventions can mitigate. These impacts are psychological, social, behavioural, forensic, academic and vocational in nature.
- Psychological impacts may take the form of depression, anxiety and low self-esteem, while social impacts include social isolation and withdrawal and reduced friendship networks.
- Behavioural impacts include disruptive and challenging classroom behaviour in children and aggressive behaviour in adults with communication disability in the presence of dementia. If there is rule transgression, damage to property and harm to individuals, the communication disorder has a forensic impact.
- Academic impacts of communication disorders include poor performance in reading and spelling and limited school and college qualifications. Poor academic attainment limits the occupational roles that are available to individuals with communication disorders. Reduced employment opportunities are a vocational impact of these disorders.
- There is an economic imperative to study SLT, as the interventions that SLT can offer help to reduce the massive costs of communication disorders. These costs are incurred in several ways. There is reduced

economic productivity in individuals with communication and swallowing disorders. There needs to be state support of these individuals and their dependants. Family members may leave employment to care for individuals with communication and swallowing disorders.

1.3 What Do SLT Students Need to Learn?

The knowledge and skills that SLT students must acquire in order to practise competently and safely are very wide-ranging in nature. They include knowledge of a number of linguistic, medical and scientific disciplines. In order to characterize communication breakdown in children and adults, SLTs must understand, and accurately apply, terms and concepts in each of the following linguistic disciplines: phonetics; phonology; morphology; syntax; semantics; pragmatics; and discourse. In isolation, knowledge of these linguistic disciplines cannot achieve an accurate characterization of a communication disorder. SLTs must additionally understand the medical causes of a communication disorder (**aetiology**), how prevalent the disorder is (**epidemiology**), the presence of any malformation of the organs of speech (**anatomy**) and any impairment of their movement or function (**physiology**). Knowledge of other medical disciplines is needed in order to understand the clinical features of mental illnesses such as **schizophrenia (psychiatry)**, the neurological basis of motor speech disorders like **dysarthria (neurology)** and the vocal pathologies that can cause dysphonia (**otolaryngology**). This extensive linguistic, medical and scientific knowledge can only be pressed into action by SLTs who also have a range of clinical skills. These skills include technical abilities that are required to undertake speech and language analysis and to operate instruments and equipment in assessment. These skills also include clinical problem-solving and decision-making in everything from performing a differential diagnosis of a speech disorder to deciding when it is appropriate to discharge a client from therapy. In this section, we examine in brief the knowledge and clinical skills that students of SLT must learn in preparation for a more detailed treatment of these topics in later chapters.

Students of SLT will tell you that they spend a lot of time taking modules in linguistics. And so they should. Linguistics is well and truly a cornerstone of SLT. It is simply not possible to understand the **hypernasal speech** of a child with a **cleft lip and palate** in the absence of knowledge of speech sound production in **phonetics**. **Phonology** is used to characterize the sound and syllable simplifications (e.g. **stopping**, **consonant cluster reduction**) that occur in the speech of normally developing children and in children with **phonological disorders**. SLTs must understand **morphology** and **syntax** in order to characterize the morphosyntactic deficits of children with specific language impairment (e.g. *He fall off*) and the limited expressive syntax of **agrammatism** in aphasia. **Semantics** is used to characterize a range of deficits in adults with **Down**

syndrome including impaired knowledge of semantic fields (e.g. *fruit* and *transport*) and **lexical relations** between words such as hyponymy (e.g. *bird – eagle*) and antonymy (e.g. *hot – cold*). To understand why children and adults with ASD struggle to understand sarcastic utterances and figurative language such as **metaphors** (e.g. *The children were angels*) and **idioms** (e.g. *Jack spilled the beans*), SLTs must have a sound knowledge of each of these aspects of **pragmatics**. Poor **cohesion** and **coherence** in the narratives of adults who sustain a TBI and the egocentric language of adults with right-hemisphere damage are only meaningfully explained by SLTs who are well versed in **discourse**. Each of these linguistic disciplines will be explored further in Chapter 2.

Alongside modules in linguistics, students of SLT are equally committed to the study of a number of medical and scientific disciplines. The structures that produce speech and voice and that make hearing possible are studied in anatomy while the function of these structures is examined in physiology. It is one thing to know the different palatal clefts that can occur in a child (anatomy), and quite another thing to know how clefting can affect the function of the **velopharyngeal port** (physiology). Knowledge of the **central nervous system** and **peripheral nervous system** in neurology is the basis upon which SLTs understand language disorders such as aphasia and motor speech disorders like dysarthria. Otorhinolaryngology (or ENT medicine) is the medical discipline that SLTs draw upon to understand voice disorders and the organic conditions that can cause conductive and sensorineural hearing loss. SLTs must also understand methods of assessment in **audiology** (e.g. **pure tone audiometry**) and techniques that are used to achieve **amplification** for clients with different types of hearing loss. The medical discipline of **gastroenterology** is of increasing relevance to SLTs as the link between **gastroesophageal reflux disease** and **laryngeal cancer** has become increasingly clear. With the exception of disorders such as specific language impairment, the epidemiology of communication and swallowing disorders is still relatively under-investigated. Yet, knowledge of the incidence and prevalence of these disorders is important both for the planning of SLT services and for what it can reveal about the aetiology of these disorders. Each of these medical and scientific disciplines will be examined further in Chapter 3.

SLT students must also study a number of psychological disciplines alongside linguistic and medical disciplines. Clinicians must know the stages at which normally developing children achieve certain milestones in order to judge if a particular child's development deviates markedly from the normal pattern. These milestones, which include motor and cognitive achievements, are investigated within **developmental psychology**. Paediatric SLTs frequently work alongside **educational psychology** services. It is educational psychologists who undertake assessments of intellectual functioning and **dyslexia** in children. Given the proximity of these areas to the remit of SLT, students of SLT must have a sound knowledge of the work of educational psychologists. **Cognitive psychology** is also studied by students of SLT. Cognitive psychological theories of language processing have influenced certain diagnostic tools and interventions used by SLTs. For example, a cognitive psychological approach is used in the assessment and intervention of adult acquired aphasia (e.g. *Psycholinguistic Assessments of Language Processing in Aphasia (PALPA)* (Kay et al., 1992); Whitworth et al., 2005). **Neuropsychology** and **clinical psychology** are also important psychological disciplines for SLTs. The language and communication difficulties of clients who sustain a TBI are explained in large part by **executive function** deficits in areas such as attention, planning and working memory. It is neuropsychologists who assess these cognitive deficits. Clinical psychologists work alongside SLTs in the management of clients with voice disorders and psychiatric conditions. These various branches of psychology are examined further in Chapter 4.

Finally, the knowledge that is gleaned from these linguistic, medical and psychological disciplines is insufficient by itself to produce SLTs who are able to assess and treat clients with communication and swallowing disorders. A number of clinical skills must also be acquired by students of SLT. These skills include the technical abilities that are needed to undertake phonetic transcription and perform linguistic analysis. Technical abilities are also required to use equipment appropriately during assessment and treatment. For example, technical abilities are needed to use a **nasometer** safely and effectively to supplement perceptual assessments of nasality and to use **electropalatography** to modify tongue–palate contact during articulation therapy. Other clinical skills are more cognitive than technical in nature. SLTs must use clinical problem-solving skills to establish why a particular intervention was not effective with a client when it is known to be effective in other clients with similar communication impairments. Problem-solving skills are also used by SLTs to address issues that may be reducing a client's compliance with an intervention or a spouse's failure to make communicative adjustments when conversing with her aphasic partner. Decision-making is another key cognitive clinical skill. SLTs must make decisions about which standardized test to use to examine a child's phonology and about which group of sounds to target first in phonological therapy. Decisions must also be made about the intensity of therapy (once or twice weekly), the mode of therapy (individual versus group therapy) and when to terminate therapy. Each of these clinical skills must be developed by students of SLT alongside knowledge of linguistic, medical and psychological disciplines.

> **KEY POINTS: What Do SLT Students Need to Learn?**
>
> - Linguistic disciplines form a key part of the knowledge base of SLT. These disciplines are phonetics, phonology, morphology, syntax, semantics, pragmatics and discourse.
> - Medical and scientific disciplines also underpin the work of SLT. Included among these disciplines are anatomy and physiology, neurology, psychiatry and otorhinolaryngology (ENT medicine).

- Several psychological disciplines are also relevant to SLT. They include developmental psychology, educational psychology, cognitive psychology, neuropsychology and clinical psychology.
- Knowledge of disciplines sits alongside clinical skills in SLTs. These skills include a range of technical abilities as well as cognitive clinical skills in areas such as problem-solving and decision-making.

1.4 SLT and Clients with Communication and Swallowing Disorders

So far, there has been little direct examination of clients who have communication and swallowing disorders. These clients and their disorders will be the focus of this section. In addressing these disorders, a distinction will be made between a developmental and an acquired communication and swallowing disorder. Developmental communication and swallowing disorders have their onset during the **developmental period**, while acquired disorders arise after the time when speech, language and swallowing skills are normally acquired. According to this distinction, it is possible for a child to have an **acquired communication disorder** (e.g. a teenager with dysarthria following a TBI) and for an adult to have a **developmental communication disorder** (e.g. an adult who has stuttered since early childhood). A second distinction to be examined in this section is that between an expressive and a receptive language disorder. An **expressive language disorder** arises when a child or adult has difficulty formulating spoken and/or written language. When there is an impairment of the comprehension of language, SLTs diagnose a **receptive language disorder**. Although it is possible for a child or adult to have only one of these language disorders (e.g. expressive SLI), clients with language disorders often have a combination of receptive and expressive impairments. The third distinction to be addressed is that between a speech disorder and a language disorder. For most people, any impairment of communication is straightforwardly a speech disorder. However, when SLTs talk about a speech disorder, they use this label to refer only to a breakdown in motoric (non-symbolic) aspects of communication. All three distinctions will be examined subsequently.

As a route into these distinctions, let us consider the following scenarios:

(A) Sally is 15 years old. Six months earlier, she sustained a severe TBI in a road traffic accident. Following the accident, she had emergency neurosurgery to remove a subdural haematoma and to reduce intracranial pressure. When Sally emerged from her coma, she was completely mute and disoriented to time and place. Her understanding of even short, simple sentences was impaired. After a number of weeks, Sally's **mutism** had resolved and her speech was dysarthric. Her understanding of language was still impaired but displayed signs of improvement. Two months after surgery, Sally was able to answer a set of 30 yes–no questions with 100% accuracy.

(B) Sammy is 45 years old. He has aphasia following a cerebrovascular accident that has caused a lesion in his left cerebral hemisphere. His expressive language is severely impaired as he is only able to produce one- or two-word utterances. His understanding of language is superior to his expression of language but is also impaired. Sammy is receiving non-oral feeding because his swallowing has been assessed to be unsafe. When Sammy was at school, he was seen by an SLT for the treatment of **childhood apraxia of speech**. His speech at school was highly unintelligible and limited his social interactions with his peers.

(C) Billy is 7 years old. He was born prematurely and had a number of medical complications in the neonatal period (e.g. **cytomegalovirus**). At six months old, Billy developed **meningitis,** which caused sensorineural hearing loss. His speech and language development are delayed. The SLT assesses Billy's speech, which is moderately dysarthric. His unintelligibility limits social interaction with his peers. The teacher reports that Billy does not understand instructions in class. Recently, Billy has displayed hoarseness, which has necessitated a referral to the ENT department of his local hospital. A direct **laryngoscopy** reveals bilateral **vocal nodules** and **hyperadduction** of the vocal folds.

In scenario (A) Sally has both a speech disorder and a language disorder. Her language disorder is receptive in nature – she has impaired understanding of short, simple sentences – although her motor speech difficulties are probably masking a severe expressive language disorder also. Sally has the speech disorder dysarthria. Because the onset of her speech and language disorder occurred when Sally was a teenager, that is, after the point at which fully mature speech and language skills are acquired, they are both acquired communication disorders. In scenario (B) Sammy has aphasia, which has compromised his expressive and receptive language. He also has a swallowing disorder (dysphagia) following his cerebrovascular accident. Because his language and swallowing skills were intact prior to his stroke, Sammy has an acquired communication disorder and swallowing disorder, respectively. However, his difficulties do not end there. When Sammy was at school, he was diagnosed with childhood apraxia of speech. This speech disorder has its onset in the developmental period and is, therefore, a developmental communication disorder. In scenario (C) Billy has a hearing, speech, language and voice disorder. His sensorineural hearing loss is related to meningitis, which he developed at six months of age. This is within the developmental period and so Billy's hearing loss is a developmental communication disorder. Two other sequelae of meningitis, the speech disorder dysarthria and a receptive language disorder (Billy does not understand instructions in class), are also developmental communication disorders. Additionally, Billy has a voice disorder, which is related to the presence of organic lesions (vocal nodules).

In these scenarios, we have seen examples of speech, language, hearing, voice and swallowing disorders. Among these disorders, we have also distinguished between developmental and acquired communication and swallowing disorders and receptive and expressive language disorders. But we can say more about clients with communication disorders. In some language disorders, there is a primary impairment of language in that language is not impaired in consequence of other factors. An example of a primary impairment of language is **pragmatic language impairment** where pragmatic difficulties are not related to any linguistic deficit even though such deficits may exist. In other language disorders there is a secondary impairment of language in that cognitive and linguistic factors account for the language disorder – the language disorder is secondary to these factors. In so-called cognitive-communication disorders, language difficulties are related to the presence of cognitive deficits. This occurs in TBI, **right-hemisphere damage** and the dementias where executive function deficits and other cognitive impairments (e.g. visual-perceptual deficits) give rise to language difficulties. But linguistic factors can also be a cause of secondary language disorders. For example, adults with aphasia may not be able to use the syntactic and semantic structures that are needed to produce **indirect speech acts** (e.g. *Can you open the window?*) and other non-literal forms of language. Children with specific language impairment may lack the linguistic structures (e.g. conjunctions) that are needed to achieve cohesion in a narrative. In both these cases, the pragmatic and discourse disorders of these clients are secondary to structural language impairments. In order to illustrate this final distinction, consider the following scenario:

> (D) Alice is 65 years old and has **Alzheimer's dementia**. As her memory and other cognitive abilities have declined, so too have her language skills. Although her phonological and syntactic skills are still relatively intact, her semantic and pragmatic abilities are significantly disrupted. Alice is unable to understand idioms, metaphors and other non-literal forms of language. She often fails to appreciate **humour** in conversation and misinterprets sarcastic and other remarks. Typically, she tends to veer towards a literal interpretation of these linguistic utterances. Moreover, her comprehension of idioms appears to correlate with scores on tests of executive function.

The question we want to address is: Does Alice have a primary language and communication disorder or a secondary language and communication disorder? Given that her language deterioration occurs in the context of significant decline in her cognitive skills, it is clear that Alice has a secondary language and communication disorder. Like clients with TBI and right-hemisphere damage, Alice has a cognitive-communication disorder. As we begin to learn more about the cognitive basis of cognitive-communication disorders, it appears likely that increasingly sophisticated classifications of these disorders will begin to emerge.

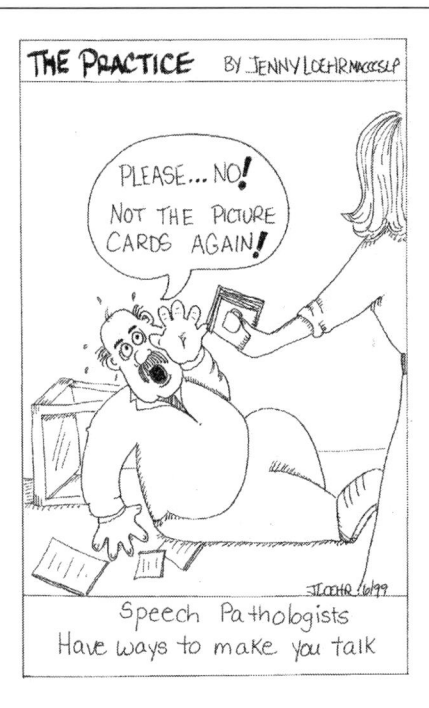

GROUP EXERCISE: Applying Clinical Distinctions

In a small group, make a list of as many people as possible with communication disorders that you have encountered at different points in your life. Your list may include children in your class at school who stuttered or had hearing loss. It may also include a sibling who had a speech disorder related to cleft palate or a grandparent with language problems as a result of a stroke. For each disorder that you identify, indicate if it is a developmental or an acquired communication disorder. Then also indicate if it is a speech, language, hearing, voice or fluency disorder. To check that your understanding of the disorders on your list is accurate, report each one and its classification to the rest of the class in the presence of an instructor.

KEY POINTS: SLT and Clients with Communication and Swallowing Disorders

- SLTs use a number of distinctions to help them talk in a precise, meaningful way about communication and swallowing disorders. Four such distinctions are: *developmental* versus *acquired* communication disorders; *receptive* versus *expressive* language disorders; *speech* versus

> *language* disorders; and *primary* versus *secondary* language and communication disorders.
> - If a communication disorder has its onset in the developmental period, it is described as a developmental communication disorder. If the onset of a disorder occurs after speech and language skills have been acquired, a communication disorder is acquired in nature.
> - In an expressive language disorder, the production or expression of language is impaired. In a receptive language disorder, the understanding or comprehension of language is impaired.
> - In a speech disorder, motoric or non-symbolic aspects of communication are compromised (i.e. **motor speech programming** and **motor speech execution**). In a language disorder, symbolic aspects of communication are disrupted (i.e. **language encoding** and **language decoding**).
> - In a primary language or communication disorder, language is not impaired in consequence of other factors. In a secondary language or communication disorder, language is impaired on account of the presence of cognitive and linguistic deficits.

1.5 SLT and Families and Carers

Children and adults with communication and swallowing disorders do not exist in social isolation from others. They are parents, siblings, children and spouses to other people. These people are integral to the work of SLT. In this section, we consider several, important roles of families and carers in SLT. First, family members and carers are a vital source of information about clients with a communication or swallowing disorder. This information might include a child's developmental history, reports about how an adult with dysphagia copes with food of different textures at home, or information about how a client with aphasia communicates in a range of social settings. Second, family members and carers can act *in loco* of therapists by implementing interventions outside of the clinic. This might involve undertaking semantic exercises with the adult who has aphasia or ensuring that the dysfluent child uses stretched or smooth speech at home. Third, family members and carers may be directly targeted in an SLT intervention. The spouse or other conversational partners of an adult with aphasia may be directly instructed in how their own conversational behaviours can be modified to facilitate communication with the adult. Fourth, family members and carers may need to be trained in the use of specialist equipment, technology and techniques. Children with Down syndrome will gain little from the use of Makaton signs and symbols if all relevant others in their environment – parents, siblings, teachers and carers – receive no training in the use of the Makaton programme. Fifth, family members and carers can provide much needed psychological and emotional support to clients. This is necessary in order to ensure compliance with SLT intervention and the continued use of techniques after discharge from therapy. These five roles will be examined further in the rest of this section.

SLTs bring vast clinical expertise to the assessment and treatment of clients with communication disorders. However, this expertise can amount to very little in the absence of the type of information that only family members and carers can provide. It is these individuals who observe a client's communicative functioning in contexts that cannot be readily accessed by clinicians. The information that can be obtained about a child's or adult's ability to communicate at home, at school or in the workplace can substantially extend the spatial reach of clinicians. But aside from a spatial dimension, there is an important temporal function served by the information that only family members and carers can provide. It is not uncommon, for example, for adults with neurodegenerative conditions such as motor neurone disease to experience some deterioration of speech later in the day when fatigue is most acute. Through their continual contact with clients, spouses and carers are best placed to report on the effects of fatigue and other factors (e.g. daily activities, illnesses) on communication skills. This temporal function can, of course, be extended beyond the changes in communication observed in a 24-hour period to include the observation of communication skills over a period of months or years. The development of communication skills in young children can often be reported by parents in considerable detail during the taking of a child's history. Also, the spouse of an adult with Alzheimer's dementia may be able to describe subtle changes in this client's communication skills long before the point where a clinical diagnosis is made. In short, family members and carers can extend the spatial and temporal reach of clinicians into contexts and time periods that are otherwise inaccessible to SLTs.

Another key role of family members and carers is to undertake interventions *in loco* of therapists. It should be emphasized that this role does not see family members and carers replacing clinicians. It is still SLTs who must decide on the nature of a particular intervention and on how an intervention may be best implemented. Rather, this role recognizes that the required treatment dose in many communication disorders exceeds that which can be delivered even in well-resourced SLT centres. Highly motivated and well-informed parents can prove to be a considerable asset in the treatment of children with speech sound disorders where continual modelling, feedback and articulatory exercises are required to bring about significant speech gains. An aphasia intervention that is administered for 30 minutes once or twice weekly is unlikely to secure any improvement in a client's communication skills if a spouse or other family member is not supplementing efforts in the clinic with additional input at home. As well as increasing the amount of treatment input, family members and carers can also plan that input to occur at times that are likely to be maximally effective. A scheduled clinic appointment cannot always take account of the time of day when a client is likely to be most receptive to speech and language exercises.

Of course, the increased treatment dose that family members and carers can provide is only possible under certain conditions. Relatives and carers must be educated about a client's communication difficulties and trained in specific intervention techniques. Clinicians must be prepared to impart certain knowledge and skills to relatives and carers and engage in regular monitoring of a client's progress outside of the clinic via telephone consultations or other means. This can be and is successfully achieved in many cases.

As well as supplementing clinic-based treatment, family members and carers may also be directly targeted in SLT intervention. This role of relatives and carers acknowledges that communication involves two or more participants and that a client's communication disorder may be most effectively addressed by modifying the conversational behaviour of other participants. This approach is used in the treatment of clients with aphasia. Two interventions of this type that are based on **conversation analysis** are the Conversation Analysis Profile for People with Aphasia (Whitworth et al., 1997) and Supporting Partners of People with Aphasia in Relationships and Conversation Analysis (Lock et al., 2001). It has been widely documented among clients with aphasia that opportunities for communication are frequently constrained by the behaviour of conversational partners. It has also been documented that even small modifications of conversational behaviour on the part of spouses and carers can significantly improve the overall experience of communication for these clients (see section 6.3.1 in Cummings, 2009, for discussion). Aside from aphasia, family members and carers are also the focus of intervention in the treatment of other communication disorders. Indirect treatments for young children who stutter are targeted at parents with no attempt made to treat the speech of these children. Rather, efforts are undertaken to modify parental interaction with these children with the aim of increasing their fluency. Also, parents are instructed in how to reduce stressors in a child's environment that may be contributing to dysfluency (see Yaruss, 2014, for discussion of these treatments). As with aphasia, it is parents and carers who are the focus of intervention rather than the child who stutters.

Family members and carers assume a further important role in SLT intervention. Some interventions with clients involve the use of specialist techniques, equipment and technology. This is particularly the case in the use of augmentative and alternative communication (AAC) with clients. For a client to use a communication board or Makaton signs effectively, family members and carers must also receive training in the use of these systems. Although communication boards are low-technology communication aids, their successful use still requires considerable skill on the part of not just the AAC user but also communicative partners. High-technology communication aids can also pose challenges to communicative partners who must receive training not only in their technical features but also in their use in communication. These skills are acquired through direct practice with the AAC system often in the presence of SLTs. Clinicians must also be available for the purposes of troubleshooting when difficulties arise for AAC clients and their families. Clearly, there are significant resource implications for any SLT service that is charged with providing this level of support and aftercare to AAC users and their families. However, the importance of this long-term support cannot be overstated. In a systematic review of the potential barriers and facilitators to continued use of high-technology AAC, Baxter et al. (2012) found that the perceptions and attitudes of family members were a highly significant factor in the successful implementation of an AAC system. An AAC system is more likely to be abandoned by its user if family members do not feel adequately trained and supported in its use. At least as far as AAC users are concerned, direct training and support of family members and carers are an essential component of any intervention.

Finally, family members and carers also play a vital role in providing psychological and emotional support to clients in SLT. Many clients who enter SLT do so following traumatic events in their lives. They may have been diagnosed with cancer, which necessitates a **laryngectomy** or a **glossectomy**. They may have sustained a TBI or had a first-ever stroke. They may have a progressive neurodegenerative disease such as motor neurone disease. All these events and illnesses cause considerable distress to clients and their families. For most of them, a long period of rehabilitation follows the event or illness that hospitalized the client. The support of family members and carers is particularly important during this time when progress in SLT can appear slow to clients and a return to good functioning can seem unattainable. There is also an elevated risk of depression in clients who sustain a head injury or develop a stroke (Barker-Collo et al., 2015; Schöttke and Giabbiconi, 2015). Depression can reduce a client's motivation to participate in SLT or to see a course of SLT intervention through to a successful outcome. As well as encouraging clients to comply with SLT intervention, family members and carers provide much needed support to clients after they have been discharged from therapy. This is a time when the support of clinicians is no longer available and there is a risk that clients will fail to maintain communication gains from therapy. The support of family members and carers is particularly important at this time to prevent a loss of skills and to ensure continual reinforcement of behaviours targeted in therapy. From entry into SLT to eventual discharge, the psychological and emotional support of family members and carers can ensure compliance with intervention and the long-term maintenance of skills.

KEY POINTS: SLT and Families and Carers

- SLTs involve family members and carers in their work with clients who have communication and swallowing disorders. Relatives and carers perform five roles: they provide information about clients; they implement interventions outside of clinic; they may be the focus of an intervention; they may receive training in the use of specialist equipment; and they provide emotional and psychological support to clients.

- *Provide information:* Family members and carers can provide SLTs with important information such as a child's developmental history and the factors that can influence a client's communication skills (e.g. fatigue, daily activities).
- *Implement intervention:* Family members and carers can implement interventions such as speech and language exercises under the guidance of SLTs.
- *Focus of intervention:* Family members and carers may be directly targeted in an intervention. They may receive instruction in how to modify their own conversational behaviours to facilitate communication in clients with aphasia.
- *Receive training:* Family members and carers must be trained and supported in the use of specialist equipment, techniques and technology. In the case of AAC users, this is necessary in order to ensure continued use of a system.
- *Provide support:* Family members and carers provide emotional and psychological support to clients. This support increases compliance with SLT interventions and the maintenance of skills after discharge from therapy.

CASE STUDY: Clients and their Families

Michael is a 49-year-old business executive. Six months ago, he sustained a severe TBI in a road traffic accident on his way to work. In the weeks following his accident, Michael was mute. Mutism gradually gave way to severe dysarthria. To facilitate communication between Michael and medical staff and family members, Michael was encouraged to point to letters and symbols on a communication board. This was difficult and inefficient at first, as Michael's neurological injury compromised some of his gross motor movements and his right arm was badly fractured in the accident. However, bedside training by the SLT improved the ease with which Michael was able to use this system of alternative communication. After two months in the hospital's neuro-rehabilitation unit, Michael's medical condition had stabilized sufficiently to allow him to be discharged into a nursing facility near his home. Michael spent a further three months undergoing rehabilitation in this facility. After this time, his progress was judged to be sufficiently good to warrant his returning home.

Michael's dysarthria continued to improve and he became less reliant on his communication board to communicate his needs. As Michael was able to use more spoken language to communicate, it became increasingly apparent to family members that his conversational skills had not returned to their pre-morbid state. Michael's wife reported considerable conversational difficulties with him at home. His communication style before his accident was described as animated, lively and engaging. However, his wife reported that following his accident, Michael did not appear to be motivated to communicate, even to his children. When he did engage in conversation, he was repetitive and unable to express ideas in a clear, logical manner. He often had difficulty retrieving words. Michael displayed poor topic maintenance and was often under-informative. He assumed his listener had knowledge of people and events when this was not the case. For example, he often used personal pronouns in the absence of preceding referents. He also became irritable at his listener's lack of comprehension and frustrated by his failure to repair conversational breakdown.

Following his accident, Michael was no longer able to work. His wife reported that he had become increasingly isolated from his social network. She believed his poor conversational skills were the reason for his isolation. On hearing these reports, the SLT decided to examine a video-recording of Michael in conversation with his wife at home. The examination confirmed many of the observations about conversation made by Michael's wife. He was repetitive in conversation. He did display word-finding problems that disrupted the flow of conversation. Michael struggled to repair conversational breakdown. However, the examination also revealed that Michael's wife employed a number of conversational behaviours which exacerbated his difficulties. Michael was most repetitive when his wife failed to acknowledge that she understood what he was communicating. Repetition was often used as a means of reiterating a point. Michael's wife did not use cues to facilitate his retrieval of words. The repair of conversational breakdown led to protracted exchanges when much shorter repair sequences would have sufficed. Having observed these behaviours, the SLT decided to institute an intervention based on conversational partner training.

Questions

(1) Michael's wife played a number of important roles in his communication rehabilitation. One of these roles was to provide the SLT with information that is relevant to the management of his case. Identify two ways in which this takes place.
(2) Family members play a vital role in providing psychological, emotional and social support to clients with communication disorders. Is this support required in Michael's case?
(3) In some SLT interventions, it is family members and carers who are the target of intervention. Is an intervention of this type adopted in Michael's case?
(4) Aside from conversational partner training, are Michael's family members able to contribute in any other way to his communication intervention?
(5) Michael is often repetitive during conversation. This appears to be related to a failure on the part of his wife to signal her understanding of what he is saying. Describe one way in which Michael's wife can be encouraged to signal more effectively her understanding of his message.

1.6 SLT and Public Health

As well as serving individuals with communication and swallowing disorders, and working with their families and carers, SLTs are increasingly being called upon to fulfil an important public health role. In the UK, the involvement of SLT for the first time in the health of populations has been ushered in by a new focus on public health in the Health and Social Care Act 2012. However, in reality, SLT has always intervened on the health of populations. This is because communication disorders are highly prevalent in the general population and are closely associated with social disadvantage and inequality. This is clearly evident in a wide-ranging survey of historical and contemporary data concerning workforce distribution and the epidemiology of speech, language, hearing and voice disorders in the United States. Ruben (2000) reported that communication disorders in the USA are estimated to have a prevalence of 5% to 10%. Moreover, people with communication disorders are more economically disadvantaged than those with less severe disabilities, while people with severe speech disabilities are more often found to be unemployed or in a lower economic class than people with hearing loss or other disabilities. Given these findings, the conclusion of this study is certainly warranted: 'The economic cost and the prevalence rates of communication disorders in the United States indicate that they will be a major public health challenge for the 21st century' (Ruben, 2000: 241). In this section, that challenge is examined by considering some of the ways in which communication disorders can impact negatively on the health of populations. SLT can, and frequently does, intervene successfully on the health of populations. Some of the ways in which this is achieved will also be addressed.

That communication disorders have the capacity to compromise health and create social exclusion and deprivation in populations is demonstrated by a number of studies. Law et al. (2009) followed a birth cohort of 17,196 children in the UK from school entry to 34 years of age. Literacy, mental health and employment at 34 years were found to be significantly associated with receptive language problems at 5 years. This relationship held over and above common demographic markers (e.g. gender). Beitchman et al. (2014) found that a cohort of children with language disorders who were followed from 5 years of age had poorer self-rated physical health at 31 years than controls with no language disorders. McAllister et al. (2012) reported a significant association between stuttering at age 16 and the socioeconomic status of occupation at age 50 in a British birth cohort dataset of 15,911 members. Cohort members who had been reported to stutter had lower-status jobs. Kobayashi et al. (2015) found that early-onset hearing loss was associated with psychological distress in a household survey of 136,849 Japanese men and women aged 20 to 39 years. In a cross-sectional survey of 461 individuals aged 50 years and older, Merrill et al. (2011) found that individuals with a history of voice disorder had significantly poorer physical and mental health than individuals with no history of voice disorder. The prevalence of language and communication disorders in the prison population is substantially elevated relative to the general population (Bryan et al., 2007). These disorders put males in particular at an increased risk of offending behaviour, which serves to perpetuate social deprivation and exclusion in the communities in which they live.

That communication disorders have adverse consequences for the health and well-being of populations is clear enough. But what is also clear is that SLT can intervene effectively on these disorders to avert some or all of these consequences. In a report commissioned by the Home Office in the UK, Moseley et al. (2006) found that reconviction rates fell sharply in prisoners who participated in oral communication courses. In the first year after release from prison, the reconviction rate among prisoners who had taken courses in oral communication was 21%. This compares with a national average for all offenders of 44%. Cooper et al. (1998) reported significant language gains in children as a result of a community-based speech and language intervention in a socially disadvantaged area of Plymouth, England. The intervention included a nursery programme called Wise Words for Nursery and parenting groups for the parents of preschool children. Between 1993 and 1997, a battery of language tests was used to collect data from consecutive year groups that entered a single primary school. The battery contained four standardized tests that assessed lexical development, word finding, narrative skills, sentence length and syntactic development, and a rating scale that recorded phonological development. There was a significant difference between the 1993 and 1997 intakes in lexical development, narrative skills and receptive grammar, a finding that was taken to support the effectiveness of the intervention. Although there was no significant difference in speech clarity or word finding, change occurred in the direction of improvement. Average sentence length remained unchanged, a finding that the authors described as a dialectal characteristic that is resistant to change.

The positive results of Cooper et al.'s intervention have more recently been replicated in a multi-agency approach to children's speech and language problems that was adopted in Stoke-on-Trent in England. The so-called 'Stoke Speaks Out' initiative will be examined in the end-of-chapter questions. The success of these community-wide projects with an emphasis on speech, language and communication is forcing SLTs to rethink how they deliver their services to the public. Planning in this direction is already under way (e.g. Law et al., 2013). However, it is clear that much work remains to be done if SLT is to embrace fully its public health role.

KEY POINTS: SLT and Public Health

- Communication and swallowing disorders are highly prevalent in the general population. By intervening on these disorders, SLTs are improving the health of populations and serving an important public health role.
- Children and adults with communication and swallowing disorders incur social and economic disadvantage. They also experience psychological distress. SLT interventions that reduce or eliminate these adverse consequences play an important role in improving opportunities for people.

- That SLT plays a significant role in enhancing the life chances of people with communication and swallowing disorders is supported by studies that demonstrate improved vocational, educational and social outcomes in individuals who receive SLT services. Re-offending rates among prisoners are also reduced when prisoners receive SLT interventions.
- The communication-related health of populations can be improved by community-wide and multi-agency approaches to intervention in the early years. These approaches make effective communication a health goal for all practitioners who deliver services in the early years.

WEBSITE: Introduction to Speech and Language Therapy

After reading the chapter, visit the website and test your knowledge of speech and language therapy by answering the short-answer questions for this topic.

Suggestions for Further Reading

Pring, T., Flood, E., Dodd, B. and Joffe, V. 2012. 'The working practices and clinical experiences of paediatric speech and language therapists: a national UK survey', *International Journal of Language & Communication Disorders* 47:6, 696–708.

This article examines the working practices of paediatric SLTs in the UK. It is based on an online survey that was completed by 516 clinicians. The article describes the settings that these clinicians work in, their different duties, and how much time is spent working with clients with a range of disorders. The views of respondents on the impact of healthcare reform on SLT are also addressed.

Kersner, M. and Parker, A. 2012. 'Developing as a speech and language therapist', in M. Kersner and J. A. Wright (eds.), *Speech and language therapy: the decision-making process when working with children*, London and New York: Routledge, 16–27.

This chapter examines the skills and knowledge that are required of SLTs in the workplace. Different learning models that are relevant to key skills in SLT are described. The process of learning and professional development that allows SLTs and therapists-in-training to make decisions is discussed.

Wright, J. A. and Kersner, M. 2004. *A career in speech and language therapy*, 3rd edn, London: Metacom Education.

This volume introduces readers to the wide-ranging work of speech and language therapy. The skills needed by SLTs are examined along with the profiles of therapists who work in a range of contexts (acute hospital, child development centre, etc.). Readers receive guidance in how to apply for SLT courses. The experience of being an SLT student is addressed as well as professional life after qualification.

QUESTIONS: Introduction to Speech and Language Therapy

(1) The roles of the SLT are many and varied. Each of the following statements captures one of these roles. Identify the role in each statement:
  (a) The SLT conducts a systematic review of the effectiveness of SLT interventions in childhood dysarthria.
  (b) The SLT attends a careers event at a local school where he or she talks to pupils and their parents about SLT.
  (c) The SLT completes the Children's Communication Checklist (Bishop, 2003a) on a 5-year-old boy with suspected ASD.
  (d) The SLT meets with students on clinical placement to review the management of clients.
  (e) The SLT identifies the problematic communication skills of a client as a case of **right-hemisphere language disorder**.
  (f) The SLT uses semantic judgement tasks with a stroke client who has aphasia.
  (g) The SLT expresses the wishes and views of a client with **motor neurone disease** at a case review meeting.

(2) Each of the following statements describes an impact of a communication or swallowing disorder. For each statement, identify the impact that is related to the disorder:
  (a) A year after his stroke, a 60-year-old man with aphasia no longer attends his local history group or goes out for meals with friends. He feels his limited expressive language restricts his participation in these events.
  (b) A woman who experiences dysphonia with the onset of the menopause reports significant loss of confidence and poor self-esteem as a result of her voice disorder.
  (c) An adult with dysarthria related to **cerebral palsy** reports that he has been prevented from moving into customer-facing roles within his workplace and has been denied several promotions where jobs involve these roles.
  (d) A 7-year-old boy with speech sound disorder is at the bottom of his class in scores in **literacy**. A classroom assistant is assigned to him to undertake work on his poor reading skills.
  (e) A 10-year-old boy with poor expressive language skills displays defiant behaviour to teachers in class. At home, he reacts to conflict with his parents with outbursts of temper and has physically threatened them on several occasions.
  (f) A teenager with a history of speech and language difficulties regularly misses school and engages in antisocial behaviour in his local community. He has appeared in juvenile courts on charges relating to car thefts and the use of illicit substances.

(3) Each of the following statements describes an aspect of the knowledge of SLTs. Relate each statement to a particular linguistic, medical, scientific or psychological discipline:
   (a) A child with **fragile X syndrome** cannot sort pictures according to the categories *furniture* and *transport*.
   (b) A 55-year-old woman with hoarseness is shown to have a **vocal polyp** on her left vocal fold.
   (c) A child referred to SLT is reported to have been delayed in crawling, walking and sitting without support.
   (d) A child with a cleft palate uses the glottal stop [?] in place of oral plosives.
   (e) An adult who has a stroke experiences facial weakness on account of damage to cranial nerve VII.
   (f) **Delusions** and hallucinations are positive symptoms of schizophrenia.
   (g) An adult with ASD cannot understand the utterance *Bill kicked the bucket*.
   (h) A child's statement of special educational needs shows that he has verbal IQ of 65 and a non-verbal IQ of 85.
   (i) An investigation of an adult's hypernasal speech reveals that there is limited elevation of the velum.
   (j) The prevalence rate of specific language impairment in monolingual English-speaking kindergarten children is 7.4%.

(4) (A) Communication disorders were examined in this chapter according to the distinctions *developmental* versus *acquired* communication disorder and *speech* versus *language* disorder. Use these distinctions to classify each of the following communication disorders, e.g. aphasia (acquired language disorder):
   (a) childhood apraxia of speech
   (b) specific language impairment
   (c) right-hemisphere communication impairment
   (d) stroke-induced dysarthria
   (e) childhood dyslexia

(B) Classify each of the following statements according to the distinctions between a *receptive* versus *expressive* language disorder and a *primary* versus *secondary* language disorder:
   (a) Joan has aphasia and cannot understand passive voice constructions.
   (b) Bill sustained a TBI and produces repetitive language during conversation.
   (c) Tom has **frontotemporal dementia** and cannot comprehend idioms.
   (d) Olive exhibits agrammatism following a CVA in the left hemisphere.
   (e) Jack has right-hemisphere damage and uses egocentric language when asked to explain the meaning of a metaphor.

(5) There is close involvement of family members and carers of clients in SLT. This involvement can take a number of forms. Each of the scenarios below describes one of these forms. Use the following terms to characterize the particular involvement indicated by the scenario: *provide information*; *implement intervention*; *focus of intervention*; *receive training*; *provide support*.

(a) The mother of a 5-year-old boy with phonological disorder practises production of /s/ in word-initial position in a sound game with him at home.
(b) The wife of a 60-year-old man with aphasia is instructed in how she can modify her cueing behaviour to aid his retrieval of words during conversation.
(c) A 75-year-old man has feeding and swallowing problems following a stroke. His self-reported quality of life is poor and he has depression. His daughter takes advice from a dysphagia therapist and dietician and encourages her father's compliance with their recommendations. With his daughter's support, the man is able to continue oral feeding.
(d) A 65-year-old woman with Alzheimer's dementia is admitted to hospital. A SLT arrives on the ward to assess her. The woman's husband is able to tell the therapist in some detail about the decline of his wife's verbal communication skills.
(e) The parents of a non-verbal child with autism spectrum disorder are instructed in the use of the Picture Exchange Communication System by an SLT.

(6) Examine the information below about an initiative that was established in Stoke-on-Trent in England in 2004 to address the high incidence of language delay in young children. Then identify three aspects of this initiative that qualify it as a speech and language intervention which fulfils a public health role:

> *Stoke Speaks Out* was established as a city-wide strategy to encourage children's communication development. In 2002, local research indicated that many children in the area were starting school with poor language skills. In 2004, this was estimated to be as high as 64%. The initiative involved everyone in Stoke-on-Trent who works with children. All practitioners who work with children under 7 years of age and their families were offered training and support in issues relating to speech, language and communication. A practitioner network was established to discuss and develop ways in which children with speech, language and communication needs could be supported. In local communities 'communication ambassadors' were recruited to share messages about early communication development. Schools and other settings were accredited with a quality mark, a 'communication friendly' award. Since the initiative was established in 2004, over 4,500 practitioners have received training in speech and language development among other areas. By 2010, the number of children who entered nursery with a language delay had dropped to 39%. Communication development is now one of five priorities in Early Years in Stoke-on-Trent.

2 Linguistic Disciplines

2.1 Introduction

The study of speech and language therapy at university and college is a tightly regulated process, and necessarily so. In order to function competently as clinicians, graduates of SLT degree courses must emerge from their studies with certain skills and knowledge. One key area of knowledge is linguistics. In the UK, three bodies oversee the education and training of SLT students. These bodies are the Royal College of Speech and Language Therapists (RCSLT), the Quality Assurance Agency for Higher Education (QAA) and the Health & Care Professions Council (HCPC). Each of these bodies has a particular role to play in SLT education. The RCSLT provides curriculum guidelines and sets good practice guidelines for the education and training of SLTs and for their continuing professional development. The QAA provides subject benchmarks for SLT. These benchmarks stipulate baseline outcomes that a graduate in SLT will have achieved at the time of graduation. The HCPC is the statutory regulatory body for SLTs and a range of other healthcare professions. It specifies standards of education and training for SLTs among a range of other standards (e.g. standards of conduct, performance and ethics). Linguistics is so integral to SLT education that each of these bodies makes significant reference to it within their respective requirements for education providers. Within its guidelines for pre-registration SLT courses in the UK, the RCSLT states that:

> The content of the linguistics and phonetics strand of the curriculum should facilitate an understanding of those concepts and constituents of Linguistics which underpin speech and language therapy theory and practice. The curriculum should address both typical/atypical patterns and processes of linguistics and phonetics. Study in this area must include linguistics (phonetics/phonology, semantics, lexicon, morphology/syntax and pragmatics), psycholinguistics, neurolinguistics, sociolinguistics and multilingualism. (2010: 34)

In its benchmark statement for SLT, the QAA requires the SLT award holder to have knowledge of the following:

- Normal processing at sub-lexical, lexical, grammatical, discourse/text and conversational levels

- The relevant aspects of linguistics, including phonetics and the application of such knowledge to normal and impaired communication at both theoretical and practical analytical levels
- Sociolinguistics: knowledge of how language and communication are used in social contexts
- Psycholinguistics: normal development and processes in the perception, comprehension and production of spoken, written and gestured messages in both monolingual and multilingual communication.

(QAA, 2001: 10)

The HCPC's standards of education and training require those who successfully complete an SLT programme to meet the standards of proficiency for SLT. The standards of proficiency state that SLTs must understand the key concepts of the knowledge base relevant to their profession. Specifically, they must 'understand linguistics and phonetics, psycholinguistics, sociolinguistics and all levels of typical processing' (HCPC, 2013: 12).

In this chapter, the linguistic disciplines that are described in these various standards will be introduced and examined. These disciplines include all the branches of linguistics that are needed to give a complete description of normal and disordered language: phonetics, phonology, morphology, syntax, semantics, pragmatics and discourse. Several applied disciplines in linguistics that are relevant to the work of SLT will also be addressed. These disciplines include sociolinguistics, psycholinguistics, neurolinguistics and child language acquisition. Although a comprehensive treatment of each of these disciplines is beyond the scope of the current chapter, a number of key linguistic concepts will be introduced. To illustrate the application of these concepts to SLT, specific examples of their use in the analysis of disordered language in children and adults will be given. For each linguistic discipline, additional sources of reading will also be provided.

2.2 Phonetics

On entering an SLT course, students very quickly become aware that the analysis of speech sounds in phonetics is a fundamental part of the linguistic toolkit of therapists. The structure and function of the organs of speech production from the generation of a pulmonary airstream in the lungs to the valving and shaping of that airstream by the larynx and articulators (e.g. lips and tongue) is an early lesson in any phonetics module. Although the anatomy, physiology and neurology of these processes is the subject of scientific and medical modules, a module in phonetics should introduce students to the valving action of the velopharyngeal port that distinguishes nasal sounds (open port) from oral sounds (closed port) and to the **adduction** (closing) and **abduction** (opening) of the vocal folds whereby **voicing** is achieved. A precise characterization of speech sounds in terms of their place and manner of articulation is an essential component of articulatory phonetics. Students must understand how sounds can be distinguished by means of their **place of articulation** so that alveolar sounds such as [t] and [d] depend on an **active articulator** (the tongue tip) making contact with a **passive articulator** (the alveolar ridge), while velar sounds such as [k] and [g] require the back of the tongue to make contact with the **velum**, or soft palate. Each of these sounds is a plosive or stop, a type of **manner of articulation** in which two articulators make direct contact with each other and achieve a complete blockage of the airstream. Fricative sounds such as [f] and [s] involve a different manner of articulation in which there is a constriction of the airstream. Early in a phonetics module, students will be introduced to the chart of all symbols for consonant speech sounds from the International Phonetic Association (see the Appendix).

Consonant speech sounds can be difficult for many children and adults with speech disorders to articulate. For example, the child who has cerebral palsy and dysarthria may be unable to achieve lip closure for the production of the bilabial sounds [p] and [b]. An adult who sustains a TBI and has acquired dysarthria may be unable to achieve closure of the velopharyngeal port for the production of oral consonant sounds. This adult will exhibit hypernasal speech as a result. Aside from consonant sounds, the production of vowel sounds can also be compromised in individuals with speech disorders. Unlike consonants, which can be voiced or voiceless, vowels are always voiced. Vowels are further described in terms of their backness (front – centre – back), openness (high – medium high – medium low – low) and roundness (lip position is spread – neutral – round). (Alternative terms for 'high' and 'low' are 'close' and 'open', as shown in the Appendix.) In this way, [iː] in _bead_ is a front, high, unrounded vowel, while [ɒ] in _hot_ (Standard Southern British pronunciation of English) is a back, low, rounded vowel. The colon symbol in [iː] indicates that this is a long vowel. Long vowels are divided into **monophthongs** (or 'pure' vowels) in which the tongue is relatively steady, and **diphthongs** in which the tongue exhibits a degree of movement. For example, during the articulation of [aI] in _pie_, the tongue rises to a higher position in the mouth. Other examples of diphthongs are [ɔI] in _boy_ and [eI] in _plane_. Although the production of any vowel sound can be compromised in a speech disorder, the additional articulatory complexity of diphthongs can put these vowels at particular risk of phonetic deviance. Pollock and Hall (1991) examined five children aged 8;2 to 10;9 years with developmental apraxia of speech. All five children had difficulty with the production of diphthongs. Diphthong reduction (e.g. [a] for /aI/) was a common error pattern.

As well as the study of articulatory phonetics, a phonetics module must also introduce SLT students to the physical properties of speech sounds (acoustic

The Practice by Jenny Loehr M.A. CCC/SLP

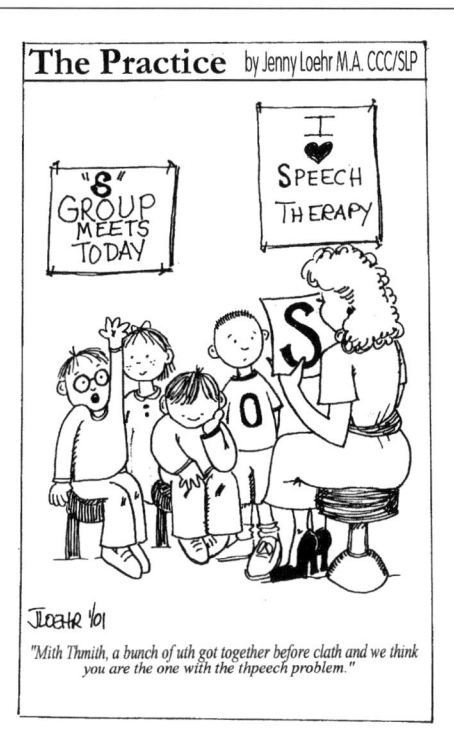

"Mith Thmith, a bunch of uth got together before clath and we think you are the one with the thpeech problem."

phonetics) and how speech sounds are perceived (speech perception). The RCSLT guidelines for pre-registration SLT courses state that acoustic phonetics should include 'the nature of sound (waveforms, amplitude, frequency and duration); spectra of speech sounds and spectrograms of speech; and instrumentation and software for acoustic measurement'. Sound waves may be characterized in terms of amplitude, frequency and wavelength. Amplitude describes the 'height' of a sound wave and is a measure of the energy in the wave (see Figure 2.1a). The frequency of a wave is the number of wave crests that pass a fixed point in a certain time interval. Frequency is usually measured in cycles per second, or hertz (Hz). Amplitude and frequency are related to the loudness and pitch of sound, respectively. Wavelength describes the distance from one wave crest to the next wave crest. Amplitude and frequency are represented on a spectrogram, which is constructed from a sequence of spectra. On a spectrogram, time is shown along the horizontal axis, frequency along the vertical axis, and the amplitude of a signal at a given time and frequency is shown as a grey level. Parts of a spectrogram shown in black indicate most acoustic energy, while white is used to signal least acoustic energy (see Figure 2.1b). An understanding of acoustic phonetics is essential for the interpretation of the results of acoustic assessments. For example, Visi-Pitch IV (KayPENTAX) contains a real-time spectrogram that may be used for voice 'typing' of clients with dysphonia. Visi-Pitch IV also contains a motor speech profile that can be

38 LINGUISTIC DISCIPLINES

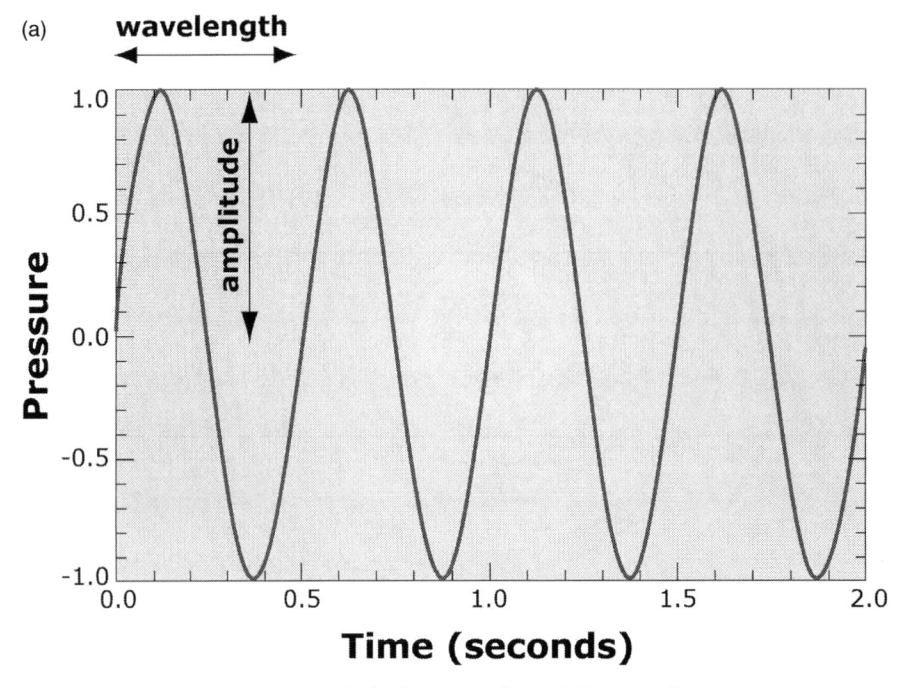

(a)

Figure 2.1a *Diagram of sound wave showing amplitude, frequency and wavelength (reproduced with kind permission of Woods Hole Oceanographic Institution)*

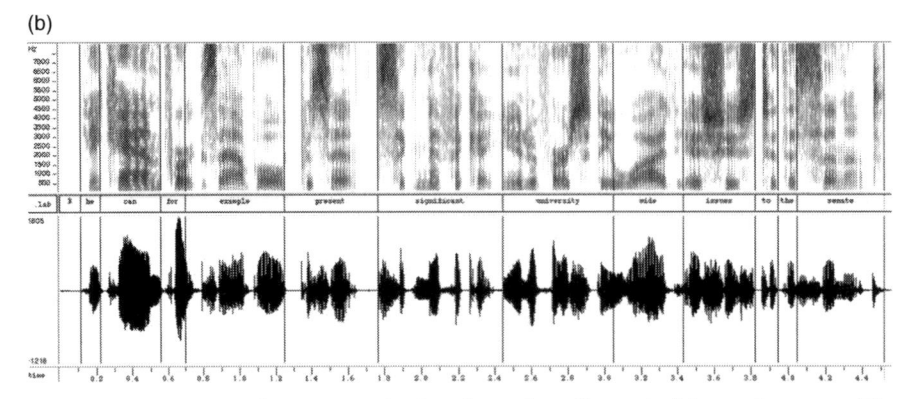

(b)

Figure 2.1b *Spectrogram (top) and waveform (bottom) of the read sentence 'He can, for example, present significant university wide issues to the senate' (reproduced with kind permission of Mark Liberman, Christopher H. Browne Distinguished Professor of Linguistics, University of Pennsylvania)*

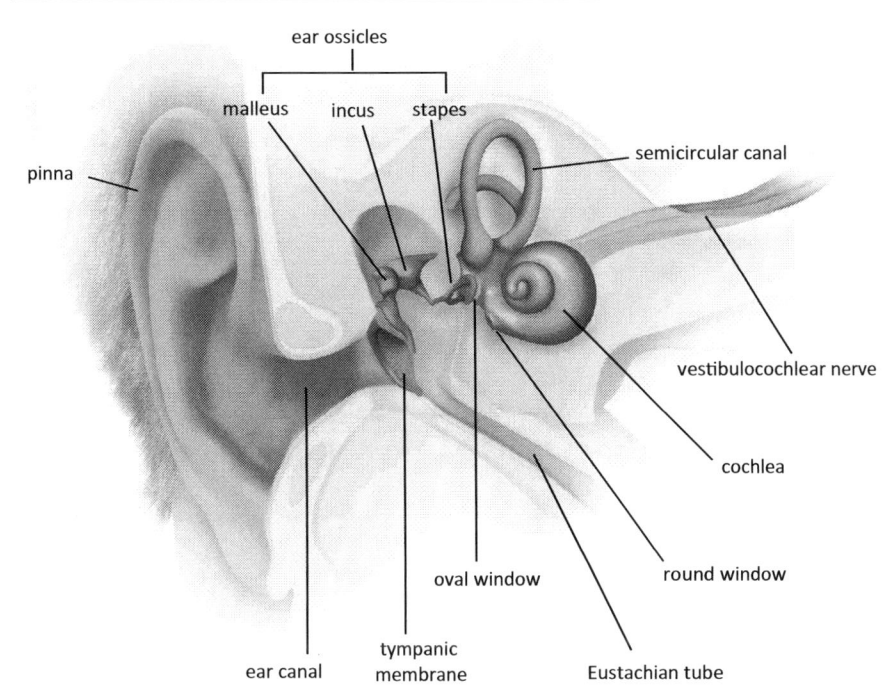

Figure 2.2 *Structure of the ear (Image reproduced with modification by kind permission of MED-EL)*

used to undertake an acoustic assessment of the speech of clients with motor speech disorders such as dysarthria.

The RCSLT guidelines for pre-registration courses also require SLT students to be introduced to hearing and speech perception in phonetics. Hearing involves peripheral and central processing, which takes place in the ear and auditory cortices of the brain, respectively. Sound waves travel through the **ear canal** or external auditory meatus (see Figure 2.2). The canal is 2.35cm in length and amplifies sound an average of 10–15 dB in the 2500–4000 Hz frequency range (Ackley, 2014). When sound waves make contact with the ear drum or **tympanic membrane**, it responds by moving inwards and outwards. This movement is transmitted through the middle ear by means of the mechanical vibration of the ear **ossicles**. The ossicles – the malleus, incus and stapes – are the smallest bones in the human body. The plunging movement of the stapes against the oval window achieves propulsion of a fluid in the **cochlea** called perilymph. The wave-like motion of this fluid displaces the stereocilia of hair cells in the **organ of Corti**. Each hair cell is tuned to a particular frequency of sound. High-frequency sounds stimulate hair cells at the base of the cochlea and low-frequency sounds stimulate cells at the apex. Displacement of the cilia triggers an exchange of potassium ions between the endolymph and the hair cells (endolymph is a potassium-rich fluid that surrounds the hair cells). The movement of ions into the hair cells triggers an action potential in the **vestibulo-cochlear nerve** (cranial nerve VIII). A nervous impulse is propagated along this nerve to a sensory nucleus (cochlear nucleus) located at the junction of the pons and medulla in the **brainstem**. The final destination of this nerve is the auditory areas in the brain, the so-called post-central gyrus and the superior temporal auditory cortex.

When nervous impulses from the hearing mechanism reach the auditory areas of the brain, the process of speech perception can begin. Although hearers can glean much information from an acoustic speech signal including the age, regional dialect and gender of the speaker, speech perception is generally taken to refer to the perceptual mapping of the acoustic signal to some linguistic representation such as phonemes, syllables and words. Speech perception does not use auditory information alone but draws extensively on visual information also. Hearers use visual information about the position of the lips, degree of jaw opening and position of the tongue in the dental/alveolar region of the oral cavity to aid perception. This is as true of individuals with normal hearing as it is of children and adults with **hearing loss** who make use of lip-reading. There are also top-down influences in speech perception. **Top-down processing** is where meaning and context, information about the speaker and rules of language contribute to the perception of speech. For example, when hearers listen to the sentence *Jack fell and _ut his knees*, they have no difficulty in perceiving the [k] of 'cut' because their perception is influenced by the meaning of the rest of the sentence. Other issues addressed in speech perception include categorical perception. This is where changes in a variable along a continuum, for example 10 ms increases in the **voice onset time** of the plosive in *buy* [baI], reach a point where the perception switches from [baI] to [paI]. Perception proceeds in terms of discrete categories with no intermediate percepts between [b] and [p]. Speech perception also addresses the redundancy of acoustic cues. This is where more acoustic information is present than is necessary to distinguish phonetic events. Redundancy allows hearers to perceive speech sounds under adverse listening conditions (e.g. environmental noise).

KEY POINTS: Phonetics

- Phonetics must be studied by all SLT students. Its inclusion in SLT curricula is stipulated by the three bodies that oversee the education of SLT students (i.e. RCSLT, QAA and HCPC).
- In articulatory phonetics, students are introduced to terms such as voicing and the place and manner of articulation of consonant speech sounds. The symbols that are used to represent these sounds in the IPA chart are examined.

- Also in articulatory phonetics, a description of vowels is given in terms of their backness, openness and roundness. The difference between monophthongs and diphthongs is considered. Students are introduced to the vowel quadrilateral of the IPA.
- In acoustic phonetics, sound waves are described in terms of their amplitude, frequency and wavelength. Spectrograms and the instrumentation that is used to conduct acoustic assessments of normal and disordered speech are examined.
- Hearing is examined at both a peripheral level and a central level. How speech sounds are converted from sound waves in the ear canal to a series of electrophysiological responses in the cochlea is studied.
- Speech perception considers the top-down and bottom-up influences on the recognition of phonemes, syllables and words. Other issues addressed in the speech perception component of a phonetics module include categorical perception and cue redundancy.

2.3 Phonology

Phonology is an essential linguistic discipline for students of SLT. Phonologists examine the **contrastive function** of phonetic distinctions in a language. For example, in English voicing is contrastive for consonants. So, in the pairs *chin* [ʧIn] and *gin* [ʤIn], the phonetic distinction between the voiceless and voiced affricates at the beginning of these words is contrastive in that it serves to distinguish these words in English. The contrastive function of voicing is also seen in the following **minimal pairs** in English: *pike* [paIk] and *bike* [baIk]; *time* [taIm] and *dime* [daIm]; and *leaf* [lif] and *leave* [liv]. Place of articulation also has a contrastive function in English as is illustrated by the minimal pairs *like* [laIk] and *light* [laIt], and *gun* [gʌn] and *done* [dʌn]. The significance of the contrastive function of phonetic distinctions such as voicing and place of articulation is best seen by considering what happens to the **intelligibility** of children and adults who are unable to use these phonetic features to distinguish between words in a language. Children with cleft palate use the glottal plosive [ʔ] in place of the oral plosives [t], [d], [k] and [g], which are difficult for them to articulate. So words such as *light* [laIt] and *lied* [laId] may be realized as [laIʔ] while *came* [keIm] and *game* [geIm] may be realized as [ʔeIm]. The loss of voicing in these realizations means that children with cleft palate are not able to distinguish certain words in language. This has an adverse effect on their intelligibility. When one considers that there is also a loss of place of articulation in words such as *day* [deI], *Kay* [keI] and *gay* [geI], all of which may be realized as [ʔeI], then the reduction in intelligibility is more severe still. An understanding of the contrastive function of phonetic distinctions is necessary in order to appreciate the reduced intelligibility that is experienced by children and adults with phonological disorders.

Some phonetic differences between sounds are non-contrastive in that they do not distinguish between different words in a language. In English, for example, the lateral approximant [l] may be pronounced as a velarized lateral approximant [ɫ] when it occurs before a consonant as in *silk*. It may be pronounced as a voiced velarized dental lateral approximant [ɫ̪] when it is produced before a dental fricative like [θ] in *wealth*. The lateral approximant may also be pronounced as a voiced nasalized and velarized alveolar lateral approximant [ɫ̃] when it occurs before [n] and [m] in words and phrases such as *all night* and *elm*. [l], [ɫ], [ɫ̪] and [ɫ̃] are described as **allophones** of the phoneme /l/ in English. Allophones of the same phoneme are in **complementary distribution**. This means that they do not appear in the same environments. Allophones are more than simply an important concept in phonology. They are directly relevant to the clinical management of clients by SLTs. A bilingual or multilingual client may have difficulty distinguishing phonemes in English because the sounds in question are allophones in the individual's primary language. When undertaking an assessment of a child who is suspected of having a speech sound disorder, SLTs must take into account phonemic and allophonic variations of the language(s) and/or dialect(s) used in the child's community and how these variations influence the determination of a disorder in a particular case. Ball (2012: 40) remarks that 'a child with speech sound disorder may realize a target sound with the wrong allophone of the phoneme concerned, with a sound that belongs to a different phoneme of the target language variety or with a sound from outside the target system altogether'.

To this point, we have presented the phoneme as the basic unit of analysis in phonology. However, the phoneme itself can be described in terms of a matrix of **phonological features**. By bringing these features together in various combinations, it should be possible to classify all the sounds in a language. Features are binary in that they can have plus (+) and minus (−) values. So, for example, vowels are [+ voice] while the voiceless plosives /p/, /t/ and /k/ are [− voice]. Another phonological feature is continuant, which describes a sound during whose production the air stream is not blocked in the oral cavity. Fricatives such as /s/ and /f/ are [+ continuant] while stops or plosives are [− continuant]. The phonological feature of sonorant describes a sound produced with a vocal tract configuration in which spontaneous voicing is possible. So vowels are [+ sonorant] while plosives, fricatives and affricates are [− sonorant]. If the tongue blade is raised during the articulation of a sound, it is [+ coronal]. Alveolar sounds are [+ coronal] while labials and velars are [− coronal]. Combining these four phonological features, we can arrive at a feature matrix for /t/: [− continuant, − sonorant, + coronal, − voice]. Phonological features are of relevance to SLTs because they allow therapists to characterize the phonological errors that are produced by children.

Consider the following single-word productions of a 4-year-old child with a phonological disorder who was reported by Yavaş (1998: 77):

[tʌn] 'sun'   [tɔk] 'sock'
[du] 'zoo'   [pit] 'feet'
[paɪb] 'five'   [nod] 'nose'
[bɛri] 'very'

This child has made four sound substitutions: /s/ → [t]; /z/ → [d]; /f/ → [p]; /v/ → [b]. However, these four substitutions can be characterized in terms of difficulty with just two phonological features. The features in question are [+/− continuant] and [+/− strident]. (The strident feature describes fricatives that are produced with high-intensity fricative noise, e.g. /f, s/.) This child with a phonological disorder is replacing target sounds that have the features [+ continuant] and [+ strident] with sounds that have the features [− continuant] and [− strident]. As well as characterizing phonological errors, phonological features may also be directly targeted in therapy. On the basis of the above productions, this 4-year-old child lacks the continuant feature in his phonological system. Velleman (2004) explains how this feature may be introduced during therapy and generalized to other sounds in the child's system as follows:

> A child who produces no fricatives lacks the continuant feature, so distinctive features therapy would focus on this feature. In theory, establishing a continuant in any place of articulation (e.g., [s]) would lead to the child's generalization of the feature to other, untrained fricatives. Once the feature is included in the child's feature inventory, it can be combined with other features (e.g., voice, palatal) to yield the remaining English fricatives. (198)

Phonological errors can also be characterized in terms of a number of **phonological processes**. These sound and syllable simplification processes occur in the speech of normally developing children and children with speech sound disorders. Paul and Norbury (2012) describe these processes as 'rule-governed attempts, which apply across a class of sounds or syllable structures, to make pronunciation easier' (294). Syllable simplification processes include consonant cluster reduction, initial consonant deletion and final consonant deletion. In each of these processes, syllable shape is simplified as a result of the process:

Consonant cluster reduction: 'green' [gin] CCVC → CVC
Initial consonant deletion: 'duck' [ʌk] CVC → VC
Final consonant deletion: 'dog' [dɔ] CVC → CV

There are phonological processes that alter the number of syllables in a word. In doing so, they change the shape of a word. Weak syllable deletion is an example:

Weak syllable deletion: 'banana' [nænə] CVCVCV → CVCV

Sound simplification processes are also evident in children's speech. Although target sounds are substituted by other sounds in these processes, the shape of the syllable in which these substitutions occur is unaffected. There are several different types of these processes:

Velar assimilation: 'wagon' [gægən] *Velar fronting:* 'key' [ti]
Nasal assimilation: 'sun' [nʌn] *Palatal fronting:* 'ship' [sIp]
Labial assimilation: 'tub' [bʌb] *Backing:* 'toy' [kɔI]
Stopping: 'sing' [tIŋ] *Gliding of fricatives:* 'food' [wud]
Prevocalic voicing: 'toes' [dos] *Cluster simplification:* 'black' [bwæk]
Devoicing: 'pig' [pIk] *Deaffrication:* 'juice' [ʒus]
Gliding of liquids: 'rabbit' [wæbIt] *Affrication:* 'shoe' [tʃu]

Phonological processes are drawn upon extensively in SLT to characterize the phonological errors of children with speech sound disorders and to decide which errors to target in therapy. For example, some phonological processes (e.g. stopping) may reduce a child's intelligibility more than other processes (e.g. deaffrication) and may be a priority for intervention for this reason. The chronology of phonological processes may also influence intervention decisions, with early-resolving processes targeted before late-resolving processes. For example, the persistence of prevocalic voicing, which normally resolves by 3 years of age, may make this process a priority for intervention over the gliding of liquids, which can be present in the speech of normally developing children up to 5 years. Whatever treatment decisions are motivated by a child's specific and sometimes idiosyncratic phonological processes, it is clear that this phonological concept is of considerable significance to SLT.

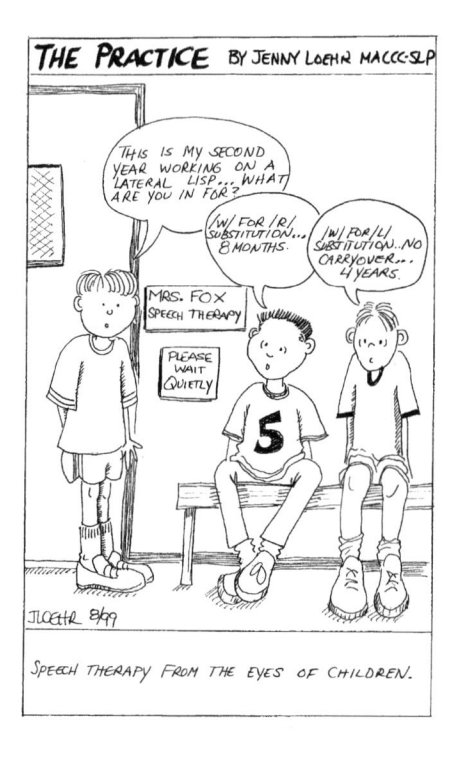

> **KEY POINTS: Phonology**
> - A number of phonological concepts are integral to the work of SLTs. These concepts must be understood both on their own terms and in terms of their relevance to the assessment and treatment of clients with speech sound disorders.
> - Phonology is the study of the contrastive function of phonetic distinctions. If a child is unable to use certain phonetic distinctions, the system of contrasts is reduced along with the child's intelligibility.
> - Not all phonetic differences between sounds are contrastive. The allophones of a phoneme are non-contrastive. SLTs must be aware of the allophones of phonemes in a bilingual or multilingual client's primary language.
> - Phonemes may be characterized in terms of phonological features that have binary values. Three such features are continuant, sonorant and coronal. The phonological errors that children make may be characterized in terms of phonological features.
> - Phonological errors may also be characterized in terms of one or more simplification processes. These processes can change the shape of words (e.g. weak syllable deletion) and the structure of syllables (e.g. consonant cluster reduction). They can also involve sound substitutions in word initial, medial and final position.
> - Both phonological features and phonological processes may be used to analyse the speech of children with speech sound disorders and are the basis of a number of speech sound interventions.

2.4 Morphology

Many clients who are assessed and treated by SLTs have problems with one or more aspects of morphology. Morphology is the study of the internal structure of words and the principles and patterns that underlie their composition (Schmid, 2015). **Morphemes** are the focus of analysis in morphology. In general, morphemes are the smallest meaningful units of a word. Some morphemes coincide with simple words or lexemes, e.g. *daughter* contains one morpheme that means 'female child'. Other morphemes are parts of complex words or lexemes. For example, *miner* contains two morphemes, the verb *mine* and the nominalizing suffix *-er* that means 'someone who does something'. The study of morphology is pursued in two main areas: inflectional morphology and word-formation. Markers of grammatical categories such as case, number, tense and aspect are examined in **inflectional morphology**. These morphemes attach to lexical stems and create new word-forms rather than new words. For example, *walk* is the base form to which *-s* is added (*walks*) to mark agreement with a third-person singular subject, *-ed* is added (*walked*) to indicate the past tense or a past participle and *-ing* is added (*walking*) to encode the progressive aspect.

Unlike inflectional morphology, **word-formation** is the study of the rules and patterns that guide the formation of new words. Word-formation includes **derivational morphology**. In the word *unhelpful*, for example, the derivational morphemes *un-* and *-ful* attach to the base *help* in a process of **prefixation** and **suffixation**, respectively. As well as derivational morphology, word-formation includes **compounding** (e.g. *council estate*) and other word-formation types that do not use morphemes as their building blocks (e.g. **blending** in *brunch* from *breakfast* and *lunch* and **clipping** in *exam* from *examination*).

The relevance of these morphological concepts and processes to SLT is best illustrated by examining examples of how their use is impaired in children and adults with language disorders. Inflectional morphology is often markedly disrupted in children with specific language impairment (SLI). These children may use incorrect inflectional suffixes on nouns and verbs or use no suffix at all when one is required. The extracts below illustrate these different morphological errors. Extracts in (a) and (b) are from Bliss et al. (1998). Extracts (c) to (f) are from Schuele and Dykes (2005).

(a) Boy with SLI aged 9;3 years: 'I flied and then I jumped down'
(b) Boy with SLI aged 9;3 years: 'I just broke my leg and I just fall down on my bike'
(c) Child with SLI aged 5;9 years: 'it's long ways to go'
(d) Child with SLI aged 5;9 years: 'let me see he work'
(e) Child with SLI aged 6;7 years: 'he need catched up'
(f) Child with SLI aged 7;10 years: 'if you just shoot it [...] it's still a points'

In (c) and (f), children with SLI have used the inflectional suffix *-s* for a plural noun when this suffix is not required. In terms of verb morphology, several errors occur. In (a), the inflectional suffix *-ed* for the past tense is used in 'flied'. This child's morphological knowledge does not include the irregular past tense form of *to fly* in English (*flew*). In (e), the inflectional suffix *-ed* is used when the infinitive form of the verb is required (*to catch*). Also in (e), the inflectional suffix *-s*, which is needed to mark agreement with the third-person singular subject 'he', is omitted. This same morphological error occurs in (d) in the verb *work*. Finally in (b), there is an absence of past tense verb morphology in 'I just fall down on my bike'.

Adults with language disorders can also have marked difficulty with noun and verb morphology. In (g) and (h) below, which are taken from Barr et al. (1989), the responses of an adult with schizophrenia during a **confrontation naming** task are presented. The utterance in (i) is taken from Chaika (1982):

(g) *Stimulus items:* octopus, cactus   *Client response:* 'octatoos'
(h) *Stimulus items:* noose, nozzle   *Client response:* 'noosle'
(i) 'I am being help with the food and medicate'

The client with schizophrenia, who produced the responses in (g) and (h) above, is making inappropriate use of blending. The source of the blend 'octatoos' in (g) can be represented as follows: (octo)pus x cac(tus) → octatoos. A similar blending error occurs in (h) and is represented as follows: (noos)e x nozz(le) → noosle. The adult with schizophrenia in (i) has difficulties with both inflectional and derivational morphology. This adult omits the inflectional suffix *-ed* in 'help' and does not use the derivational suffix *-ion* in 'medicate' to form the noun *medication*.

Clearly, SLTs must have an understanding of morphological concepts in order to characterize the errors above. But they must also have some appreciation of key milestones in morphological development. A seminal study by Brown (1973) of children's morphological development is still used today by SLTs to assess the extent of delays in this aspect of **language development**. Brown reported that the inflectional suffix for progressive aspect *-ing* is typically acquired between 28 and 36 months when children's **mean length of utterance** in morphemes (MLUm) is 2.25 (Stage II). At around the same stage, the suffix for plural nouns *-s* also emerges. Irregular past tense verb forms emerge between 36 and 42 months when mean MLUm is 2.75 (Stage III). The genitive form in *woman's dress* emerges at this same stage in development. At 40 to 46 months, when typically developing children have a mean MLUm of 3.5, the regular past tense suffix *-ed* is acquired (Stage IV). This is also the stage when children begin to use the suffix *-s* to mark agreement with a third-person singular subject. The child with SLI in (d) above, who at 5;9 years (69 months) is still not using *-s* to mark agreement with the third-person singular subject in 'let me see he work', is clearly displaying a considerable delay in his morphological development according to Brown's stages. Morphological development is one aspect of **child language acquisition,** which will be examined further in section 2.12.

> **KEY POINTS: Morphology**
> - Morphology is the study of the internal structure of words and the principles and patterns that underlie their composition. SLTs must have a sound working knowledge of morphology in order to assess and treat clients with language disorders.
> - SLT students need to understand inflectional morphology and be able to identify a range of inflectional suffixes (e.g. *-s, -ed, -ing*). These suffixes give rise to new word-forms rather than new words.
> - SLT students must also be able to identify derivational prefixes and suffixes in words such as *discoverable, fortunate, kindness, misunderstanding, disappear, unattractive, impossibility, incomprehensible* and *ponderable*. The processes of prefixation and suffixation that use these **affixes** to generate new words are examined in derivational morphology.
> - Besides derivational morphology, SLT students must be introduced to other word-formation processes such as compounding (e.g. *dog food*), blending (e.g. *info(rmation) x (enter)tainment → infotainment*) and clipping (e.g. *(in)flu(enza) → flu*).

> - SLT students must also have knowledge of the emergence of inflectional morphemes during normal language development and be able to apply this knowledge to an assessment of delayed morphology in disorders such as specific language impairment.

GROUP EXERCISE: Linguistic Disciplines and SLT

Using evidence to support your claims, discuss the following statement from McAllister and Miller (2013: 2) in a small group:

> Understanding the structure and function of language systems is as fundamental to the job of an SLT as understanding the structure of the human body is to the job of a doctor.

2.5 Syntax

A key component of all curricula in linguistics for SLT students is syntax. Syntax is the study of how phrases and sentences are constructed. In no natural language do words occur in a random order. Regardless of the language in question, there is always a clear order on the occurrence of words in sentences. Linguists who work in syntax aim to reveal that order and uncover the rules of the grammar of a language that make that order possible. According to the approach to syntax taken by Noam Chomsky, our internalized grammar of language – so-called **linguistic competence** – is what permits us to judge that the sentence in (a) below is ungrammatical, the sentence in (b) is ambiguous and the sentence in (c) is a paraphrase of the sentence in (d):

(a) She lived to next the church.
(b) He saw Big Ben flying over London.
(c) The dog attacked the postman.
(d) The postman was attacked by the dog.

To pursue Chomsky's ideas a little further, it is his contention that as children we are exposed to linguistic data which is degenerate in quality and limited in extent. Yet, as adults we all display the same knowledge of the grammar of our language, which permits judgements of the type illustrated in (a) to (d) above to be made. According to Chomsky, the only way to explain this gap between exposure to impoverished linguistic data and the mastery of the grammar of a language is to posit the existence of an innate **universal grammar**. This universal grammar undergoes **particularization** to the grammar of the language of the speech community in which the child lives. For the child exposed to English, this particularization leads him or her to acquire a grammatical rule about the order of adjectives and nouns in a noun phrase. This rule stipulates that adjectives must precede nouns in noun phrases, e.g. *the old man*. For the child exposed to French, a different grammatical rule is acquired as a result of the particularization of the universal grammar. This rule states that some adjectives precede nouns in noun phrases (e.g. *la jolie femme* 'the pretty woman'), while other adjectives follow nouns in noun phrases (e.g. *le chat noir* 'the black cat'). Other grammatical rules stipulate the order of occurrence of words in *yes–no* interrogatives, *wh*-interrogatives and passive voice constructions, as the sentences in (e) to (g) below illustrate:

(e) *Yes–no interrogative*, e.g. 'Are you going to the party?' (subject-auxiliary inversion)
(f) *Wh-interrogative*, e.g. 'What did you put in the cupboard?' (*wh*-movement)
(g) *Passive voice*, e.g. 'The robber was arrested by the police' (subject-object inversion)

The study of syntax in an SLT curriculum aims to provide students not only with the concepts and terms that are needed to give a full grammatical description of language but also with an understanding of the grammatical rules by means of which syntactic constructions are generated. Even a brief examination of the syntactic errors of children and adults with language disorders shows that there is a need for both components to be taught in syntax. Consider the utterances in (h) to (k) below; (h) and (i) are taken from Moore (2001) and (j) and (k) are taken from Schuele and Dykes (2005):

(h) Child with SLI aged 3;11 years: 'Her painting'
(i) Child with SLI aged 4;9 years: 'Why he fall in the car?'
(j) Child with SLI aged 5;9 years: 'lemme see looks like'
(k) Child with SLI aged 5;9 years: 'I don't know that is'

The child with SLI in (h) exhibits two syntactic errors. He uses the third-person object pronoun 'her' in place of the subject pronoun *she*. Additionally, he omits the auxiliary verb *is*, which should precede the main or lexical verb 'painting'. In the utterance in (i), the child with SLI forms a *wh*-interrogative by placing 'why' in front of a declarative sentence. This is an immature interrogative form which reflects the child's limited knowledge of the grammatical rules that are needed to form a *wh*-interrogative. Specifically, the child does not use the auxiliary verb *did*, which needs to be present in order for subject-auxiliary inversion to occur. In the utterances in (j) and (k), the child with SLI is unable to form *wh*-clauses in 'lemme see [what it] looks like' and 'I don't know [what] that is'. None of these syntactic problems can be adequately described, let alone assessed and treated, by SLTs who lack knowledge of the syntactic structures that are impaired in these children. The same is true of the syntactic errors produced by adults with language disorders. The following extract of language was produced by an aphasic client called

Roy who was studied by Beeke et al. (2007). Roy sustained a left-hemisphere cerebrovascular accident while waterskiiing seven years before this extract was recorded:

> um ... so s- er skiing ... er waterskiing ... yeh uh Greenbridge ... yeah? uh Kent ... uh ... uh ... four of them ... uuuhh ... blokes y'know ... uh ... uhhh ... boat ... and ... anyway ... sort of ... waterskiing ... and strange! ... sort of ... and then ... ur ... bang! [mimes falling over] ... funny ... and all of a sudden ... bang.

Roy's expressive syntax is severely disrupted as a result of his stroke. He exhibits a condition called agrammatism in which words from certain syntactic categories are retained while words from other syntactic categories are lost. Nouns (e.g. Kent, blokes, boat) and adjectives (e.g. strange, funny, sudden) are retained in Roy's verbal output. However, articles (definite and indefinite) and pronouns are completely omitted. Prepositions (with the exception of 'of'), conjunctions (with the exception of 'and') and verbs (with the exception of 'waterskiing') are also not present. As well as characterizing syntactic impairments in clients, knowledge of the syntax of language is also needed by SLT students in order to assess aspects of receptive and expressive syntax. Most formal language assessments contain one or more sub-tests relating to syntax. One assessment, which examines the comprehension of 20 different syntactic structures, is the *Test for Reception of Grammar – Version 2* (TROG-2; Bishop, 2003b). The TROG-2 contains the following stimulus items:

(l) The cow is chased by the girl.
(m) The duck is bigger than the ball.
(n) The elephant pushing the boy is big.
(o) The cup is in the box that is red.
(p) The man sees that the boy is pointing at him.

SLT students must be well versed in syntax in order to understand that the sentence in (l) is testing the comprehension of a reversible passive construction ('is chased by'), the sentence in (m) the comprehension of a comparative adjective ('bigger'), the sentence in (n) the comprehension of a post-modified subject ('the elephant pushing the boy'), the sentence in (o) the comprehension of an object relative clause ('the box that is red') and the sentence in (p) the comprehension of pronoun binding ('The man sees that the boy is pointing at him'). Interventions that target aspects of receptive and expressive syntax can only be competently implemented by clinicians who have a sound knowledge of syntax. For example, Hsu and Bishop (2014) used an intervention that trained children with SLI to understand reversible sentences such as 'The ball is above the cup', where the spatial configuration in the sentence depends on word order. It emerges that clinicians cannot describe, assess or treat clients with grammatical disorders in the absence of knowledge of a range of syntactic structures and the syntactic operations that generate these structures.

KEY POINTS: Syntax

- Syntax is central to the linguistics curriculum of SLT students. Students must understand the structure of phrases and sentences and the grammatical principles and operations that govern and generate this structure. Theoretical approaches to syntax (e.g. Chomsky) should be introduced.
- SLT students must be introduced to the terms and concepts that are needed to provide a full grammatical description of language. This includes terms such as *conjunction* and *preposition* at word level, *premodifer* and *head* at phrase level, *relative clause* and *subordinate clause* at clause level and *imperative* and *interrogative* at sentence level.
- SLT students must also understand the syntactic operations by means of which structures such as passive voice sentences and *wh*-interrogatives are generated.
- SLT students require extensive practice in performing syntactic analyses of disordered language in children and adults. This practice ensures accurate characterization of syntactic deficits in clients.
- The assessment and treatment of syntactic impairments in clients demands a sound working knowledge of all of the aforementioned aspects of syntax.

2.6 Semantics

Semantics is the study of word and sentence meaning. Because both aspects of language meaning may be disrupted in clients with language disorders, semantics is a significant component in the linguistics curriculum of SLT students. Concepts that are fundamental to the study of semantics include reference and sense. The notion of **reference** captures a fundamental intuition about language meaning. Briefly, that intuition is that at least part of the meaning of linguistic expressions derives from the use of these terms to refer to people, objects and events in the external world. The referential relation that hooks aspects of language onto features of the external world is reflected in the use of the term *referential meaning* in semantics (also known as denotational meaning or extensional meaning). However, not all aspects of language meaning can be captured in terms of referential relations between language and the external world. Expressions in a language can also derive meaning – their **sense** – from their place in a system of semantic relationships with other terms or expressions in the language. A number of these so-called sense relations or **lexical relations** have come to occupy a focal position in discussions of **lexical semantics**. They include the following six lexical relations:

synonymy (e.g. *liberty – freedom*): two words have the same or similar meaning
hyponymy (e.g. *bird – eagle*): relation of inclusion
antonymy (e.g. *empty – full*): relation of opposition
meronymy (e.g. *book – chapter*): part-whole relation
polysemy (e.g. 'drive', *drive a nail – drive a car*): related senses of a word
homonymy (e.g. 'lap', part of body – circuit of a course): unrelated senses of a word

Antonymy can be further characterized as *binary* or *complementary* in nature where the positive of one term implies the negative of another term (e.g. *dead – alive*), *gradable* where terms can be arranged along a continuum (e.g. *hot – cold*), *converse* where a relation between two entities is described from alternate viewpoints (e.g. *employer – employee*) and *reverse* where one term describes movement in one direction and the other term describes movement in the opposite direction (e.g. *ascend – descend*). Knowledge of lexical relations is needed in order to characterize certain lexical errors that are produced by children and adults with language disorders. The data below was obtained from a 74-year-old right-handed woman, known as JT, who was studied by Buckingham and Rekart (1979). JT displayed clinical symptoms that were typical of **Wernicke's aphasia** after she sustained a left parietal cerebrovascular accident. The utterances below were produced during conversation and picture naming. The target lexeme in each case is indicated in brackets:

(a) 'Well, that's the fingers (knuckles) . . .'
(b) 'It wasn't cold (hot) for me'
(c) 'My brother brought me an apple (cherries) today'

In the utterance in (a), the relation of meronymy explains JT's lexical error – the target word 'knuckles' is a meronym of 'fingers'. The lexical error in the utterance in (b) can be characterized in terms of antonymy – 'cold' is a gradable antonym of 'hot'. In the utterance in (c), JT makes a lexical error based on hyponymy – 'apple' and 'cherries' are both hyponyms of *fruit*. These errors are known as **semantic paraphasias**. They suggest that as part of her stroke-induced aphasia, JT has experienced significant disruption of her lexical semantic knowledge.

In the same way that phonemes can be characterized in terms of a number of phonological features, words in semantics can be characterized in terms of **semantic components** or primitives. Saeed (2016) states that 'some semanticists have hypothesized that words are not the smallest semantic units but are built up of smaller components of meaning which are combined differently (or lexicalized) to form different words' (259). Semanticists who examine these components do so within an approach to semantics called **componential analysis**. In this way, the meaning of the word *spinster* may be characterized in terms of three components: [FEMALE] [ADULT] [UNMARRIED]. With a larger number of components, the analysis of word meaning can become cumbersome and unwieldy. Componential analysts rely on binary features and redundancy rules to achieve a more economic characterization of the components that apply in a particular case. In terms of binary features, an individual component may have plus (+) and minus (−) values. So rather than using two separate components to represent the meaning of *spinster* [UNMARRIED] and *wife* [MARRIED], a single component with plus and minus values can be used instead, i.e. *spinster* [−MARRIED] and *wife* [+MARRIED]. Redundancy rules permit further economy by reducing the number of components that apply in a particular case. For example, the following redundancy rule can be applied to the word *wife*: [MARRIED] → [ADULT]. This rule removes the need to list [ADULT] as a separate component of *wife* – this component is simply assumed to apply as a result of the redundancy rule attached to [MARRIED].

Semantic components also have direct relevance to the work of SLTs. Impairments of **semantic memory** in conditions such as dementia and aphasia have often been reported to involve specific components such as *abstract/concrete* and *living/non-living*. In this way, clients with aphasia or dementia may display a selective naming or comprehension deficit for words such as *justice*, *trust* and *love* that share the component [ABSTRACT], or words such as *woman*, *dog* and *boy* that share the component [ANIMATE]. Alternatively, these clients may struggle to produce or comprehend words that share the [CONCRETE] component or the [INANIMATE] component. The presence of deficits that involve specific components or primitives receives support from the findings of clinical studies. Bonner et al. (2009) examined semantic memory for concrete and abstract verbs in patients with **semantic dementia** using a two-alternative, forced-choice measure of lexical semantic associative knowledge. These patients had significantly greater difficulty with concrete verbs than with abstract verbs. Papagno et al. (2009) reported a subject with semantic dementia in which there was also sparing of abstract word processing and impairment of concrete words. However, this effect was restricted to nouns. Proper names (people and landmarks) were severely damaged, while among common names living entities were severely impaired relative to non-living entities. The preservation of abstract word processing over concrete words in these patients with semantic dementia is the reverse effect of that reported in neurologically healthy subjects and in adults with aphasia (Sandberg and Kiran, 2014).

It is also important for SLT students to have an understanding of sentence semantics. One aspect of sentence semantics of particular relevance to clinicians is the use of **semantic roles** to describe various entities in a situation. These roles are associated with the **argument structure** of verbs. A number of semantic roles are described below (Saeed, 2015: 182). Their use is illustrated in sentences (d) to (f):

    AGENT: initiator of some action, typically capable of acting with volition

    PATIENT: entity undergoing the effect of some action, typically undergoing a change of state

THEME: the entity which is moved by an action, or whose location is described
EXPERIENCER: an entity aware of the action or state described by the predicate but not in control of it
BENEFICIARY: the entity benefiting from some action
INSTRUMENT: the means by which an AGENT causes something to come about
LOCATION: the place in which something is situated or takes place
GOAL: the entity towards which something moves
SOURCE: the entity from which something moves
STIMULUS: the entity causing an effect in the EXPERIENCER

(d) The teenager$_{AGENT}$ threw stones$_{THEME}$ from the balcony$_{SOURCE}$.
(e) The tremor$_{STIMULUS}$ terrified the tourists$_{EXPERIENCER}$.
(f) The lorry driver$_{AGENT}$ stirred the coffee$_{PATIENT}$ with a spoon$_{INSTRUMENT}$.

Some semantic roles are obligatory in the argument structure of verbs while others are optional. For example, in the sentence in (d) the AGENT is an obligatory role while the SOURCE is optional. Obligatory semantic roles are often used erroneously or omitted altogether by children with SLI and other language disorders. Andreu et al. (2013) investigated the formulation of verb argument structure in Catalan- and Spanish-speaking children with SLI and typically developing age-matched controls. As verb argument complexity increased, these investigators found that children with SLI made more errors of obligatory arguments, especially of themes, than typically developing children. SLT interventions may target the semantic or **thematic roles** of noun phrases in verb argument structures. Thompson et al. (2013) trained individuals with chronic **agrammatic aphasia** to produce three-argument verbs (verbs which have three thematic roles) in active sentences (e.g. 'The boy is giving the flowers to the woman'). This training emphasized argument structure and thematic role mapping. It was found to be effective for improving verb and sentence production in these individuals with aphasia.

KEY POINTS: Semantics

- Semantics is the study of word and sentence meaning. Because semantic aspects of language are often impaired in clients with language disorders, semantics must be part of any linguistics curriculum for SLT students.
- SLT students should be introduced to semantic concepts such as reference and sense. These concepts capture basic intuitions about meaning – the idea that expressions in language have meaning by virtue of a referential relation to people, objects and events in the world

- (reference) and by virtue of their relationship to other expressions in language (sense).
- The study of word meaning in lexical semantics includes an examination of lexical relations: synonymy (*regal – royal*), hyponymy (*dog – spaniel*), antonymy (*old – young*), meronymy (*eye – retina*), polysemy (fork: *fork in road – item of cutlery*), and homonymy (bark: *cry of a dog – outer layer of tree*). Additionally, antonymy has binary (*present – absent*), gradable (*rich – poor*), converse (*pupil – teacher*), and reverse (*fill – empty*) forms.
- SLT students should be introduced to theoretical approaches to semantics. One approach, known as componential analysis, seeks to examine word meaning in terms of a number of semantic components or primitives. Components are needed to conceptualize impairments of semantic memory in clients with conditions such as aphasia and dementia.
- Sentence semantics is also relevant to SLT students. Clinicians need to understand the various semantic roles that can represent different entities in a situation. These roles, which include AGENT, PATIENT and THEME, are part of the argument structure of verbs. Obligatory semantic or thematic roles may be used erroneously or omitted altogether by clients with language disorders.

2.7 Pragmatics

An account of language meaning is not complete by studying semantics alone. To understand what someone means by an utterance, we frequently have to look beyond the meanings of words and sentences and consider utterances within the contexts in which speakers use them. The study of the meaning of utterances in context is the essence of pragmatics. In recent years, there has been increased interest in pragmatics in SLT. This increase has seen the emergence of **clinical pragmatics** as a distinct sub-discipline of linguistic pragmatics and a new emphasis on pragmatics in the clinical education of SLT students (Cummings, 2009, 2014a). Among the pragmatic concepts included in the linguistics curriculum of SLT students are speech acts. The concept of a **speech act** originated in the work of a group of philosophers of language (e.g. John L. Austin) who recognized that language could be used to do more than describe states of affairs in the world. Specifically, language can be used to make promises, to issue warnings and threats, to convey orders and to make apologies. Examples of these speech acts are shown below:

(a) 'I will be at the meeting' (*promise*)
(b) 'The river has broken its banks' (*warning*)
(c) 'Big Jim wants to see you' (*threat*)

(d) 'Finish your homework!' (*order*)
(e) 'I'm so terribly sorry' (*apology*)

While a number of speech acts are explicitly indicated by the use of a **performative verb** (e.g. *I baptize this child Peter Brown*), many other speech acts are not signalled through specific lexemes or grammatical constructions. For example, the following utterances are all ways in which a speaker may make a request to be given the time:

(f) Can you tell me the time?
(g) It must be nearly midday
(h) Do you know the time?
(i) I left my watch in the office
(j) What time is it?

Many children and adults with language disorders struggle to produce and comprehend speech acts. The subject-auxiliary inversion that is needed to produce the utterance in (f) may exceed the syntactic skills of children with SLI or adults with aphasia. These clients may exhibit a limited repertoire of speech acts on account of their expressive language difficulties, although they may still be able to produce specific speech acts through other linguistic and non-linguistic means (e.g. a speaker can request the time by pointing at a person's watch). The comprehension of speech acts may be impaired in children and adults with autism spectrum disorder. This is illustrated in a study by Loukusa et al. (2007) in which a 9-year-old boy with **Asperger's syndrome** is shown a picture of a mother and a girl. The girl has a dress on and she is running. There are muddy puddles on the road. The girl has just stepped in the puddle and the picture shows the mud splashing. The researcher reads the following verbal scenario aloud and then asks the boy a question:

The girl with her best clothes on is running on the dirty road. The mother shouts to the girl: 'Remember that you have your best clothes on!' What does the mother mean?

The boy with Asperger's syndrome replies: 'You have your best clothes on.'

The response of this boy is little more than a repetition of the mother's utterance. It indicates that he has failed to comprehend the type of speech act which this utterance performs. The speech act is clearly a warning to the girl to keep her clothes clean.

SPECIAL TOPIC: Autism Spectrum Disorder

Persistent deficits in social communication and social interaction, and restricted, repetitive patterns of behaviour, interests or activities set children with autism spectrum disorder (ASD) apart from their typically developing peers. For those children with ASD who develop language, there can be marked difficulties in the pragmatics of language. Impaired pragmatic language skills are a significant barrier to establishing social relationships and performing occupational roles. Among the pragmatic deficits of clients with ASD are the following behaviours:

- Domination of conversation with topics that represent a restricted interest of the child or adult with ASD
- Literal interpretation of indirect speech acts and other non-literal forms of language such as idioms, metaphors and sarcasm
- Difficulty establishing the gist of a story or the temporal and causal relationships between events in a story
- Use of impolite and other socially inappropriate utterances during conversation
- Use of repetitive, tangential and over-informative discourse
- Impaired use of non-verbal pragmatic skills such as gesture and eye gaze

Each of these pragmatic anomalies can be explained by a cognitive deficit in theory of mind (ToM) in children and adults with ASD (also see section 4.2 in Chapter 4). ToM is the ability to attribute cognitive mental states (e.g. knowledge, beliefs) and affective mental states (e.g. fear, happiness) to the minds of other people. The child or adult with ASD who cannot attribute mental states to others pursues topics of conversation which are not of interest to the hearer, produces discourse which exceeds the informational needs of the listener and cannot establish the communicative intention which motivates a speaker to utter an indirect speech act such as *It's warm in here* – the speaker wants the heating to be turned off. As well as communicative difficulties, children with ASD and impaired ToM have limited appreciation of the emotional states of others. This is clearly demonstrated in the responses to an experimental task of a 7-year-old boy with Asperger's syndrome, who was studied by Loukusa et al. (2007). The boy is shown a picture of a boy sitting on the branch of a tree. A wolf is underneath the boy at the bottom of the tree. The wolf is growling at the boy. A man with a gun is walking nearby. The researcher reads the following verbal scenario aloud and then asks a question:

The boy sits up in the tree and a wolf is at the bottom of the tree. How does the boy feel?

Response of boy with Asperger's syndrome: 'Fun because he climbs up the tree. I always have fun when I climb up a tree.'

The boy with Asperger's syndrome has failed to attribute the correct emotional or affective mental state (namely, fear) to the boy in the picture.

Utterances can also convey a range of implicated meanings. These so-called **implicatures** were first characterized by H. Paul Grice. Grice proposed a regulative principle (the **cooperative principle**) which he took to apply to all forms of rational behaviour and not only to verbal communicative behaviour. Grice (1975) formulated this principle as follows: 'Make your conversational contribution such as is required, at the stage at which it occurs, by the accepted purpose or direction of the talk exchange in which you are engaged' (45). The cooperative principle is fleshed out through four sub-maxims which Grice called quality ('Do not say that which you believe to be false or that for which you lack adequate evidence'), quantity ('Do not contribute more information than is required but also do not contribute less information than is required'), relation ('Be relevant') and manner ('Be brief and orderly; avoid obscurity of expression and ambiguity'). The role of the cooperative principle and **maxims** in the generation and recovery of implicatures is illustrated in the exchange below between Bill and Jill:

> BILL: Do you want pasta and fish for dinner?
> JILL: I want fish.

Jill explicitly states that she wants fish for dinner. But in doing so, she also implicates that she does *not* want pasta for dinner. How does Bill recover this particular implicature of Jill's utterance when that utterance makes no mention of pasta? Bill sets out from the assumption that Jill is observing the cooperative principle. In other words, Bill believes that Jill is attempting to be truthful, informative, relevant and unambiguous to the best extent possible in her verbal exchange with him. It is with this assumption of cooperation in mind that Bill proceeds to process Jill's utterance. That utterance is under-informative – Jill has been asked a question about two types of food (pasta and fish), but her response only mentions one type (fish). Bill uses Jill's under-informative reply to recover the implicature that Jill does not want pasta.

The inferential steps which take Bill from Jill's utterance to the **communicative intention** that motivated that utterance continue to fascinate pragmatists. However, these steps still evade a fully satisfactory explanation (Cummings, 2005). What is clear is that while individuals with intact pragmatic language skills can effortlessly establish the implicatures of utterances, the recovery of these implicated meanings is anything but effortless for a large number of children and adults with pragmatic disorders. Individuals with pragmatic disorders frequently misinterpret non-literal language such as **irony** and **metaphor**. In producing an ironic utterance, a speaker overtly flouts the maxim of quality – the speaker says X when it is clear that he believes not-X. Only hearers who can establish the belief of the speaker are able to interpret the speaker's use of irony. Irony was one of a number of pragmatic phenomena examined by Colle et al. (2013) in a study of linguistic and extra-linguistic pragmatic functioning in 17 adults with schizophrenia. In one stimulus presentation, subjects with schizophrenia were shown the following videotaped scenario:

> A boy and a girl are eating a disgusting soup. The boy smacks his lips with a gesture meaning 'It's very good!'
>
> *Question:* 'What did the boy mean by that?'
>
> *Subject's response:* 'He meant to say that she cooked a delicious soup.'

The subject with schizophrenia who produced this response has failed to grasp the ironic intent which motivates the boy's non-verbal behaviour in this scenario. In the same study, subjects with schizophrenia also displayed difficulty with the interpretation of irony in linguistic utterances. These findings are replicated in other clinical studies of implicature across a range of clients with pragmatic disorders (see Cummings, 2014a, for a review). These studies confirm the need to introduce SLT students to different types of implicature as part of a comprehensive curriculum in linguistics.

SLT students must also have a sound knowledge of **deixis**. Speakers use deictic expressions to refer to the people present in a conversation (*personal deixis*), to capture aspects of the social relationship between speaker and hearer (*social deixis*) and to reflect spatial aspects of context in utterances (*spatial deixis*). Deictic expressions may also be used to locate an utterance in time (*temporal deixis*) and to refer to aspects of spoken and written texts (*discourse deixis*). These five uses of deixis are illustrated in the utterances in (k) to (o):

(k) 'I want to leave early' (*personal deixis*)
(l) 'Wie heiβen Sie?' (*social deixis*)
(m) 'Jack really wants to live here' (*spatial deixis*)
(n) 'John arrived yesterday' (*temporal deixis*)
(o) 'This view of grammar is discussed in the next chapter' (*discourse deixis*)

As these utterances demonstrate, a range of linguistic expressions fulfil a deictic function in language. They include personal pronouns (*I, we, you*), verbs (*bring, take*), adverbs (*here, there*), adjectives (*next, last*), demonstratives (*this, that*) and calendrical terms (*yesterday, tomorrow*). Also, a single expression can assume two or more deictic functions. For example, the underlined expressions in utterances (p), (q) and (r) use the demonstrative determiner *this*. In the utterance in (p) 'this way' is a form of spatial deixis, in (q) 'this week' is an instance of temporal deixis and in (r) 'this chapter' is a form of discourse deixis:

(p) 'I want to walk home this way' (*spatial deixis*)
(q) 'I want to see the movie this week' (*temporal deixis*)
(r) 'I want to present an opposing view in this chapter' (*discourse deixis*)

Deixis is often disrupted in children and adults with language disorders. Chapman et al. (1998) examined the retelling of fables by adults with **fluent aphasia**. In one fable, a raven painted his feathers white so that he could get access to the pigeon coop and share in the pigeons' food. However, when he started to crow, the pigeons realized he was an imposter and chased him away. The raven then returned to his own kind. But because his feathers were painted white, the other ravens did not recognise him and also chased him away. This is how one adult with fluent aphasia retold the fable:

> This was a story of the raven that ... painted his feathers white. And got over, to get over the pigeons and they caught him and made him get away. But he left, let me see, some of them was still <u>there</u> but the pigeons got them all out of the way. *(E: Some of who were still there?)* The pigeons – the ravens, the ravens was <u>there</u>. But they finally got them all out. They all uh had uh yellow-yellow-no white, the was painted white. *(E: And how did the pigeons know ... that this was a raven and not a pigeon?)* Because they s – I don't know, it's, they sounded different (laughs).

This adult's retelling of the fable is particularly difficult to follow. This difficulty is related in part to the use of deictic expressions for which there are no clear referents. On two occasions, this speaker with aphasia uses spatial deixis in the form of the adverb *there*. However, there is no obvious **referent** of either use of this expression – *there* could refer to the pigeon coop, an area where the ravens congregate or some other location in the mind of the speaker.

Finally, SLT students must also understand the pragmatic concept of **presupposition**. Presuppositions are assumptions or inferences that are implicit in particular linguistic expressions. Speakers can represent shared or background knowledge with hearers in the presuppositions of an utterance. In doing so, considerable efficiency can be achieved by reducing the amount of explicit language that speakers need to produce during communication. Specific lexical items and syntactic constructions are used to represent the presuppositions of an utterance. These so-called presupposition triggers include the lexemes and constructions shown in the utterances in (s) to (w) below:

(s) '<u>It was</u> the teenager who vandalized the bus shelter' (*cleft construction*)
(t) '<u>The house on the hill</u> is for sale' (*definite description*)
(u) 'Mary <u>regretted</u> getting divorced' (*factive verb*)
(v) 'The prisoner escaped <u>again</u>' (*iterative*)
(w) 'The doctors <u>managed</u> to save the baby's life' (*implicative verb*)

The presuppositions of these utterances are that *someone* vandalized the bus shelter (s), that there *exists* a house on the hill (t), that Mary *did* get divorced (u), that the prisoner escaped *before* (v), and that the doctors *tried* to save the baby's life (w). A characteristic of presupposition is its capacity for **constancy under negation**. This feature sets presupposition apart from **entailment**. The utterance in (x) entails that *Sally groomed a dog*. However, this entailment is cancelled if the original utterance is negated, as in (y). But the presupposition of the utterance in (z) – that Fred is sexist – holds even when the original utterance is negated:

(x) 'Sally groomed a King Charles spaniel' *entails* Sally groomed a dog.
(y) 'Sally did *not* groom a King Charles spaniel' *does not entail* Sally groomed a dog.
(z) 'Bill is as sexist/is not as sexist as Fred' *presupposes* Fred is sexist.

The use of presupposition may be impaired in children and adults with pragmatic disorder. McTear (1985) examined a 10-year-old boy with pragmatic disorder. In the exchange below, an adult (A) is introducing a communication task to the boy (C). The task, which is described by the adult as 'games', is unfamiliar to the boy:

A: now do you want to see if you can play some games with me?
C: yes
A: they're very easy games um (1.0)
C: they are indeed
A: well we'll see

The child's second turn is an utterance which presupposes that the child has some familiarity with the games in question. However, this is not the case and so the presupposition is false. The failure of this child with pragmatic disorder to make appropriate use of presupposition serves to illustrate why SLT students must be introduced to this important pragmatic concept as part of their curriculum in linguistics.

KEY POINTS: Pragmatics

- Pragmatics is the study of meaning in context. This form of meaning is also described as implied or intended meaning, speaker meaning and utterance meaning.
- Language may be used to do more than describe states of affairs in the world. Language can be used to make promises, issue threats and express condolences. These different uses of utterances are speech acts.
- Utterances can also convey implicated meanings or implicatures. The implicatures of utterances can be recovered by means of the cooperative principle and maxims: quality, quantity, relation and manner.
- Deixis is an important pragmatic concept for SLT students. Deictic expressions can refer to the people present in a conversation (*personal deixis*), to spatiotemporal aspects of context (*spatial and temporal deixis*), to the social relationship between speaker and hearer (*social deixis*), and to parts of spoken and written texts (*discourse deixis*).
- Presuppositions are inferences and assumptions which are implicit in utterances. They represent shared or background knowledge between speakers and hearers. Specific words and linguistic constructions can trigger presuppositions (e.g. cleft constructions, factive verbs). Presupposition differs from entailment in that it displays constancy under negation.

2.8 Discourse

Increasingly, SLT students must have an understanding of what discourse is and how it can be analysed. Linguists who study discourse are less concerned with the internal structure of sentences and are more interested in how one sentence or utterance relates to other sentences and utterances in extended spoken and written texts. The context for a **discourse analysis** of language in SLT is typically narrative production tasks (monologic discourse) and conversation (dialogic discourse). As with other disciplines in linguistics, SLT students need to have a sound knowledge of certain concepts in discourse. One such concept is **cohesion**. Speakers and narrators use a range of linguistic devices to achieve cohesion between sentences and utterances. These devices provide essential links between one event, idea or information unit and the next. They are the means by which hearers and readers are able to establish causal and temporal relations between events and are able to impose logical order on what would otherwise be a sequence of disconnected ideas. Several cohesive devices are illustrated by the sentences in (a) to (e) below:

(a) Jack bought new boots. They were very expensive.
(b) Verity ordered a large cocktail even though she had already had one.
(c) A: Who would like gravy? B: I would.
(d) Dan decided to remove the elm in the back garden. The tree had fungal disease.
(e) It was raining. So we went to the cinema.

The two sentences in (a) are linked through **anaphoric reference** – the referent of 'they' is the preceding noun phrase 'new boots'. The cohesive device in (b) is one of **substitution**, with 'one' acting as a substitute for the noun phrase 'a large cocktail'. The second utterance in (c) is an example of **ellipsis**. B's response omits 'like gravy' which B knows A can effectively supply. The sentences in (d) are an example of **lexical reiteration** in which cohesion is achieved through 'elm' and its superordinate term 'tree'. Finally, the conjunction 'so' in (e) expresses a meaning of 'in consequence'. This conjunction makes it clear that one event (a visit to the cinema) occurred in consequence of another event (a downpour of rain).

Cohesion is often impaired in children and adults with language disorders. In the following exchange between a teacher (T) and a child called Adam (A) who has attention deficit hyperactivity disorder, there are a number of problems with cohesion. These problems have an adverse effect on the comprehensibility of Adam's account of snow tubing. Adam is 7;10 years at the time of this study by Peets (2009):

T: Can you tell us about snow tubing?
A: Snow tubing is is freaky.
T: Freaky. Tell us what it's like. What do you do?
A: They uh they have a machine that will they have a hooks that will pull you back up and then you have eight tickets you give one of them to (th)em then you got hold onto a rope they have like a little round thing and then you go they put the put the hook inside and then and then it pulls you back up and then you slide down they put they maybe the if you want to stay straight you tell my parents from up there if you want a spin they he spins you.

Adam exhibits significant difficulties with the use of reference. He makes repeated use of pronouns in the absence of any referent of those pronouns in an earlier part of his discourse. Examples include the underlined expressions in 'they have a machine', 'they have like a little round thing' and 'he spins you'. He also makes repeated use of 'and then' to link clauses. The predominance of this somewhat immature form of conjunction limits the range of relationships that exists between clauses to one of addition (*and*) and temporal order (*then*).

An individual can produce cohesive spoken and written discourse and yet still relate an incoherent narrative, for example. **Coherence** is another important discourse concept for SLT students. Notwithstanding the ease with which we can identify incoherent discourse, a generally accepted definition of coherence remains somewhat elusive. Hoey (1991) states that coherence is 'a quality assigned to text by a reader or listener, and is a measure of the extent to which the reader or listener finds that the text holds together and makes sense as a unity' (265–6). If we hear a story in which the narrator fails to relate individual episodes to the purpose or goal in telling the story, we are left with the sense that the narrative is incoherent. Other impressions of incoherence arise when we cannot establish the motivations of characters in a story or how one event leads to another event. Equally, the narrator who omits key episodes or digresses significantly cannot be said to have produced a coherent narrative. Given the wide range of ways in which narratives and other forms of discourse may be incoherent, it should not be surprising to discover that there is no core set of linguistic features which constitute coherent discourse. The coherence of narrative and conversational discourse is often impaired in children and adults with cognitive-communication disorders. This is evident in the following exchange between an examiner (E) and a 36-year-old man called Warren (W). Warren has **AIDS dementia complex**. His problems with pragmatics and discourse were examined by McCabe et al. (2008):

> E: What would be the longest job you had?
> W: Oh, when I had the business, cleaning the building
> E: mm and that was for how many years?
> W: 8 years, like I said I was spoiled
> E: And that was when you were in your twenties?
> W: Twenty two. (Name) was the only person who had total faith in me. There was an intelligent person in there that, um, he said I've got more common sense. I like that idea 'cause there's nothing common about this little black duck and if I am on my way to prove that I'm not. My great grandmother was born into a family that was indentured to a castle near Salisbury, Newcastle. Well she was supposed to be a house servant. She sort of looked at then at the age of 17 and said 'Do I look like a peasant girl to you? I don't think so, I'm jumping on a boat and going to Australia ...' [continued in same vein for six more utterances]

Warren's third turn in this exchange displays marked incoherence. This turn deviates markedly from the **topic** of Warren's prior jobs. There is intrusion of bizarre detail and the entire turn has a confabulatory quality. The events which Warren relates are almost completely incomprehensible within the context of this particular discourse. Warren's problems with coherence occur alongside relatively intact structural language and cohesion.

KEY POINTS: Discourse

- Increasingly, SLTs are making use of techniques that require a sound knowledge of the features of different types of discourse. Discourse is now an essential component of the linguistics curriculum of SLT students.
- Narrative, conversational and procedural discourse may be examined in a clinical context. Narrative production tasks are often used to elicit discourse in clinic.
- Cohesion is often disrupted in clients with language and communication disorders. Grammatical and lexical cohesion may be achieved through reference, ellipsis, substitution and lexical reiteration among other forms.
- Coherence is another important discourse concept. While language users can readily distinguish coherent from incoherent discourse, it is less easy to capture the essence of this notion.
- A conversation or narrative may be judged to be incoherent if it deviates markedly from topic, if information is missing or is presented in an illogical way, or if there is no apparent purpose or goal to which events relate.
- There is no well-defined set of linguistic features which constitute the coherence of a text, either spoken or written.

CASE STUDY: Linguistic Disciplines in Action

This case study is designed to make you think about some of the linguistic disciplines which are part of the knowledge base of SLTs. Read the case study carefully. Then, individually or in a group, answer the questions that follow it.

A 6-year-old boy called Jake is referred to a child development unit by an educational psychologist who is concerned about his limited language skills. He attends an initial assessment with his mother. The SLT takes an extensive case history. This reveals that Jake was pre-term and was delivered by caesarean section. According to his mother, he was a 'late talker' and did not produce his first words until 20 months. His motor development appeared to be normal. Jake's mother reports that he has some social interaction difficulties with other children. The SLT engages Jake in conversation during play. She observes poor turn-taking, lack of eye contact and poor topic maintenance. The SLT records the following utterances which Jake produced spontaneously during play:

'Doggie bad' 'He falling' 'Two mouses' 'man car' 'Now he eated'
To test Jake's auditory verbal comprehension, the SLT asks him to respond to a number of commands. Jake's only correct response was to the first of these commands. His understanding of the items used in these commands – ball, spoon, etc. – was tested beforehand and was intact:

> 'Show me the ball'
> 'Put the cup beside the spoon'
> 'Give me the large cup'
> 'Put the pencil on top of the box'
> 'Show me the pencil and give me the spoon'

The SLT uses her observations of Jake's receptive and expressive language skills to plan a comprehensive language assessment which will be conducted at the next appointment.

Questions

(1) Which verbal behaviour(s) suggest(s) that the SLT may need to assess Jake's pragmatic language skills and discourse skills in more detail?
(2) Which commands suggest that Jake may have limited lexical semantic knowledge of prepositions?
(3) Give one example of an immaturity in Jake's use of noun morphology and one example of an immaturity in his use of verb morphology.
(4) Is there any evidence that the genitive form is still not part of Jake's knowledge of expressive syntax?
(5) One of Jake's errors stems from the misapplication of a syntactic rule. Which error is it? What name is given to this error?

2.9 Sociolinguistics

Sociolinguistics and bilingualism are essential components of the linguistics curriculum of SLT students. The RCSLT guidelines for pre-registration courses in the UK require SLT students to have an understanding of:

> **Sociolinguistics and current language change:**
> Regional and social dialects and accents
> Gender- and age-related variation in speech and language
> Styles and registers
>
> **Bilingualism:**
> Theoretical models of bilingualism
> Varying dimensions of bilingualism
> Bilingual language acquisition, speech production and perception
> (RCSLT, 2010: 36)

SLTs work with children and adults who live in communities where a range of **accents** and **dialects** are spoken. These accents and dialects reflect the regional identity of speakers. The use of the 'for to' infinitive by speakers of Northern Irish English (e.g. *I want for to meet them*) is an example of grammatical variation (Henry, 1992). The presence of this infinitive in the language of a client does not signal grammatical deviance which requires intervention by SLTs. Speakers of **Estuary English** can use l-vocalization in consonant clusters at the end of a syllable, e.g. *milk* /mɪʊk/ (Beal, 2010). These speakers are simply displaying normal phonetic variation and do not have a speech sound disorder which should raise clinical concern. SLTs must be aware of these regional variations in speech and language in order to avoid mistaken diagnoses and inappropriate intervention. Published assessments may also need to be adapted to reflect the accents and dialects of the clients that SLTs serve. There are also gender- and age-related differences in the use of speech and language. In English, there are gender differences in the pronunciation of the inflectional suffix *-ing* in words such as *running* and *talking*. This ending may be pronounced as /ɪn/ or /ɪŋ/. Studies have consistently shown that girls and women tend to use higher levels of the /ɪŋ/ pronunciation than boys and men (Schilling-Estes, 2006). There are also age-related differences in the use of language. Adolescent speakers from all social classes in a wide range of urban communities are observed to use a significantly higher number of socially stigmatized variants than do speakers of other ages (Cheshire, 2004). An example is the use of **multiple negation** as in the utterance *She don't want nothing*. As with regional variation, gender- and age-related differences in the use of speech and language are not a cause for clinical concern and do not require SLT intervention.

In addition to variation in accordance with attributes of speakers, language can also vary to reflect changes in situation or context. This type of variation is called **register** variation. (Some linguists use the term *register* more narrowly to refer to the specific vocabulary that is used by different occupational groups, e.g. legalese by lawyers.) As speakers switch between registers, they must make linguistic choices to reflect different audiences, purposes and circumstances. For example, the linguistic choices that are made in writing a letter of complaint to a retailer are quite different from those which are appropriate in completing an academic assignment. In terms of spoken language, speakers often use expressions in conversation with a friend which would not be appropriate during conversation with an employer. Because clients with communication disorders can make inappropriate linguistic choices in different situations and contexts, it is important for SLTs to have a sound understanding of register. In the following extract, a client with schizophrenia has been asked how he comes to be living in a certain US city. The client's unflattering description of the interviewer's tie and use of questions reveal a register which is not appropriate in a doctor–patient interview:

> Then I left San Francisco and moved to ... where did you get that tie? It looks like it's left over from the 1950s. I like the warm weather in San Diego. Is that a conch shell on your desk? Have you ever gone scuba diving?   (Thomas, 1997: 41)

There can also be intra-speaker language variation. Known as speech **style**, this type of variation reflects attention paid to speech, at least on one prominent account (Labov, 1972). Speakers increase the monitoring of their speech with increased levels of formality, according to Labov. Greater attention paid to speech leads to an alteration of speech style. The **vernacular** is a speaker's most casual style in which there is minimal attention paid to speech. On another account (Bell, 1984), speakers shift their style to be more like the person to whom they are talking. The essence of style on this account is that speakers are responding to their audience. Regardless of the particular approach taken to style, this sociolinguistic concept has considerable relevance to SLTs. Therapists need to be aware, for example, that how a client articulates a list of words in clinic, when there is increased attention paid to speech, is unlikely to resemble the articulation of these same words in casual speech where there is minimal attention paid to speech. These shifts in style according to formality are accommodated to a large extent by therapists when they assess a client's speech and language production both in single-word production tasks in clinic and in connected speech with a familiar communication partner outside of clinic. The emphasis on audience in Bell's account serves as an important reminder to SLTs that their presence may also induce a shift in a client's speech style. In general, therapists need to be aware that the speech and language which they record and analyse in clinic may differ in significant ways from the speech and language that clients use outside the clinic and in more informal settings.

Bilingualism and **multilingualism** are common and sometimes the norm in communities served by SLTs. To this end, SLT students must be introduced to issues that are raised by bilingualism and multilingualism as part of their clinical training. These issues include patterns of language development in bilingual and multilingual children. There is evidence, for example, that bilingual language development is not the same as monolingual language development. Brebner et al. (2016) found very different rates and patterns of verb-tense marking in English in English–Mandarin bilingual children depending on whether English was a first or second language. Thordardottir (2015) reported that bilingual children can perform similarly in terms of morphosyntactic development to monolingual peers in each language if they receive equal exposure to both languages and that poorer performance is observed when there is unequal exposure to both languages. Also, SLTs must be aware of how first, second and third languages may be impaired by conditions such as aphasia. Clinicians must consider if both languages are equally disrupted in speakers with **bilingual aphasia**, if there is cross-linguistic generalization to untreated languages when treatment is delivered in one language and if there is parallel or non-parallel recovery across languages. Kambanaros and Grohmann (2011) observed non-parallel language recovery in a Greek–English bilingual speaker with aphasia. Croft et al. (2011) reported naming treatment effects in both languages and cross-linguistic generalization from L1 to L2 in clients with aphasia who were bilingual in English and Bengali. The theoretical frameworks which explain these different findings must also be addressed in the linguistics curriculum of SLT students.

Bilingual children and adults create a number of challenges for SLTs. One of the key challenges is that most SLTs, at least in the UK, are monolingual English speakers. Ideally, bilingual clients should be assessed and treated by bilingual SLTs. Where this is not possible, monolingual SLTs may work alongside bilingual interpreters or assistants. A further challenge is that most formal language assessments use normative data from monolingual, English-speaking populations. There is a dearth of published assessments in languages other than English. Even where these assessments do exist, they also use normative data from monolingual populations. There is nothing to be gained by comparing the performance of bilingual children to data obtained from non-English, but still monolingual populations. Another factor that SLTs must be aware of during assessment in bilingual clients is the use of code switching. Code switching is a common, normal behaviour in bilingual speakers and is not a sign of poor language skills (Stow and Dodd, 2003). There are risks associated with basing an assessment of a client's language skills on just one of the speaker's languages. If the assessment examines the language that the client is most proficient at using, general language skills may be overestimated. Alternatively, if the assessment examines the language that the client is least proficient at using, there may be an underestimation of language skills. These factors and other considerations require considerable expertise on the part of the assessing clinician. With so few bilingual therapists in service – Stow and Dodd report only 48 therapists in the Bilingualism Special Interest Group of the Royal College of Speech and Language Therapists – this expertise is often lacking.

KEY POINTS: Sociolinguistics

- SLTs must understand when a speech or language feature is a characteristic of a regional accent or dialect and is not a sign of speech delay or language deviance.
- There is also considerable gender- and age-related variation in language. This affects pronunciation of words, lexical choices, grammatical usage and aspects of conversation.
- Language variation can also reflect changes in situation or context. Clients with language disorders can often exhibit difficulties with register variation.
- Style captures intra-speaker language variation. A speaker's style can reflect attention paid to speech (Labov) or an attempt to respond to audience (Bell).

- Bilingualism and multilingualism are very common and even the norm in some communities. SLTs must have an understanding of how language development differs in monolingual and bilingual speakers. There must also be an awareness of the effects of aphasia on first, second and third languages in bilingual and multilingual speakers.

2.10 Psycholinguistics

Psycholinguistics is the study of the mental processes that underlie the use of language. It is a broad discipline which encompasses many different enquiries, not all of which are relevant to SLT students (e.g. characteristics of animal communication). To get a sense of the parts of the field that have relevance to SLT, one need only consult the RCSLT guidelines for pre-registration SLT courses. These guidelines require students to have an understanding of the following:

> Current psycholinguistic frameworks and their clinical application, including: comprehension of language; expression of language; speech production; speech perception.
> Extension of psycholinguistic models to other communicative modalities.
> (RCSLT, 2010: 35)

Three topics in psycholinguistics which have particular relevance to SLT are models of the storage of words in the mind, and of language comprehension and production. For language production and comprehension to occur, there must be a store of words in the mind. This store is called the mental lexicon. The lexicon contains entries (lexical entries) for all the content and function words in language. Individual lexical entries contain information relating to the form and meaning of the word. Form refers to the spoken and written forms of words as language users must be able to access both in order to process spoken and written language. Within the meaning component of entries is information relating to semantic features of the word (e.g. that MOTHER is a 'female parent') and the syntactic environment in which the word may be used (e.g. that the verb *give* must be followed by a direct object and an indirect object). Entries in the lexicon must be accessed during language comprehension and production. During comprehension, lexical entries permit hearers and readers to assign meanings to the words that they hear and read in spoken and written utterances. During production, lexical entries permit speakers and writers to select words that most closely express the particular thoughts and ideas that they want to convey. The issue then is how language users proceed to identify the particular lexical entries that they need from among the very large number of entries that are present in the mental lexicon.

The criteria that guide the search of the lexicon have been the focus of debate for many years by psycholinguists. If we confine ourselves to word recognition during language comprehension, there is widespread agreement that hearers and readers do not attempt to match whole words to entries in the lexicon. Rather, they use various pieces of evidence to guide their search of the lexicon. For written words, this evidence might take the form of the curves and straight lines that make up individual letters and the order of letters in a word. For spoken words, this evidence might be the number of syllables in a word and whether the syllables are stressed or unstressed. Of course, these pieces of evidence may be consistent with several words as a possible match for the spoken or written target word. The letters L, V and G occur in the same order in the written words LIVING, LOVING and LEAVING, and each of the following spoken words contains three syllables with the second syllable stressed in each case: BANANA, MAJESTIC and INSIPID. On the basis of these rather limited pieces of evidence, a potentially large number of words could be contenders for the target word. However, as more and more pieces of evidence are considered, each contender to be the target word achieves different levels of activation. Eventually just one of these words achieves a certain threshold of activation and is identified as the target word. It is the competition between different contenders for the target word that finds this model of word recognition described as a competition model.

Within the mental lexicon, it appears likely that words are grouped together according to phonological and orthographic similarities. Some of the linguistic errors that speakers produce tend to support this idea. For example, a speaker who is trying to retrieve the word MIGRATION may end up producing INFLATION (phonological similarity), or for MINE might say MINT (orthographic similarity). Alongside word groupings based on form, there are also word groupings in the lexicon that are based on meaning. Psycholinguistic studies that have shown quicker reaction times to words that have a semantic relationship to a target word support the role of lexical relations like synonymy and hyponymy in how words are organized in the lexicon. For example, subjects who are presented with the word DOG and are asked to press a button when they hear an actual word rather than a non-word will have a quicker reaction time to POODLE (a hyponym of DOG) than to a semantically unrelated word like CAR. A similar effect occurs when presented with the word COLD. Subjects will display quicker reaction times to HOT (an antonym of COLD) than to the semantically unrelated word HOSPITAL. The **semantic relations** between words in the mental lexicon have a facilitative effect during language comprehension. The spreading activation that occurs between a word like DOG and semantically related terms like POODLE and KENNEL allows hearers and readers to anticipate certain words, and more quickly integrate them into their mental representation of a spoken or written text.

Psycholinguistic models of word storage in the mind are supported by errors that are made by subjects with language disorders. Adults with aphasia are often observed to produce semantic paraphasic errors in which there is a close semantic relation between the target word and the word that clients say or write. An adult with aphasia may say *I used to run this cycle* when they intended to say *I used to ride this cycle*, or *I cannot hear with this eye* instead of *I cannot hear with this ear*. Other semantic paraphasias are clearly based on the lexical relations that were examined in section 2.6. So an adult with aphasia may say *It wasn't cold for me* instead of *It wasn't hot for me* where 'cold' and 'hot' are gradable antonyms. The competition model has been used to investigate problems with word recognition in clients with language disorders. Titone and Levy (2004) examined lexical competition in word recognition in patients with schizophrenia. Patients with schizophrenia were less able to identify words from high lexical competitor environments than controls. A similar pattern was not observed in low lexical competitor environments. Spreading activation between terms in a **semantic network** was used by Kreher et al. (2008) to explain loose associations in clients with schizophrenia and **thought disorder**. In clients with schizophrenia who have positive thought disorder, activation in a semantic network was observed to spread further within a shorter period of time than in schizophrenic clients with no thought disorder. In each of these cases, psycholinguistic models of lexical storage are supported by the impairments of clients with language disorders.

Of course, lexical storage and access are contributing ultimately to language production and comprehension. For ease of explanation, the discussion below will address spoken language only. However, readers should be aware that similar stages can be identified in the production and comprehension of written language. Psycholinguists use information-processing models to explain the stages in language production. At the *conceptualization* stage, a speaker formulates an intention (thought or idea) that he wants to communicate to a hearer. These intentions represent a speaker's reason or motivation for communicating which is why they are called 'communicative intentions'. For the most part, speakers are adept at selecting the thoughts that should become communicative intentions and inhibiting those that for social, moral or other reasons should not be expressed. A communicative intention is an abstract notion that must undergo several other stages of processing before it can be expressed by a speaker. Having decided on a message to be communicated, speakers must set about selecting a linguistic code for the expression of that message. During the *language encoding* stage, a grammatical frame for an utterance is established. It is into this frame that words from the mental lexicon will be inserted. A key component in the frame is the verb, as it is around the verb that the rest of the spoken utterance will be structured. For example, the verb *put* has three slots (or argument places) that must be filled in the frame. One of these slots is for the subject in the sentence (the person who is doing the putting). A second slot is for the direct object of the verb (the thing that is put). The third and final slot in the frame is filled by an adverbial, typically a prepositional phrase, which tells us where the direct object is put (*Bill put milk in the fridge*, for example).

During language encoding, certain semantic restrictions on the use of words also come into play. For example, degree adverbs like *very* and *really* can only be modifiers of certain types of adjectives. So, while *very tired* and *really poor* are acceptable, an adjective phrase like *very equal* is not. It is also during language encoding that words can end up in the wrong slots in grammatical frames. This leads to errors called spoonerisms, in which the positions of two words in a sentence or utterance are reversed, e.g. *Sally mounted the car in the pavement*. Once the grammatical frame has been filled with words from the lexicon, the still abstract linguistic code must be converted into speech. During the *motor planning* stage, phonemes are selected and arranged in the order that will be required to produce a spoken utterance. The arrangement of phonemes during planning can also go awry, producing spoonerisms such as *The mechanic changed the blake fruid*. Also during motor planning, the word that will carry the primary stress in the utterance is identified. The location of this stress can alter the meaning of the sentence as in *Paul did not build the boat with <u>wood</u>* (he built it with something else) and *Paul did not <u>build</u> the boat with wood* (he repaired it with wood). During the *motor execution* stage, nervous impulses are sent to the muscles that are responsible for articulation. These are the muscles of the lips, tongue, soft palate, jaw, larynx and diaphragm, the contraction of which will result in the production of speech sounds. If motor execution proceeds smoothly, an intelligible spoken utterance will be produced and the journey from conceptualization to speech is complete.

These different stages of language production are displayed in Figure 2.3. Although this diagram is a flowchart, information in the model does not always pass in one direction from higher to lower levels. It is possible for lower levels in the model to influence higher levels. The reason speakers can still produce intelligible utterances even when they are chewing gum or holding a cigarette between their lips is because the conditions under which motor execution occurs can lead to adjustments in motor planning. These adjustments permit speech intelligibility to be maintained even under adverse speaking conditions. Feedback between lower levels and higher levels is possible at every stage of language production. It requires language users to monitor (subconsciously, of course) their language production and use that information to alter the processing of earlier stages in the model.

Psycholinguists have also characterized the comprehension of spoken and written language in terms of stages in an information-processing model. As with language production, the discussion below will focus on the comprehension of spoken language. The input to comprehension is the speech signal that is generated by the speaker's laryngeal mechanism and articulators. This signal may be degraded in quality if the speaker has a speech disorder or is speaking under adverse environmental conditions (e.g. loud background noise). During the *sensory processing* stage, the signal that reaches the ears of the hearer is

2.10 Psycholinguistics

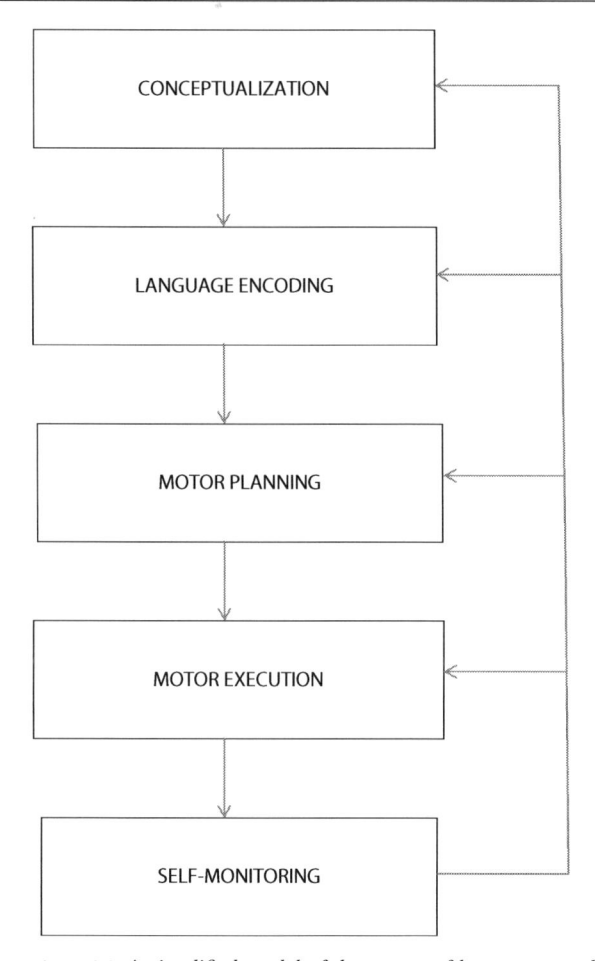

```
        ┌──────────────────────┐
        │  CONCEPTUALIZATION   │◄──────┐
        └──────────┬───────────┘       │
                   ▼                   │
        ┌──────────────────────┐       │
        │   LANGUAGE ENCODING  │◄──────┤
        └──────────┬───────────┘       │
                   ▼                   │
        ┌──────────────────────┐       │
        │    MOTOR PLANNING    │◄──────┤
        └──────────┬───────────┘       │
                   ▼                   │
        ┌──────────────────────┐       │
        │    MOTOR EXECUTION   │◄──────┤
        └──────────┬───────────┘       │
                   ▼                   │
        ┌──────────────────────┐       │
        │    SELF-MONITORING   │┄┄┄┄┄┄┄┘
        └──────────────────────┘
```

Figure 2.3 *A simplified model of the stages of language production*

converted by means of a series of mechanical and electrophysiological processes into nervous impulses. These impulses travel from the cochlea in the inner ear to the auditory cortices of the brain where the process of speech perception begins. During the *speech perception* stage, phoneme identification takes place. This process is not as straightforward as it might at first seem given that phonemes are variously realized in different phonetic contexts (e.g. /n/ is realized differently in *ten pins* [tɛm pɪnz] and *ten kings* [tɛŋ kɪŋz] on account of the bilabial and velar places of articulation, respectively, of the consonant sounds that follow /n/). The phonemic structure of words is integral to the identification of words in the mental lexicon, as lexical entries contain phonemic as well as syntactic and semantic information. During the *language decoding* stage, parsing of the grammatical structure of an utterance takes place. This structure varies between different types of sentence and conveys important information about the semantic relations between parts of a sentence. For declarative sentences such as *Bill sold the car*, the subject-verb-object word order tells us that Bill is the subject of the sentence and undertook the action of the verb, while the car is the object and received the action of the verb.

At the stage of language decoding, the hearer still has some way to go until the communicative intention that prompted the speaker to produce the utterance has been established. For example, the hearer has to establish the referents of personal pronouns (*she, they*) and deictic expressions (*next week, there*), resolve any lexical or grammatical ambiguities and determine what speech act the speaker has performed (e.g. the speaker who utters *I will be at the party* may be making a promise or conveying a threat). Some of these aspects of language processing are more closely related than others to the structure and propositional meaning of a sentence and, it appears likely, are performed during language decoding. In order to arrive at the propositional meaning of a sentence, for example, it is necessary to resolve ambiguities and determine the referents of terms like *she* and *there*. However, other aspects of this processing are pragmatic through and through, and require the interpretation of an utterance in context. It is context, for example, that leads a hearer to conclude that the speaker who utters *What a delightful child!* in the presence of a disruptive 5-year-old is being sarcastic. By accessing the mental lexicon, language decoding can tell us what *child* means. But it cannot tell us the specific child to whom the speaker is referring in this particular utterance. An additional stage of *utterance interpretation* as well as language decoding is necessary in order to arrive at these meanings of the speaker. It is only when an utterance has been fully interpreted in its context of use that a hearer may be said to have established the communicative intention that prompted a speaker to produce it. Language comprehension terminates in the same conceptual processes – intentions, thoughts and ideas – from which language production set out.

These five stages of language comprehension are displayed in Figure 2.4. As with language production, there is considerable interaction between the stages. Psycholinguists use the term *top-down processing* to describe how world knowledge and knowledge of the context in which an utterance is produced may influence earlier stages in language comprehension such as speech perception and language decoding. Hearers can supply missing or degraded phonemes in an incoming speech signal when that signal is conveying a well-rehearsed social greeting such as *Good morning!* or word combinations such as *fish and chips* and *salt and pepper*. Linguistic, social and other expectations make such phoneme identification possible. Similarly, the resolution of lexical ambiguities is effortlessly achieved for most hearers based upon their knowledge of the world, the topic of conversation and the setting in which a conversation is taking place. This is only possible because higher levels in the language comprehension model are able to influence lower levels which are involved in the perceptual and linguistic processing of the utterance. The work of psycholinguists has been vital in understanding top-down processing and the constructive comprehension that it makes possible.

2.10 Psycholinguistics

```
                    INPUT
          (speech signal, printed text)
                      │
                      ▼
          ┌─────────────────────────┐
          │   SENSORY PROCESSING    │◄───────┐
          └─────────────────────────┘        │
                      │                      │
                      ▼                      │
          ┌─────────────────────────┐        │
          │    SPEECH PERCEPTION    │◄───────┤
          └─────────────────────────┘        │
                      │                      │
                      ▼                      │
          ┌─────────────────────────┐        │
          │    LANGUAGE DECODING    │◄───────┤
          └─────────────────────────┘        │
                      │                      │
                      ▼                      │
          ┌─────────────────────────┐        │
          │ UTTERANCE INTERPRETATION│◄───────┤
          └─────────────────────────┘        │
                      │                      │
                      ▼                      │
          ┌─────────────────────────┐        │
          │    CONCEPTUALIZATION    │────────┘
          └─────────────────────────┘
```

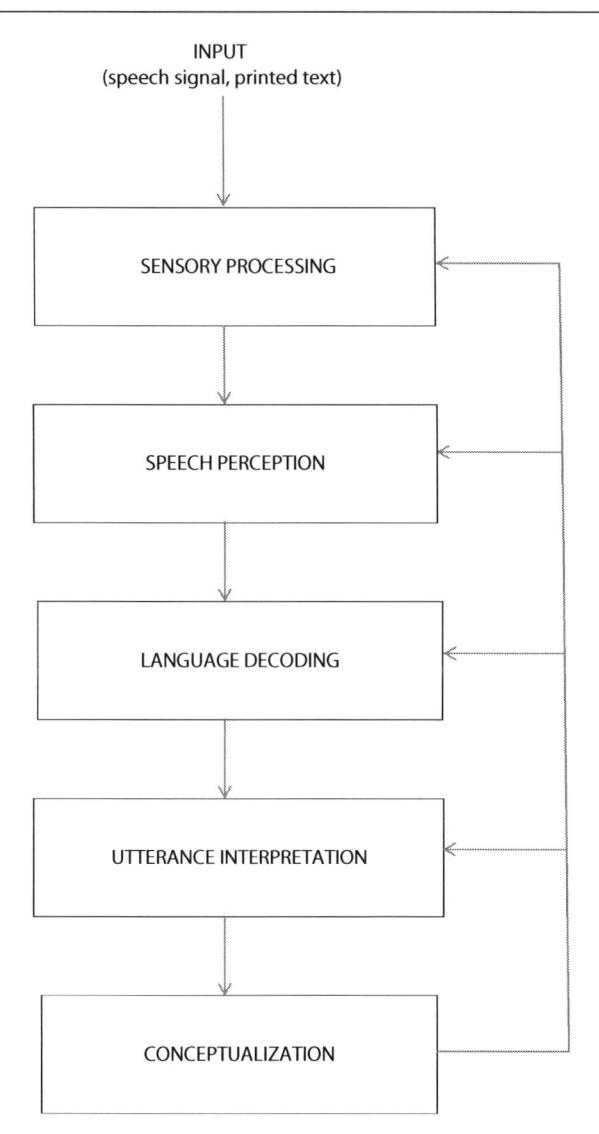

Figure 2.4 *A simplified model of the stages of language comprehension*

KEY POINTS: Psycholinguistics

- Psycholinguistics is the study of the mental processes that are involved in the production and comprehension of language.
- The field involves many topics and areas, ranging from language storage and language processing to first and second language acquisition.
- Word recognition is investigated in psycholinguistics, with models such as the competition model used to explain this process. SLT students must also understand the word recognition effects that are related to

spreading activation through a semantic network of associations between words.
- Psycholinguists represent the production of spoken and written language in terms of the following stages in an information-processing model: conceptualization; language encoding; motor planning; and motor execution. Lower levels in the model can influence the processing of higher levels. This is achieved through self-monitoring and correction.
- Psycholinguists represent the comprehension of spoken and written language in terms of the following stages in an information-processing model: sensory processing; speech or letter perception; language decoding; utterance interpretation; and conceptualization. World knowledge and knowledge of the speaker and context can influence the linguistic and perceptual processing of utterances (top-down processing).

2.11 Neurolinguistics

Field (2015) includes neurolinguistics in the study of psycholinguistics. Ahlsén (2006: 3) states that neurolinguistics has a 'very close relationship' to psycholinguistics 'but focuses more on studies of the brain'. This is how Ahlsén defines the field more fully:

> Neurolinguistics studies the relation of language and communication to different aspects of brain function, in other words it tries to explore how the brain understands and produces language and communication. This involves attempting to combine neurological/neurophysiological theory (how the brain is structured and how it functions) with linguistic theory (how language is structured and how it functions). (2006: 3)

A primary concern of neurolinguistics, and the chief reason why this area of study is of relevance to SLTs, is the examination of the relationship between brain damage and language impairment. This is achieved through a range of methods including the use of experiments and neuroimaging techniques such as **functional magnetic resonance imaging (fMRI)** and **single-photon emission computed tomography (SPECT)**. These methods have produced an array of neurolinguistic findings about language functions such as reading and writing. For example, Vandenborre et al. (2015) investigated whether **apraxic agraphia** – a peripheral writing disorder – might result from damage to areas outside of the typical language areas such as the cerebellum or thalamus. A range of methods including functional imaging (SPECT) and neurolinguistic and neurocognitive tests was used to investigate a 32-year-old patient who developed apraxic agraphia following a bithalamic stroke. This study found the thalamus to be implicated in the neural network that subserves graphomotor processing. Other neurolinguistic studies have investigated the relationship between brain damage and specific aspects of language such as syntax and semantics. For example,

Wilson et al. (2011) examined the relationship between white matter damage and syntactic deficits in patients with **primary progressive aphasia**. Multimodal neuroimaging and neurolinguistic assessment were conducted. Deficits in comprehension and production of syntax were associated with microstructural damage to left hemisphere dorsal tracts.

Beyond the study of clients with brain damage, neurolinguistics makes a further important contribution to SLT. This linguistic discipline is shedding light on the neural processes and mechanisms that are involved in spontaneous and assisted recovery from conditions such as stuttering. Kell et al. (2009) found that assisted recovery from developmental stuttering, which was induced by a fluency-shaping therapy programme, resulted in the re-lateralization of brain activity to the left hemisphere (see section 6.5 for discussion of fluency-shaping therapy). Unassisted or spontaneous recovery was specifically associated with the activation of a brain region in the left lateral orbitofrontal cortex. In a later study, Kell et al. (2017) reported that therapy and spontaneous recovery normalize left-hemisphere speaking-related activity via an improvement of auditory-motor mapping. Long-lasting unassisted recovery is additionally supported by a functional isolation of the superior cerebellum from the rest of the speech production network. With neurolinguistics contributing to our knowledge of the type of functional reorganization that is possible through fluency interventions, it is clear that this branch of linguistics is moving beyond its research focus to become a discipline which has direct implications for the management of clients with communication disorders. Similar intervention studies in neurolinguistics have examined the effects of naming therapy in clients with the semantic variant of primary progressive aphasia (Jokel et al., 2016) and language therapy in childhood stroke-induced dysphasia (Carlson et al., 2016).

The rapid expansion of neurolinguistics has resulted in the development of a number of sub-disciplines in the field. One sub-discipline is **neuropragmatics**. Neuropragmatists use neuroimaging techniques to explore the neural basis of pragmatic phenomena such as implicature, metaphor and irony (Cummings, 2010). To date, most of these studies have been conducted in neurotypical individuals. For example, Obert et al. (2014) conducted an auditory fMRI study of the comprehension of predicative metaphors (e.g. *to kill the song*) in 22 healthy subjects. The comprehension of the literal counterparts of these metaphors was also investigated. There was bilateral activation of parietal areas (i.e. left angular gyrus and right inferior parietal gyri) for metaphorical sentences compared with literal ones as well as activation of the right precuneus. Some neuropragmatic studies have investigated the neural basis of pragmatic phenomena in individuals with neurological disorders. Downey et al. (2015) used **diffusion tensor imaging** to examine the neuroanatomical basis of **sarcasm** identification in 29 subjects with behavioural variant frontotemporal dementia and 15 subjects with semantic variant primary progressive aphasia. Both clinical groups showed similarly severe deficits for the identification of sarcasm. These deficits were correlated with white matter tract alterations which particularly affected fronto-temporal connections in the right cerebral hemisphere. There has been considerable expansion of neuroimaging techniques in recent years. As these techniques continue to develop, it appears likely that the neural basis of aspects of language will come to assume an increasingly important role in the linguistics curriculum of SLT students.

> **KEY POINTS: Neurolinguistics**
>
> - Neurolinguistics is the study of the relationship between language and aspects of brain function.
> - The relationship between brain damage and language impairment is a key concern of neurolinguistics. This aspect of the discipline has most relevance to SLTs.
> - Neurolinguists employ a range of methods. These include experiments and the use of neuroimaging techniques such as fMRI, SPECT and diffusion tensor imaging.
> - Neurolinguistic research examines neurotypical individuals and individuals with neurological disorders. It investigates language functions (e.g. writing) and aspects of language (e.g. syntax, semantics).
> - The expansion of neurolinguistics has seen the emergence of sub-disciplines. One sub-discipline is neuropragmatics. This is the study of the neural basis of pragmatic phenomena such as metaphor and irony.

2.12   Child Language Acquisition

To understand disorders of language development, SLTs must have knowledge of how normally developing children acquire speech and language. Child language acquisition, or first language acquisition, is a broad area of inquiry. It encompasses the study of theoretical approaches to language acquisition such as **nativism** and **social interactionism**. It also encompasses a description of the stages through which children pass on their way to acquiring the phonology, morphology, syntax, semantics and pragmatics of their native language. In section 2.4, some of Brown's (1973) stages of morphological development were described. These stages saw the emergence of the inflectional suffix for progressive aspect *-ing* between 28 and 36 months while the regular past tense suffix *-ed* emerges later in normally developing children, between 40 to 46 months. Similar stages have been characterized in children's phonological, syntactic, semantic and pragmatic development. SLT students require an in-depth knowledge of **phonological development** in children. Most phonological development occurs between 1 year 6 months and 4 years (Yavaş, 1998: 146). The phonological maturation that occurs during this time has been variously characterized. Ball ([1984] 2014: 117) remarks that

> The most recent, and perhaps the most insightful, way of characterizing phonological development is that termed natural phonology or phonological process theory ... Acquisition is seen as the use of certain phonological processes at certain stages of development, which are dropped or changed at a later stage.

An examination of the single-word productions of a child of 4;8 years examined by Yavaş (1998: 78–9) shows how speech may exhibit a range of phonological processes. Some of this child's productions and processes are shown below:

> *Consonant cluster reduction:* 'black' [bæk]
> *Stopping of /s/:* 'soup' [tup]
> *Palatal fronting:* 'dish' [dIs]
> *Prevocalic voicing:* 'talk' [dɔk]
> *Liquid gliding:* 'ring' [wIŋ]
> *Final consonant devoicing:* 'dog' [dɔk]

Three of these processes – palatal fronting, liquid gliding and final consonant devoicing – are known to persist after 3 years of age. Their presence in the speech of this 4-year-old child is not a cause of clinical concern. Prevocalic voicing usually disappears by 3 years of age. Its persistence in the speech of a 4-year-old child raises suspicion of a phonological disorder. This suspicion is supported by the presence of cluster reduction and stopping of /s/ which have usually disappeared by 4 years of age. It is clear from this pattern of processes that this child's phonological development is not proceeding along normal lines. Only SLTs who have knowledge of the chronology of phonological processes during normal development will be able to make this assessment.

Syntactic development is an important area of knowledge for SLTs. To understand difficulties in the use of interrogatives in children with SLI (Van der Lely and Battell, 2003), clinicians must have an appreciation of how *yes–no* interrogatives and *wh*-interrogatives are acquired by normally developing children. The following data is taken from Peccei (1999: 41–2). It shows the production of *yes–no* and *wh*-interrogatives by normally developing children across three word stages:

	Yes/No	WH
STAGE I (2–3 words)	See hole? Sit chair? Jamie water?	What that? Where Mama? What doing? Who that?
STAGE II (3–4 words)	See my doggie? That black too? I have it? You can't fix it?	What me think? Why you smiling? Where me sleep? Why not me drink it?
STAGE III (over 4 words)	Does lions walk? Will you help me? Can't you work this thing? Oh, did I caught it?	Where my spoon goed? Why the tree going? Why kitty can't stand up? What I did yesterday?

In terms of *yes–no* interrogatives, this data shows that normally developing children tend to use simple intonational questions in the first two word stages. These questions have a subject-verb-object word order ('I have it?'). It is the role of intonation to signal that these declarative sentences have the function of questions. It is not until children produce utterances of over four words that **inversion** is used to form questions. Errors at this stage include the use of the wrong auxiliary form ('Does lions walk?') and a tendency to mark tense on both the auxiliary and main verb ('Oh, did I caught it?'). The development of *wh*-interrogatives shows that only certain *wh*-words (*what, where, who*) are used to form questions initially, with *why* appearing for the first time in stage II. Auxiliaries emerge later in *wh*-interrogatives (stage III: 'Why kitty can't stand up?') than in *yes–no* interrogatives (stage II: 'You can't fix it?'). Inversion appeared in stage III for *yes–no* interrogatives ('Will you help me?') but is still not present in *wh*-interrogatives by the same stage ('Why kitty can't stand up?').

Semantic development is a key component of child language acquisition for SLTs. The two-word stage of language development typically occurs in the age range 19–26 months and is characterized by a mean length of utterance of two morphemes (range 1.75–2.25) (Berk and Lillo-Martin, 2012). This stage is significant for the semantic relations that children begin to produce. Several two-word utterances and the semantic relations that they express are shown below:

daddy kick → agent + action
throw stick → action + affected
me ball → agent + affected
sit chair → action + location
spoon table → entity + location
daddy coat → possessor + possession
kitty big → entity + attribute
that cake → nomination
more ball → recurrence
no ball → negation

These same semantic relations are found in the expressive language of children with Down syndrome at a similar mean length of utterance. However, they emerge at a significantly delayed rate in these children, as indicated by more advanced chronological age. Coggins (1979) examined two-word, non-imitated utterances of four children with Down syndrome whose mean length of utterance ranged from 1.22 to 2.06. The chronological ages of these children ranged from 3;10 to 6;3 years. Coggins reported that 'Down's syndrome children at Stage 1 of linguistic development do indeed concentrate on the same, rather small set of relational meanings as in normal children's early two-word combinations' (1979: 176). Duchan and Erickson (1976) examined the comprehension of semantic relations in children with Down syndrome and normally developing children at the one- and two-word stage of language development. For both groups of children, performance was best on the possessive relations (e.g. *Mummy hat*) than on the action-object (e.g. *throw ball*) and agent-action (e.g. *Mummy come*) relations. Poorest performance occurred on the locative relations (e.g. *sweater chair*). Clearly, SLT students must have an understanding of milestones in normal semantic development in order to appreciate the developmental trajectories of children with **genetic syndromes** and **neurodevelopmental disorders**.

Pragmatic development is the least well understood and investigated aspect of first language acquisition in children. However, a sizeable literature exists on early pre-linguistic behaviours such as eye gaze and pointing which are regarded as precursors to the emergence of pragmatic language skills in children (see Cummings 2015 for a review). Also, investigators are beginning to examine in earnest a range of linguistic pragmatic concepts. One such concept is implicature. Studies have found that children can understand a range of implicatures, but that these pragmatic inferences are still in development many years after structural aspects of language are already established. Janssens et al. (2015) investigated the understanding of conventional implicatures in 'but' utterances in children aged 8 to 12 years. These children were able to establish the conventional implicatures of utterances such as *John is obese but healthy* (implicature: it was not expected that John would be healthy), but their understanding was sensitive to the content of the arguments used. Scalar implicatures have also been investigated in normally developing children. The scalar term *some* has a semantic interpretation of 'some and possibly all' and a pragmatic interpretation of 'some but not all'. While adults invariably opt for a pragmatic interpretation of utterances such as *Some of the books were interesting* (implicature: not all of the books were interesting), normally developing children of 5 years of age adopt a semantic interpretation of such utterances (Papafragou and Musolino, 2003). Verbuk and Shultz (2010) examined so-called relevance implicatures in normally developing children. A relevance implicature is a particularized conversational implicature that arises from the flouting of the relation maxim. In the following exchange between A and B, B's utterance generates the relevance implicature that A can find a new cartridge at the pharmacy:

  A: Where can I find a new cartridge?
  B: There is a pharmacy around the corner.

Verbuk and Shultz found that normally developing children aged 5;1 to 8;1 years were significantly better at computing non-linguistic inferences than relevance implicatures, a finding which they explained in terms of the additional reasoning about language that is needed to compute implicatures. An understanding of the developmental stages through which implicatures and other pragmatic concepts pass is an integral part of child language acquisition for SLTs.

KEY POINTS: Child Language Acquisition

- In order to understand disorders of language development, SLT students must have knowledge of how normally developing children acquire their native language. This is the study of child language acquisition, or first language acquisition.
- Child language acquisition includes the study of theoretical approaches to language acquisition (e.g. nativism, social interactionism). It also includes a description of the stages that normally developing children pass through on their way to acquiring the phonology, morphology, syntax, semantics and pragmatics of their native language.
- SLT students need to know the chronology of phonological processes such as consonant cluster reduction, prevocalic voicing and stopping. Processes that persist raise a suspicion of phonological disorder in children.
- SLT students must also know the order in which morphemes emerge in normally developing children. For example, in normal language development the inflectional suffix *-ing* for progressive aspect emerges before the suffix *-ed* for regular past tense.
- Syntactic development is a crucial component of first language acquisition for SLT students. It includes the acquisition of *yes–no* interrogatives and *wh-*interrogatives.
- Semantic development includes lexical acquisition as well as acquisition of sentential aspects of semantics such as semantic relations (agent + action).
- Pragmatic development is the least well understood and investigated aspect of language acquisition. Two exceptions are the non-linguistic behaviours that are precursors of pragmatic language skills and concepts such as implicature.

WEBSITE: Linguistic Disciplines

After reading the chapter, visit the website and test your knowledge of linguistic disciplines by answering the short-answer questions for this topic.

Suggestions for Further Reading

McAllister, J. and Miller, J. 2013. *Introductory linguistics for speech and language therapy practice*, Chichester, West Sussex: Wiley-Blackwell.

This volume is a practical introduction to the aspects of linguistics that SLTs need to understand in order to use published tools for analysing clients' language abilities. It contains 17 chapters that examine words and non-words; word and sentence meaning; parts of speech; word structure; sentence structure; language in use; and narrative. Each chapter interrogates why SLTs need to have knowledge of a particular aspect of linguistics.

Cummings, L. 2013. 'Clinical linguistics: a primer', *International Journal of Language Studies* 7:2, 1–30.

This article examines a number of linguistic disciplines that are integral to the study of clinical linguistics and SLT. The disciplines in question are phonetics, phonology, morphology, syntax, semantics, pragmatics and discourse. Data from children and adults with language disorders are examined with a view to illustrating a range of linguistic concepts.

Black, M. and Chiat, S. 2003. *Linguistics for clinicians: a practical introduction*, London: Hodder Arnold.

This book provides an introduction to linguistic analysis in a clinical context. There is an emphasis on syntax and the links between syntax on the one hand and phonology and semantics on the other hand. Linguistic concepts are introduced with examples of their clinical use.

QUESTIONS: Linguistic Disciplines

(1) An understanding of articulatory phonetics is integral to the work of SLT. The following statements describe some aspect of disordered articulation in children and adults with speech disorders.

Part (A): For each statement, describe the type of error that occurs. There may be more than one error.
  (a) A 6-year-old girl with a repaired central cleft of the hard and soft palates produces [ʔaʊɴ] for 'down'.
  (b) A 41-year-old woman with **multiple sclerosis** produces [fæs] for 'fast'.
  (c) A boy of 4;11 years with developmental dysarthria produces [xɑː] for 'car'.
  (d) An adult with **apraxia of speech** produces [bɛn] for 'pen'.
  (e) A child with Down syndrome produces [glʌf] for 'glove'.

Part (B): Respond to the following questions by using the statements in (a) to (e) above.
  (a) Which client is able to produce a consonant cluster?
  (b) Which client is able to produce a diphthong?
  (c) Which client produces an error of manner of articulation?
  (d) Which clients produce voicing errors?
  (e) Which client produces an error of place of articulation?

(2) Normally developing children and children with speech sound disorders use a range of phonological processes. These processes can reduce a child's intelligibility to a significant extent. For each of the single-word productions below, identify the phonological process or processes that characterize the production:
  (a) 'duck' [gʌk]
  (b) 'cat' [tæt]

(c) 'sea' [ti]
(d) 'coat' [dut]
(e) 'lap' [jæp]
(f) 'pig' [bik]
(g) 'steps' [bɛps]
(h) 'dress' [dɛs]
(i) 'bike' [baɪ]
(j) 'snake' [neŋ]
(k) 'matches' [mæmiz]
(l) 'vacuum' [gæjum]
(m) 'sheep' [tip]
(n) 'potato' [teto]
(o) 'green' [gwin]
(p) 'jump' [zʌmp]
(q) 'sun' [tsʌn]
(r) 'seat' [hit]
(s) 'fish' [ɪʃ]
(t) 'zebra' [jiba]

(3) Normally developing children can make a number of morphological errors during language development. Several errors described by Crystal (1986) are shown below. Describe the error in each utterance:
(a) 'It's furnitures'
(b) 'We eated it all up'
(c) 'My hand's the biggest than Ben's'
(d) 'You drinked it'
(e) 'My sore's worser now'

(4) An SLT receives a referral from the school psychologist about a boy with suspected language disorder. Receptive syntax is examined as part of a comprehensive assessment of this boy's language skills. The formal language test used by the SLT contains a sub-test of receptive syntax. It requires the boy to point to pictures in response to spoken sentences. Five of these sentences are presented below. Which aspect of receptive syntax is assessed by these sentences? The underlined words serve as a clue.
(a) The tall man is <u>next to</u> the chair.
(b) The girl <u>who is crying</u> has blue shoes.
(c) The van <u>is followed by</u> the lorry.
(d) The dog <u>growling at the woman</u> is black.
(e) The circle <u>is smaller than</u> the square.

(5) Michael et al. (2012) examined the use and comprehension of verbs which differ in argument structure in nine individuals with Down syndrome aged 11;11 to 32;10 years. During a narrative task, these individuals were presented with sequences of four pictures. One utterance accompanied each picture in a sequence. Subjects were then provided with all four pictures in a sequence and were required to retell the story to the examiner. Some of the utterances that were used in this study are presented below. For each utterance (i) indicate if it contains a one-, two-, or three-argument verb and (ii) identify the semantic role of each noun phrase:

(a) Joey sweeps the floor.
(b) A boy swims in the pool.
(c) Mary gives a cookie to her friend.
(d) A girl jumps from the diving board.
(e) A boy runs in the grass.

(6) Indicate whether the utterances on the right of the following pairs are related to the utterances on the left by means of implicature or presupposition:

(a) Bob stopped smoking → Bob had been smoking.
(b) Joe is a better musician than Pip → Pip is a musician.
(c) Fran has three children → Fran has only three children.
(d) If I were president, I would end poverty → I am not president.
(e) Some of the poems were good → Not all the poems were good.
(f) A: Did you bring beer and wine? → B: I brought beer.
(g) She realized Bill had left → Bill had left.
(h) Sue helped a child into the car → The child Sue helped was not her own.
(i) The swan beside the lake is beautiful → There is a swan beside the lake.
(j) Even Larry passed the exam → It was not expected that Larry would pass the exam.

(7) McTear (1985) examined a 10-year-old boy with pragmatic disorder. An examination of conversational exchanges between this boy (C) and an adult (A) revealed that he has difficulty with aspects of discourse cohesion. Two such exchanges are shown below. Identify the type of cohesion which this boy fails to use.

Exchange 1:
    A: are they friends of yours?
    C: they are friends of mine

Exchange 2:
    A: do you play with P?
    C: yes I do =
    A: = umhmm =
    C: = play with him
    A: after school?
    C: yes
    A: umhmm
    C: I play with him after school

(8) SLTs must be aware of speech features that are attributable to a speaker's regional dialect when they assess children with suspected speech sound disorders. Harris and Cottam (1985) examined the speech of a boy of 4;11 years called Mike. Mike presented with speech unintelligibility. An articulation test revealed three features of the South Yorkshire urban vernacular to which Mike is exposed. These features were: (1) the presence of 'h-dropping' (the absence of historical /h/ in words such as *house*); (2) monophthongal realizations of the nuclei in words such as *nice* (/aɪ/ →[æ]); and (3) the loss of historical /r/ in preconsonantal and prepausal position (South Yorks vernacular is non-rhotic), e.g. *horsie, chair*. Several of Mike's single-word productions are shown below. For each production, identify one

feature of South Yorkshire urban vernacular that should not be attributed clinical significance:
- (a) 'hiss' [Iṣ]
- (b) 'car' [kʰɑ:]
- (c) 'night' [næ:ʔṣ]
- (d) 'hoop' [u:pʰ]
- (e) 'water' [wɔ:ṣə]
- (f) 'sugar' [ṣəṣə]
- (g) 'smoke' [mo:ʔṣ]
- (h) 'paper' [pʰe:ɸə]
- (i) 'hit' [Iʔṣ]
- (j) 'boat' [bo:ʔṣ]

(9) Respond with *true* or *false* to each of the following statements about psycholinguistics:
- (a) Psycholinguistics is primarily interested in language acquisition.
- (b) Words in the mental lexicon may be organized according to form and meaning.
- (c) Motor planning is the stage in language production during which words from the lexicon are inserted into a grammatical frame.
- (d) During speech perception, phoneme identification is influenced by linguistic regularities and expectations.
- (e) Spreading activation through a semantic network is aberrant in schizophrenia.

(10) Respond with *true* or *false* to each of the following statements about neurolinguistics:
- (a) Neurolinguistics is an interdisciplinary enterprise.
- (b) Neurolinguistics investigates how language is instantiated in the brain.
- (c) Neurolinguistics is the study of the real-time processing of language.
- (d) Neurolinguistics investigates only semantic aspects of meaning.
- (e) Neurolinguistic investigations may be used to examine the effect of SLT interventions on the brain.

(11) During the two-word stage of language development, children begin to express a number of semantic relations. Several two-word utterances of children are shown below. For each one, indicate the semantic relation expressed by the utterance:
- (a) man run
- (b) hide key
- (c) Mummy comb
- (d) shoe dirty
- (e) sleep bed
- (f) dolly tired
- (g) more juice
- (h) no toy
- (i) that milk
- (j) shoe cupboard

3 Medical and Scientific Disciplines

3.1 Introduction

In Chapter 2, it was described how three bodies are involved in the clinical education of SLT students in the UK. These bodies are the Royal College of Speech and Language Therapists (RCSLT), the Quality Assurance Agency for Higher Education (QAA) and the Health & Care Professions Council (HCPC). As well as emphasizing specific requirements of the linguistics curriculum for SLT students, these bodies also require SLT students to have knowledge of a range of biological and medical sciences. An examination of the specific recommendations of these bodies reveals the extent to which these scientific disciplines inform the knowledge base of SLT. The HCPC's standards of education and training require those who successfully complete an SLT programme to have knowledge of biomedical and medical disciplines. The Council's standards require such individuals to

> understand the structure and function of the human body, together with knowledge of health, disease, impairment and dysfunction relevant to their profession ... understand biomedical and medical sciences as relevant to the development and maintenance of communication and swallowing. (HCPC, 2013: 12)

In its benchmark statement for SLT, the QAA requires the SLT award holder to have knowledge of human biological sciences:

> The relevant aspects of biomedical and medical sciences including the anatomy and physiology of body systems relevant to the development of, and maintenance of, communication and swallowing. This includes disruptions to the functions of these systems. (QAA, 2001: 10)

Within its guidelines for pre-registration SLT courses in the UK, the RCSLT makes specific recommendations about the inclusion of biological and medical sciences in the SLT curriculum. These sciences should develop

> a sound understanding of the topic areas which provide the necessary underpinning for speech and language therapy practice. This strand of the curriculum should include relevant input relating to anatomy and physiology, neuroanatomy and neurophysiology. The curriculum should address systems and processes involved in typical and atypical functioning

throughout the lifespan. Content on specific pathologies should be presented in such a way that students can understand roles and responsibilities of professional specialisms, and the relevance of these specialist areas to SLT.   (RCSLT, 2010: 37)

This chapter will provide an account of each of these biological and medical disciplines as they relate to the specific learning needs of SLT students. To understand a communication disorder is to know something of its frequency and distribution in populations and the medical and other conditions that cause it. Accordingly, **epidemiology** and **aetiology** will be addressed in section 3.2. The anatomical and physiological basis of speech, language, voice and hearing are an essential part of the knowledge of SLT students and a core component of SLT curricula. The study of the structure (**anatomy**) and function (**physiology**) of organs such as the tongue, lips, larynx and lungs will be examined in section 3.3. Many communication disorders are caused by impairments of the central and peripheral nervous systems. For example, dysarthria may be caused by **cranial nerve** damage, while aphasia often arises as a result of a lesion in the language dominant **left hemisphere** of the brain. The disorders of the nervous system that cause these **neurogenic communication disorders** are studied by a branch of medicine known as neurology, which is examined in section 3.4. Communication disorders may also be related to pathologies that fall within the purview of **ENT medicine** or **otorhinolaryngology**. These pathologies include vocal nodules and polyps which cause voice disorders (dysphonias) and conductive hearing loss related to the presence of **otitis media**. A scientific discipline which works closely with ENT medicine and SLT is **audiology**. Audiologists assess and treat hearing disorders. SLTs must be acquainted with different methods of audiological assessment and aural rehabilitation. ENT medicine and audiology are discussed in sections 3.5 and 3.6, respectively.

The medical disciplines which are integral to SLT are by no means exhausted. Clients with mental health conditions such as schizophrenia and **bipolar disorder** can present with significant impairment of their language and communication skills. SLT students must have an understanding of the onset, symptoms and **prognosis** of these conditions in order to appreciate fully their impact on communication. This knowledge is examined in section 3.7 in a branch of medicine called psychiatry. Increasingly, investigators are establishing a link between gastrointestinal conditions and vocal pathologies. For example, gastroesophageal reflux disease (GERD) is linked to the development of laryngeal cancer and **reflux laryngitis**. The management of GERD in clients with voice disorders brings the discipline of gastroenterology into contact with otolaryngology and SLT. Gastroenterology will be examined in section 3.8. Hormonal imbalances during menstruation and the menopause are related to dysphonia in women. Also, **androgen therapy** used in the treatment of female-to-male (FTM) transsexual clients can induce laryngeal tissue changes and a reduction in vocal **pitch**. The management of many voice disorders brings **endocrinology** into contact with SLT and otolaryngology. This branch of medical science will be examined in section 3.8. Finally, the incidence and prevalence of several communication disorders including aphasia and dysarthria increase with advancing years. Many older people also have unique physical and cognitive challenges (e.g. dementia) that have implications for communication. The branch of medicine that studies ageing and older adults is called **geriatrics**. Geriatrics will be examined in section 3.8 of this chapter.

3.2 Epidemiology and Aetiology

SLT students must understand key terms in epidemiology in order to discuss communication disorders with accuracy. Some of these terms include the prevalence and incidence of a disorder. The **prevalence** of a disorder is the number of individuals in a population who have the disorder at a specific period of time. This is usually expressed as a percentage of the population. A commonly cited prevalence figure in the literature on communication disorders is Tomblin's prevalence rate of 7.4% for SLI. **Incidence** captures the number of individuals who develop a disease or disorder during a particular time period, usually a month or a year. In a study of Cantonese-speaking Chinese children who met the Hong Kong criterion of dyslexia, Chan et al. (2008) estimated an incidence rate of 0.66% for developmental dyslexia over a four-year period. Aside from prevalence and incidence, epidemiologists are also concerned to describe the distribution of diseases and disorders in populations in accordance with demographic variables such as sex, racial or ethnic identity and **socioeconomic status**. It is widely reported, for example, that many more boys and men than girls and women exhibit developmental stuttering. In their epidemiological study, Craig et al. (2002) reported a male-to-female ratio for stuttering of 2.3:1 across all ages. Ethnicity is a significant factor in the epidemiology of communication disorders. Duncan et al. (2012) examined the relationship of race/ethnicity to cognitive and language scores in extremely preterm toddlers at 18–22 months of age. The study population included 369 white toddlers, 352 black toddlers and 144 Hispanic white toddlers. It was reported that black and Hispanic white toddlers had lower language scores than white toddlers, even after adjustment for medical and psychosocial factors.

Socioeconomic status (SES) is variously defined in epidemiological studies. An assessment of SES may be based on family income, parental education and social networks and relationships, among other factors. Letts et al. (2013) examined the relationship between SES and language delay in 1,266 children aged 2;00 to 7;06 years. Children whose mothers had minimum years of education and children who attended quintile 1 (most deprived) schools and nurseries had higher than expected levels of language delay. In children aged 2;00 to 5;06 years, moderately delayed comprehension and production, defined as language scores between −1 and −1.5 standard deviations (SDs), were present in 17.6% and 19.0%, respectively. The percentage expected to fall in this range for a normal distribution was 9.2% for both comprehension and production. Knowledge of the social and other determinants of language and communication disorders is vital if clinicians are to intervene successfully on these disorders. Notwithstanding the importance of this knowledge, epidemiological investigations of communication disorders have traditionally been conducted infrequently in comparison to other types of research. It was with a view to addressing the paucity of epidemiological research in communication disorders that the National Institute on Deafness and Other Communication Disorders (NIDCD) in the USA hosted a workshop in March 2005. The purpose of this workshop was to stimulate more epidemiological research in NIDCD mission areas. A growing number of large-scale epidemiological studies of communication disorders and increased discussion of the epidemiology of communication and swallowing disorders suggest that this may be happening (Byles, 2005; McLeod and McKinnon, 2007).

Aetiology is the study of the medical causes of diseases and disorders. For many communication disorders, a medical cause of the disorder can be clearly identified. A child may have language disorder which is related to genetic syndromes such as **Williams syndrome** and Down syndrome. An adult may develop aphasia as a result of a cerebrovascular accident, a **brain tumour** or a viral infection like **herpes simplex encephalitis**. The dysphonia of a **professional voice user** may be related to the presence of vocal nodules. An adult may have **hypokinetic dysarthria**, which is caused by the neurodegenerative condition **Parkinson's disease**. In each of these cases, a communication disorder is caused by an illness, injury or disease. Some of these causes are proximal in nature (**proximal aetiology**) in that they act directly or almost directly to cause a communication disorder. The brain lesion that occurs in a cerebrovascular accident is a proximal cause of aphasia. Other causes are distal in nature (**distal aetiology**). These causes are found further back in the causal chain and act via one or more intermediary causes. The chromosomal abnormality in Down syndrome (**trisomy 21**) leads to neurodevelopmental anomalies. These anomalies lead in turn to intellectual disability. It is intellectual disability that causes language disorder in children with Down syndrome. In this case, the chromosomal abnormality is a distal aetiology and intellectual disability is a proximal aetiology of language disorder in Down syndrome. A similar distinction between distal and proximal aetiology applies to clients with an **organic voice disorder**. Vocal nodules (proximal aetiology) cause dysphonia. However, they arise because of a habitual pattern of **vocal abuse and misuse** (distal aetiology).

There are also many communication disorders for which a clear aetiology does not exist. These disorders include developmental stuttering and specific language impairment. To say that there is no current aetiology of these disorders is not to say that a medical aetiology does not exist. As brain imaging techniques and genetic studies increase in number and sophistication, it appears likely that communication disorders which currently lack a clear cause will come to be explained in genetic and neurobiological terms. Exactly this is happening in relation to the genetic basis of SLI (see section 5.5 in Ellis Weismer, 2014, for discussion). Where a disorder lacks a medical aetiology, it is called a functional disorder. For example, clients with dysphonia who have no organic defect of vocal fold structure and function on laryngological examination may be said to have a **functional voice disorder**. The term *functional* has often been used in SLT to describe disorders of psychogenic origin or that relate to personality variables. However, in relation to voice disorders at least, the term is now reserved for voice disorders in which there is impairment of how the vocal apparatus is used or functions, with 'psychogenic' reserved for voice disorders that are related to psychological and psychiatric factors (Connor and Bless, 2014). It is also worth noting that communication and swallowing disorders can have psychogenic and neurogenic forms. For example, **psychogenic stuttering** has some form of psychological trauma as its aetiology. In **neurogenic stuttering**, **dysfluency** is related to a known neurological trauma. This is most often a cerebrovascular accident or head injury (Yaruss, 2014).

KEY POINTS: Epidemiology and Aetiology

- Epidemiology is the study of the distribution and determinants of diseases and disorders in populations.
- Two key concepts in epidemiology are prevalence and incidence. Prevalence is the number of individuals in a population who have a disorder at a specific period of time. Incidence describes the number of people who develop a disease or disorder in a specific time period, usually a month or a year.
- Epidemiologists are also interested in how diseases and disorders in a population vary in accordance with variables such as age, sex, racial or ethnic identity and socioeconomic status.
- Aetiology is the study of the medical causes of disorders. These causes may include infectious diseases, neurological injuries and genetic and chromosomal defects.
- Aetiologies can vary depending on whether they are direct causes of a disorder (proximal aetiology) or a cause of a disorder through other, intermediary causes (distal aetiology).
- Where no organic cause of a disorder is found, a functional disorder is diagnosed. In relation to voice disorders, the label 'functional voice disorder' is reserved for dysphonias in which there is impairment of the use and function of the vocal apparatus. Where psychological factors are believed to be the cause of a voice disorder, the label 'psychogenic voice disorder' is used.
- There are other psychogenic communication disorders (e.g. psychogenic stuttering). They differ from neurogenic communication disorders (e.g. neurogenic stuttering), which are caused by neurological injuries and disorders.

3.3 Anatomy and Physiology

SLT students must have knowledge of the structure (anatomy) and function (physiology) of the organs of speech, language and hearing. The importance of these biological disciplines to SLT is reflected in their prominence in the RCSLT guidelines for pre-registration SLT courses in the UK. Under *General Anatomy and Physiology*, the guidelines state that:

> A basic level of understanding of general anatomy and physiology is needed in order to understand both normal biological processes and pathological processes which may affect speech, language, hearing and other aspects of communication. The curriculum should include: cell biology and histology; genetics; and the basic structure and function of the following systems: respiratory; cardiovascular; endocrine; nervous; musculoskeletal; and sensory.   (RCSLT 2010: 37)

Knowledge of **cell biology** includes the structure and function of the hair cells in the cochlea and how these cells may be degraded through illness (e.g. meningitis) and injury (e.g. noise exposure). The study of tissues in **histology** is necessary in order to understand vocal fold structure and function. The tissues that lie deep to the squamous epithelium of the vocal fold are known as the **lamina propria**. The three layers of the lamina propria – superficial, intermediate and deep – have different cellular and tissue contents which confer important properties on the lamina propria during vocal fold vibration. Knowledge of **genetics** is needed in order to understand genetic syndromes such as fragile X syndrome that involves a mutation of the fragile X mental retardation 1 (FMR1) gene on the X chromosome. Also, the genetic basis of conditions such as autism spectrum disorder is beginning to be revealed. A genetic explanation of the significant male: female sex ratio in this disorder – 4–5: 1 on most accounts (Lai et al., 2015) – is the imprinted-X liability threshold model (Skuse, 2000). According to this model, an imprinted X-linked gene that is expressed only on the X-chromosome inherited from the father has a protective effect by raising the threshold for the phenotypic expression of autism. Because only female offspring have a paternal X-chromosome, it is only girls who receive the protective effect of this gene. In order to understand this genetic explanation of the sex ratio in autism, SLT students must have knowledge of sex chromosomes, Mendelian inheritance, gene expression and **phenotype**. The biological sciences curriculum must address genetics in order to equip SLT students with this vital knowledge.

Knowledge of the structure and function of respiratory, cardiovascular, endocrine, nervous, musculoskeletal and sensory systems is an essential component of the clinical education of SLT students. **Respiration** is an important speech production subsystem. In children with cerebral palsy and developmental dysarthria, reduced breath support for speech can adversely affect intelligibility. Reduced vocal volume is a significant and incapacitating symptom of hypokinetic dysarthria in adults with Parkinson's disease. The cardiovascular system relates to the work of SLT in a number of ways. Children with congenital heart disease who undergo early corrective heart surgery are at risk of brain injury. These children can experience adverse neurological sequelae including speech and language problems (Hövels-Gürich et al., 2008). SLT students must understand the relationship between cardiovascular disease and cerebrovascular accidents. Specifically, the blood clots that cause strokes are produced during a process called **atherosclerosis** in which there is a build-up of cholesterol, calcium and cells following damage to the inner lining (endothelium) of arteries. The plaques that form in this process can fragment into clots. When these clots travel to a blood vessel in the brain and prevent oxygenated blood from reaching brain tissue, a stroke is the result. The endocrine system has relevance to SLT students. Hormonal changes related to the menstrual cycle and the menopause can result in altered laryngeal physiology and affect the speaking and singing voice (D'haeseleer et al., 2013; Tatar et al., 2016). These vocal changes must be understood by SLTs, as must the effect on the voice of drugs such as the oral contraceptive pill and androgen therapy in the female-to-male transsexual client (Cosyns et al., 2014; Meurer et al., 2015).

SLTs must have a sound knowledge of the structure and function of the body's nervous system. The central nervous system (CNS) includes the brain and spinal cord which are surrounded and protected by the skull (neurocranium) and vertebral column, respectively. The brain contains neuroanatomical areas related to speech and language such as the **primary motor context**, **Broca's area** and **Wernicke's area**. The peripheral nervous system (PNS) consists of 31 pairs of **spinal nerves** and 12 pairs of cranial nerves. As their name suggests, the spinal nerves originate from the spinal cord, while the cranial nerves originate from the brainstem. Cranial nerves innervate a range of muscles involved in speech production. They include the **facial nerve** (CN VII) which innervates the **orbicularis oris** (a sphincter muscle which encircles the lips), and the **vagus nerve** (CN X) which innervates the **levator veli palatini** (a pair of muscles that elevate the velum against the **nasopharynx**). Spinal nerves involved in speech production include the **phrenic nerve**, which innervates the **diaphragm** and the **intercostal nerves**, which innervate the **intercostal muscles**. The musculoskeletal system consists of bones, muscles and connective tissues. The latter tissues include cartilage, tendons and ligaments. The main functions of this system are to provide structure and support to the body and enable movement. The laryngeal mechanism involves a complex arrangement of muscles, cartilages and ligaments. SLT students must understand the structure and function of each of these parts and their role in the production of voice (**phonation**). Finally, sensory systems such as hearing, vision and **olfaction** are vital to communication and swallowing. Although hearing is most commonly associated with communication and is studied in detail by SLT students in consequence, there are many aspects of communication that depend on the ability to perceive visual stimuli such as **facial expressions** and **gestures**.

As well as an understanding of general anatomy and physiology, the RCSLT guidelines require SLT students to have knowledge of lifespan changes in anatomy and physiology. The guidelines state:

> The curriculum should provide a good grounding in typical patterns of change throughout the lifespan, with particular reference to the nervous system, orofacial and upper thoracic regions. This should include:
>
> - **embryology** and an introduction to congenital malformations
> - growth and development in childhood and adolescence; **sexual dimorphism**
> - maintenance and change during adulthood.
>
> (RCSLT, 2010: 37)

One of the most common congenital malformations encountered by SLTs is cleft lip and palate. SLT students must understand the embryological processes which are disrupted in clefting and the impact of this congenital malformation on speech, language, hearing and feeding (see section 2.2 in Cummings, 2008, for detailed discussion). Other congenital malformations with implications for speech production include **micrognathia** (a small or underdeveloped mandible) in **Treacher Collins syndrome** and **Pierre Robin syndrome**, and a large tongue (**macroglossia**) relative to the size of the oral cavity in Down syndrome and **Beckwith-Wiedemann syndrome**. SLTs must also understand growth and development in childhood and adolescence. For example, there is extensive maturation of the nervous system after birth. During the preschool period, the brain increases fourfold in size, reaching approximately 90% of adult volume by 6 years of age (Stiles and Jernigan, 2010). The development of secondary sexual characteristics during adolescence includes laryngeal changes that result in **voice mutation**. In males, the larynx descends and the dimensions of the infraglottal, sagittal and transverse planes increase. There is also an increase in the anterior-posterior dimensions of the larynx, with greater increases in the male than in the female larynx. Changes in the size and mass of the vocal folds are less for girls than for boys (Higdon and Vaughan, 2011). The pitch of the male voice drops significantly and has an average **fundamental frequency** of about 130 Hz at 18 years. At the completion of voice change, the fundamental frequency of the female voice is approximately 220–225 Hz (Davies and Jahn, 2004). SLT students must understand these laryngeal changes and their effect on voice production.

SPECIAL TOPIC: Cleft Lip and Palate

The congenital condition cleft lip and palate (CLP) amply demonstrates the importance of anatomy and physiology to the work of speech and language therapists. CLP is a relatively common embryological malformation which has an overall prevalence of 9.92 per 10,000 (IPDTOC Working Group, 2011). The birth prevalence is higher in boys than in girls, with one epidemiological study reporting a boy to girl ratio of 1.75: 1 (Matthews et al., 2015). There are also different incidence rates among different ethnicities. Saad et al. (2014) found the highest rates for any oral cleft, isolated cleft palate, and cleft lip with and without palate in the white (non-Hispanic) population of the state of California.

Children with CLP exhibit speech, language and hearing problems. Hypernasal speech is often found in children with cleft palate and is related to velopharyngeal incompetence or insufficiency. Closure of the velopharyngeal port during speech production is often not achieved for both anatomical and physiological reasons. In terms of anatomy, a surgically repaired palate may be short. The pharyngeal cavity that it is expected to occlude may also be excessively capacious. In both cases, the velum is structurally incapable of closing the velopharyngeal port. Enlarged adenoids in children with cleft palate may provide the additional structural bulk that is needed to achieve closure of the port. If an adenoidectomy is performed, a child with previously normal speech resonance may display hypernasality for the first time after surgery.

Velopharyngeal incompetence may also arise on account of physiological reasons. The paired levator veli palatini muscles are the primary elevators of the soft palate. The course and insertion of these muscles are markedly abnormal in children with cleft palate. This has implications for the contraction of these muscles and for their ability to elevate the soft palate to make contact with the posterior and lateral pharyngeal walls. The paired tensor veli palatini muscles are also abnormal in children with cleft palate. Contraction of these muscles is believed to play an important role in Eustachian tube opening and middle ear ventilation. When the function of these muscles is disrupted, the middle ear is inadequately ventilated and otitis media with effusion can develop. Abnormal physiology of the palatal muscles in children with cleft palate contributes not only to velopharyngeal incompetence but also to middle ear pathology and conductive hearing loss.

Adulthood brings changes in speech- and hearing-related anatomy and physiology. Some of these changes are part of the normal aging process. The lungs are mature by 20–25 years. After this age, there is a progressive decline in lung function (Sharma and Goodwin, 2006). Structural changes to the thoracic cage with aging can cause a reduction of chest wall compliance. This can lead to higher residual volume, as a stiff chest wall leads to incomplete emptying of the lungs. Respiratory muscle function also declines with age. A decrease of maximum inspiratory pressure can lead to inadequate ventilation and impaired clearance of airway secretions. There is evidence that age-related changes in the respiratory mechanism can affect how older adults generate subglottal pressure during speech production (Huber, 2008). Other anatomical and physiological changes in adulthood arise for reasons of pathology. The anatomy and physiology of the ossicular chain in the **middle ear** may be compromised in adulthood with the onset of **otosclerosis**. In this condition, there is the formation of new bone growth on the anterior stapes footplate, leading to the fixation of the stapes. Both genetic factors and environmental factors (e.g. fluoride, measles) are believed to play a role in the aetiology of otosclerosis (Schrauwen and Van

Camp, 2010). Otosclerosis is treated by **stapedectomy** surgery. In one large study of 1,351 patients, the mean age at surgery was 43.57 years (Niedermeyer et al., 2007). However, the age of onset of the hearing loss caused by otosclerosis occurs earlier in adulthood, principally between 15 and 40 years (Cureoglu et al., 2006). Otosclerosis is just one of many pathological conditions that can disrupt speech- and hearing-related anatomy and physiology in the adult years. Lifespan changes in anatomy and physiology are thus a key part of the knowledge of SLT students.

> **KEY POINTS: Anatomy and Physiology**
>
> - SLT students must have knowledge of the structure (anatomy) and function (physiology) of the organs of speech, language, hearing and swallowing.
> - Speech- and hearing-related anatomy may not develop normally in the pre-natal period, resulting in conditions such as cleft lip and palate, micrognathia and atresia of the ear canal.
> - Speech- and hearing-related anatomy may be impaired in adulthood through injury or illness. For example, an adult may have to have all or part of the tongue removed (glossectomy) on account of oral cancer.
> - Anatomical structures may be intact but their function may be impaired. For example, the velum may be a normal length and width. Yet it might fail to make contact with the lateral and posterior pharyngeal walls on account of limited elevation. In this case, velopharyngeal incompetence is related to a physiological impairment.
> - Physiological impairments may be congenital in nature. Velopharyngeal incompetence in a child with cleft palate is related to impaired function of the levator veli palatini muscles. Physiological impairments may also have their onset in adulthood. Stroke-induced neurological damage may lead to paresis or paralysis of the velum in an adult.
> - Often, an anatomical defect of the organs of speech and hearing may lead to a physiological defect. A benign or malignant growth on a vocal fold will adversely affect the movement of the fold during phonation.

3.4 Neurology

The study of the nervous system and its disorders is a key part of the medical knowledge of SLT students. In its guidelines to pre-registration SLT courses in the UK, the RCSLT includes neurology in a range of medical disciplines that must be addressed in the SLT curriculum. Not only does knowledge of these disciplines 'underpin SLT practice', but the medical specialists who practise these disciplines are also involved in the multidisciplinary management of clients with communication disorders. According to the RCSLT guidelines, SLT students must be introduced to the following aspects of neurology:

- Aetiological factors, presenting features and communicative consequences of developmental, acquired and progressive neurological impairments
- The principles of clinical neurological assessment
- Current neurological approaches to assessment and intervention (medical and surgical) in common neurological impairments with an impact on communication

(RCSLT, 2010: 38–9)

SLTs can encounter a large range of neurological impairments in their clinical practice. A common developmental neurological impairment that has implications for communication and swallowing is cerebral palsy. Cerebral palsy is a motor disability which has a prevalence that ranges from 1.5 to 2.5 per 1,000 live births (Paneth et al., 2006). The disorder has a number of aetiologies including abnormal neurodevelopment in the pre-natal period, hypoxia/ischaemia-related events in the perinatal and neonatal periods and infections such as congenital cytomegalovirus and neonatal meningitis. In approximately 17% of cerebral palsy cases, no abnormality is detectable by conventional MR or CT imaging (Korzeniewski et al., 2008). The pre-, peri- and post-natal events that give rise to cerebral palsy compromise the motor centres and pathways in the brain that control speech production and swallowing. This results in developmental dysarthria and dysphagia, respectively. Depending on the nature and extent of an individual's neurological impairment, language and hearing may also be compromised (Dufresne et al., 2014). Language is most impaired in individuals with cerebral palsy who have intellectual disability (Vos et al., 2014). Cerebral palsy is classified according to the type of motor impairment (e.g. **spasticity**, dyskinesia) and the distribution of that impairment (e.g. **hemiplegia, diplegia**). So, an individual with spastic hemiplegia has very tight muscle tone on one side of the body, with the arm usually affected more than the leg. SLT students must understand how different types of cerebral palsy can affect the tone, range and strength of the speech musculature in a range of dysarthrias (e.g. **spastic dysarthria, flaccid dysarthria**). The reader is referred to Hodge (2014) for discussion of dysarthria in cerebral palsy and other developmental neurological impairments.

Acquired neurological impairments are the cause of a large group of neurogenic communication and swallowing disorders in adults. Stroke-induced lesions of the brain are the most common acquired neurological impairment in adulthood. These lesions can affect cortical and sub-cortical areas and can cause aphasia, dysarthria, **apraxia of speech** and dysphagia. SLT students must understand the nature of stroke-induced brain damage and the implications of this damage for neural reorganization and recovery of language skills. There is evidence, for example, that recovery from post-stroke aphasia is associated with increased activation of undamaged areas and recruitment of perilesional tissue and homologue right language areas (Saur et al., 2006). Although the effects of stroke-induced brain lesions on language and other functions change over time, these lesions are non-progressive in nature. There are also many acquired neurological impairments that are progressive in nature. These impairments include neurodegenerative diseases such as Parkinson's disease, **multiple sclerosis** (MS), motor neurone disease (MND) and the dementias. The CNS lesions that occur in these conditions are rapidly or slowly progressive, with the result that speech, language and swallowing deteriorate over time. SLT students need to understand the course of these disorders and the implications of these different courses for the management of clients. For example, the rapidly progressive nature of MND – the median survival time from onset to death ranges from 20 to 48 months (Chio et al., 2009) – requires early consideration of augmentative and alternative communication (AAC), while a speech-based intervention may be more appropriate for clients with Parkinson's disease. Progressive neurological impairments can also have their onset in the developmental period, e.g. **Duchenne muscular dystrophy** in children.

SLT students must understand the principles of clinical neurological assessment. During an assessment, the overriding goal of the neurologist is to ascertain if the client has a neurological impairment. The neurologist will also want to establish which components of the nervous system are affected (e.g. motor, sensory, cranial nerves) and the location of any dysfunction (e.g. CNS or PNS, left or **right hemisphere** of the brain). The assessment will examine the following components: **mental status**; cranial nerves; muscle strength, tone and bulk; reflexes; coordination; sensory function; and gait. As part of a cranial nerve examination, the neurologist can test the function of the **hypoglossal nerve** (CN XII) by asking a patient to stick out his tongue and move it internally from cheek to cheek. To test the facial nerve (CN VII), a patient is asked to smile, raise his eyebrows and keep his eyes and lips closed while the neurologist tries to open them. SLT students must be aware of the clinical signs of **upper motor neuron** (UMN) and **lower motor neuron** (LMN) lesions. There is loss of strength, tone and reflexes in a LMN lesion as well as muscle **atrophy** and **fasciculations**. Among the clinical signs of a UMN lesion are increased tone, **hyperreflexia**, loss of distal extremity strength and a Babinski's sign. The **Babinski reflex** occurs in children up to 2 years old. When the sole of the foot is firmly stroked, the big toe moves upwards or towards the top surface of the foot and the other toes fan out. As children mature, the reflex disappears. Its presence in an adult is a sign of neurological damage, specifically within the **pyramidal system**. SLTs must have knowledge of the components of a neurological examination in order to assess motor speech disorders such as dysarthria. Indeed, clinical assessments of these disorders such as the *Frenchay Dysarthria Assessment – Second Edition* (FDA-2; Enderby and Palmer, 2008) draw directly on this knowledge.

Finally, SLT students must have knowledge of approaches used in neurology to assess and treat neurological disorders that have an impact on communication and swallowing. In terms of assessment, SLT students require an understanding of the imaging techniques that are used to assess brain structure and function. These techniques include clinical magnetic resonance and x-ray computerized tomography (CT) imaging as well as techniques that are used mostly, but not exclusively, in research settings: functional magnetic resonance imaging (fMRI); **positron emission tomography** (PET); **electroencephalography** (EEG); **magnetoencephalography** (MEG); **near infrared spectroscopy** (NIRS); and **transcranial magnetic stimulation** (TMS). SLT students must understand what is measured by each of these techniques as well as their limitations. EEG and MEG measure neuronal activity by measuring changes in the electrical activity of neurones as they become active (EEG) or changes in magnetic fields that are related to changes in electrical activity (MEG). However, one limitation of these techniques is that it is difficult to measure changes in electrical activity and magnetic fields in deep brain structures (Crosson et al., 2010).

Knowledge of the medical and surgical interventions that are used to treat neurological impairments includes pharmacotherapy for conditions such as Parkinson's disease. Drug treatments have relevance to SLTs as some treatments can produce side effects that have implications for communication and swallowing. For example, chronic treatment of Parkinson's disease with **levodopa** can lead to the development of motor fluctuations and **dyskinesias**, particularly in young patients (Pilleri and Antonini, 2015). Dyskinesias can further compromise speech production in clients with Parkinson's disease. A range of interventions, including **neurosurgery, cranial radiotherapy** and **chemotherapy**, are used to treat brain tumours and **primary CNS lymphoma**. These therapies can have long-term implications for individuals who receive these treatments. In some cases, language and cognitive problems are evident many years after treatment of these neoplastic conditions is complete. Correa et al. (2004) examined cognitive functioning in 28 patients with primary CNS lymphoma who were treated with whole brain radiotherapy with or without chemotherapy or with chemotherapy alone. There was more pronounced cognitive impairment, particularly in memory and attention/executive domains, among patients who were treated with whole brain radiotherapy with or without chemotherapy than in patients who were treated with chemotherapy alone. Extent of white matter disease on MRI correlated with attention/executive, memory, and language impairment. SLTs must be aware of the neurocognitive sequelae of these various interventions.

> **KEY POINTS: Neurology**
> - Neurology is an important medical discipline for SLTs. As such, it should be taught in SLT curricula. Neurologists are part of the multidisciplinary

team that assesses and treats clients with neurogenic communication and swallowing disorders.
- SLT students must understand the aetiology, clinical features and effect on communication and swallowing of developmental neurological impairments. These impairments can be static (e.g. cerebral palsy) or progressive (e.g. Duchenne muscular dystrophy).
- SLT students must understand the aetiology, clinical features and effect on communication and swallowing of acquired neurological impairments. These impairments can be static (e.g. stroke-induced brain lesions) or progressive (e.g. the CNS lesions in neurodegenerative disorders such as multiple sclerosis).
- SLT students must have knowledge of the different components of a clinical neurological assessment. This includes how to assess cranial nerve function and the significance of the presence of primitive reflexes (e.g. Babinski reflex) in adults with neurological impairments.
- SLT students must have knowledge of the techniques used by neurologists to assess neurological impairments that have an impact on communication and swallowing. This includes imaging techniques (e.g. fMRI) that are used to assess brain structure and function.
- SLT students must also have knowledge of the medical and surgical interventions that are used to treat neurological impairments. This includes pharmacotherapy, neurosurgery, cranial radiotherapy and chemotherapy. As well as treating neurological impairments, these various interventions can have adverse consequences for speech, language and cognition.

3.5 ENT Medicine

Another medical discipline of particular significance to SLT is ENT medicine or otorhinolaryngology. The RCSLT guidelines for pre-registration SLT courses require students on these courses to have knowledge of the following areas of ENT medicine and maxillofacial surgery:

- Developmental abnormalities and acquired pathologies of:
  ○ The ear and hearing
  ○ The larynx, throat, nose, oral cavity and surrounding structures, including the velopharyngeal system
- Traumatic injury to the maxillofacial and neck areas
- Current approaches to assessment and intervention (medical and surgical) in ENT and maxillofacial conditions

(2010: 39)

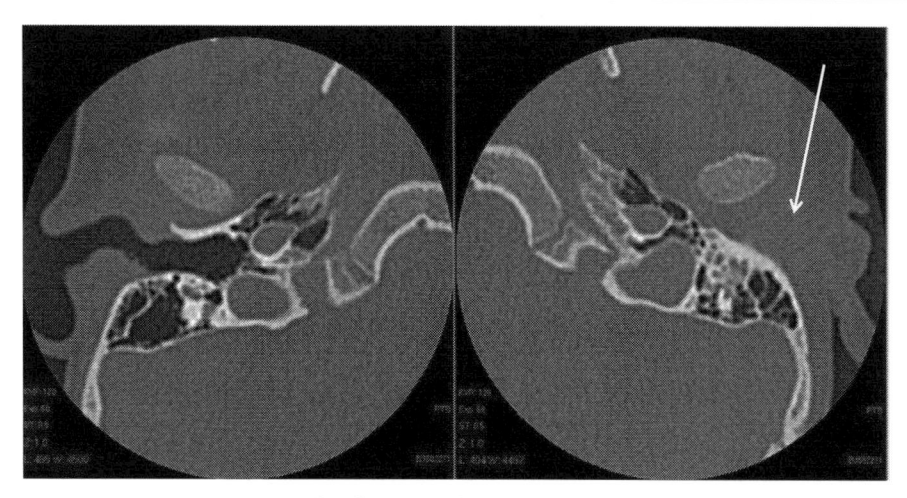

Figure 3.1 *External auditory canal atresia. CT of the temporal bones of a 3-year-old boy with a hypoplastic left external ear. There is atresia of the left external auditory canal, indicated by an arrow. The handle of the malleus in the middle ear was short or absent. (Reproduced courtesy of Dr Laughlin Dawes, Diagnostic Neuroradiologist, Prince of Wales and Sydney Children's Hospitals, Randwick)*

The ear and hearing were described in section 2.2 of Chapter 2. The focus of this description was on normal anatomy and physiology. But SLT students must also understand developmental abnormalities and acquired pathologies of the ear and their effect on hearing. Developmental abnormalities such as **atresia** of the ear canal have their origin in embryological development. In normal embryological development, the formation of the **external auditory meatus** is complete by the mid-point of gestation. The meatus is fully patent along its entire length, although the lumen is still narrow and curved, in a foetus of 16.5 weeks. In an 18-week foetus, the meatus has fully expanded to its complete form (Nishimura and Kumoi, 1992). Failure of development of the first branchial groove, starting at 8 weeks with the non-formation of the primitive auditory canal, results in a spectrum of malformations that range from minor stenosis of the external auditory canal to severe atresia (Casselman et al., 2015) (see Figure 3.1). Other anomalies can occur alongside atresia including malformation of the ossicles and **microtia** (see Figure 3.2). The syndromes most commonly associated with atresia are **VACTERL/VATER association**, **CHARGE syndrome**, Treacher Collins syndrome, Pierre Robin syndrome, **Goldenhar syndrome** and **Alport syndrome**. Unilateral atresia is three to six times more common than bilateral atresia, and the right ear is more frequently affected than the left ear (Roland and Marple, 1997). Atresia results in a 60 dB conductive hearing loss (Mikulec, 2009). Although most individuals with atresia have a conductive hearing loss only, up to 15% of people with the condition have a mixed hearing loss (Quesnel and Cohen, 2015). As one might expect, there are high rates of speech therapy

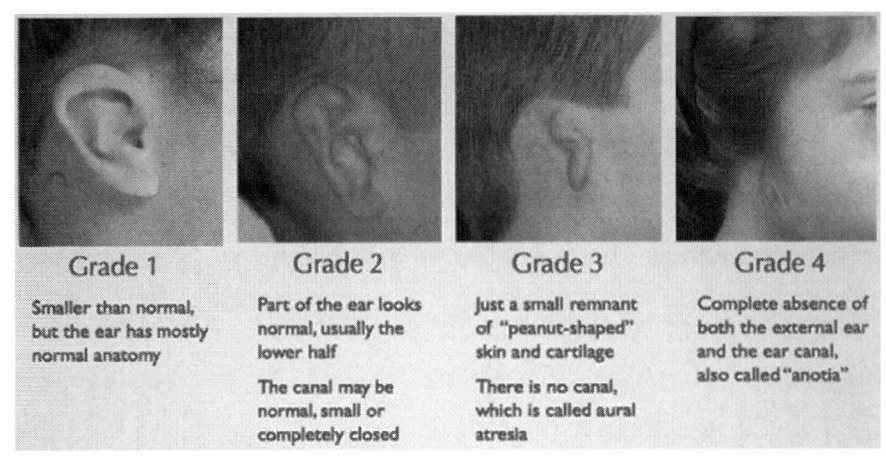

Figure 3.2 *Grades of microtia (Photograph provided courtesy of Dr Sheryl Lewin)*

among children with bilateral (86%) and unilateral (43%) aural atresia (Jensen et al., 2013).

Other abnormalities of the ear with their onset during embryological development are cochlear aplasia and hypolasia. In the fifth week of embryological development, three folds form that represent the primordial cochlear, vestibular and endolymphatic sac appendages. If there is arrested development of the cochlear bud at this stage, **cochlear aplasia** is the result. In this condition, there is a complete lack of cochlear development with preservation of the **semicircular canals** and **vestibule**, although the latter structures may not be normally developed. Arrested development in the sixth week results in a rudimentary cochlea, which may range from a small diverticulum (pouch) to a cochlear bud of several millimetres in length. This condition is called **cochlear hypoplasia**. Arrested cochlear development in the seventh week results in a small, flattened cochlea which has only 1 to 1.5 turns (a fully developed cochlea has 2.5 to 2.75 turns). This condition is known as **incomplete partition dysplasia** (Scott and Carey, 2006). Although cochlear aplasia and hypoplasia are relatively rare conditions, they are a significant cause of sensorineural hearing loss in children. Masuda et al. (2013) identified cochlear malformations in 20.3% of patients aged 0–15 years with unilateral sensorineural hearing loss. **Cochlear implantation** may be used in the **aural rehabilitation** of patients with certain cochlear malformations. Total aplasia is a contraindication to implantation, as there are no spiral ganglion cells for the implant to stimulate. However, in cases of incomplete partition, a subnormal cochlea that fails to reach 2.5 turns and mild cochlear hypoplasia (basal turn only), cochlear implantation is recommended and can achieve similar rehabilitation results as in individuals with normal **inner ear** structure (Feng et al., 2012).

SLT students must also have knowledge of acquired pathologies of the ear that can lead to conductive and sensorineural hearing loss. **Cholesteatoma** is a skin cyst which grows into the middle ear and **mastoid bone**. Although it is a non-malignant growth, it can erode the ossicles in the middle ear and lead to CNS complications such as meningitis and brain abscesses. Cholesteatomas are believed to arise from **Eustachian tube** dysfunction. Inadequate opening of the tube leads to negative middle ear pressure and the retraction of the **tympanic membrane**. Epithelial cells that are shed from the surface of the tympanic membrane may accumulate and get trapped under the membrane, causing a cholesteatoma to develop (Govil, 2015). Although there is a congenital form of the disease (Kojima et al., 2006), cholesteatomas occur more commonly in adulthood. Olszewska et al. (2004) reported the annual incidence of cholesteatoma to be 3 per 100,000 in children and 9.2 per 100,000 in adults. Conductive hearing loss typically results from erosion of the **incus** (Chole and Nason, 2009). The hearing loss is progressive and unilateral. Otolaryngologists treat cholesteatomas using surgical and non-surgical interventions. Surgical interventions involve **mastoidectomy** with or without reconstruction of the **middle ear cleft**. The two main surgical procedures – canal wall up (CWU) mastoidectomy and canal wall down (CWD) mastoidectomy – differ in respect to whether the bony posterior canal wall is preserved (CWU) or removed (CWD). Non-surgical interventions include the use of antibiotics to treat infections. Only surgical interventions are capable of eradicating cholesteatomas (Kuo et al., 2015).

Noise exposure is a significant cause of sensorineural hearing loss in adults. Hoffman et al. (2006) reported the prevalence of **noise-induced hearing loss** (NIHL) among American adults aged 20–69 years to be 15%. Prevalence increased with each decade of life except for the oldest age group (60–69 years) and was greater in males (21.8%) than in females (8.5%). In NIHL, there are morphological changes to outer hair cells in the cochlea, among a number of other pathological findings (e.g. degeneration of auditory nerve fibres). In the early stages of NIHL, the stereocilia of these cells become bent and disorganized and some can be broken or missing (Sliwinska-Kowalska, 2015). The first row of outer hair cells in the cochlea is most sensitive to noise, followed by the third row. The second row of outer hair cells and inner hair cells are most resistant to noise exposure. There are significant functional consequences of these morphological changes to cochlear hair cells. The loss of at least 30% of hair cells causes a shift in hearing threshold at frequencies related to the place of damage in the organ of Corti. In humans, the most sensitive region of the cochlea corresponds to frequencies in the range 3–6 kHz. Accordingly, an audiometric notch at high frequencies (typically 4 or 6 kHz) is the first sign of NIHL (Sliwinska-Kowalska, 2015). This notch can be seen in the **audiogram** in Figure 3.3, with better hearing at frequencies above and below 4 kHz. Individuals with NIHL exhibit poor speech understanding in the presence of background noise. They also experience **recruitment**, a perceptual phenomenon in which sounds become rapidly louder with increasing sound level. Recruitment can cause considerable

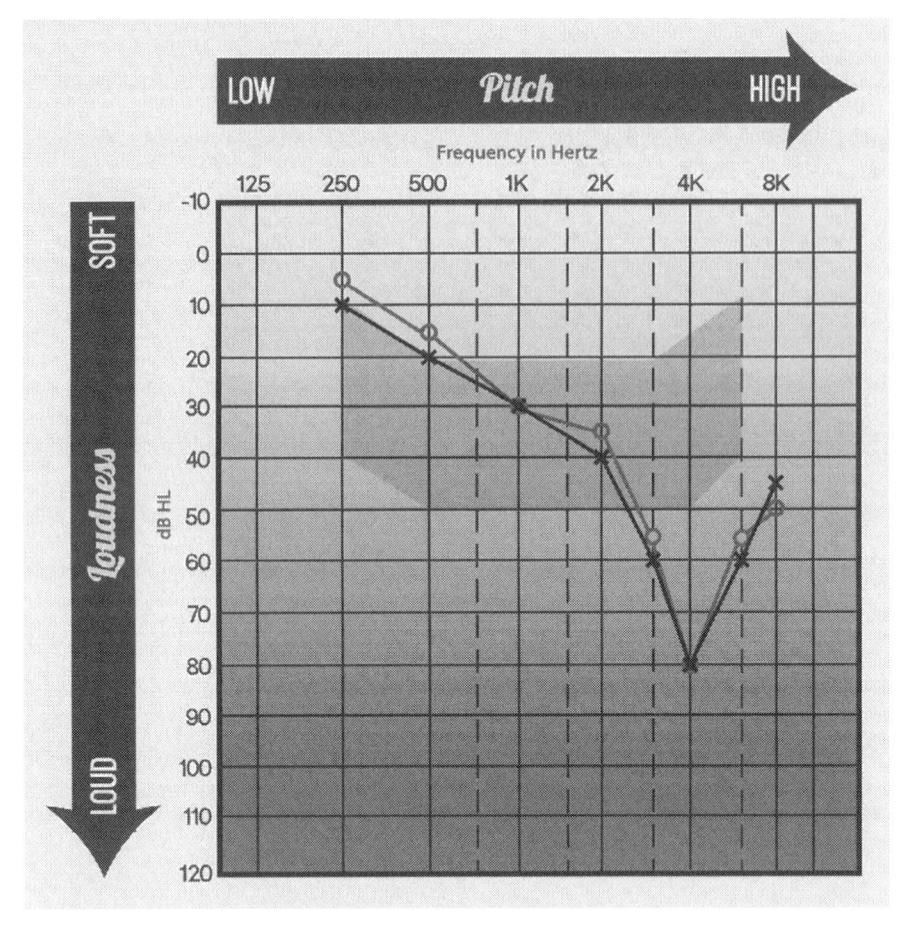

Figure 3.3 *Audiogram in noise-induced hearing loss (reproduced with kind permission of Joe Hinz and Leah Garaas)*

discomfort for patients. Another feature of NIHL is **tinnitus**, the perception of sound in the absence of an acoustic stimulus.

Otolaryngologists also assess and treat laryngeal pathologies in children and adults. SLT students must have knowledge of these pathologies and their effect on the production of voice. The most common congenital anomalies of the larynx are **laryngomalacia**, **vocal fold paralysis** and **subglottic stenosis** (Sichel et al., 2000). In laryngomalacia, supraglottic structures collapse during inspiration. This results in intermittent airflow impedance and associated inspiratory **stridor**. Children with this condition can also have feeding problems. The prevalence and incidence of laryngomalacia in the general population are unknown. In a study of 358 children with sleep-disordered breathing, the prevalence of laryngomalacia was 3.9% (Thevasagayam et al., 2010). Symptoms generally resolve within the first 24 months of life. However, for 5% to

20% of children with severe symptoms, **supraglottoplasty** may be performed (Thorne and Garetz, 2016). Vocal fold paralysis is the second most common congenital laryngeal anomaly in newborns. Its cause is often unknown, although a chromosomal translocation has been identified in cases of familial congenital bilateral vocal fold paralysis (Hsu et al., 2015). **Arnold-Chiari malformation** is the most common congenital CNS abnormality resulting in vocal fold paralysis (Ada et al., 2010). Stridor is the most common presenting symptom of vocal fold paralysis. It is more severe in bilateral paralysis, necessitating in some cases a **tracheotomy** to protect the airway. Dysphonia is usually found in unilateral vocal fold paralysis. Feeding difficulties and **aspiration** are also features (Daya et al., 2000).

Congenital subglottic stenosis is a rare anomaly in which the cricoid cartilage ring of the larynx is an abnormal size or shape. In terms of embryology, the disorder is believed to be related to anomalous proliferation of mesenchyme at the cranial end of the laryngotracheal tube in the fifth week of gestation or incomplete recanalization of the laryngotracheal lumen at the tenth week of gestation (Campisi and Busato, 2015). The more common form of subglottic stenosis is acquired in the early months of life as a result of **endotracheal intubation** in neonates. The condition may be managed conservatively by watchful waiting or through surgical intervention where the airway is compromised. A currently popular surgical procedure for the treatment of severe subglottic stenosis is **partial cricotracheal resection**. George and Monnier (2010) examined the long-term voice outcome in 77 children who underwent partial cricotracheal resection for severe subglottic stenosis. Only 14 children (18%) had normal voice. The remaining 63 children (82%) exhibited mild to severe dysphonia. Aside from congenital laryngeal abnormalities, otolaryngologists also assess and treat laryngeal pathologies which are acquired in childhood. One of the most common pathologies is vocal nodules. In a retrospective review of 646 patients in a paediatric hospital's voice centre from 1996 to 2003, Shah et al. (2005) identified 254 patients (40%) with vocal nodules. Nodules were most commonly found in males aged 3–10 years. Hyperfunction of the larynx was identified in three-quarters of patients with nodules and correlated with the size of nodules. There was a positive correlation between the severity of hoarseness, breathiness, straining and **aphonia** and the size of nodules.

Adult-onset injuries and pathologies of the larynx, pharynx, and nasal and oral cavities are assessed and treated by otolaryngologists and maxillofacial surgeons. Trauma of the laryngeal framework can result from road traffic accidents, sports injuries and violent assaults (Paluska and Lansford, 2008; Dunsby and Davison, 2011). Laryngeal injuries include dislocation of the **cricothyroid joint**, **hyoid bone** fractures, and fractures of the thyroid and cricoid cartilages. There may also be iatrogenic damage of the larynx. The **recurrent laryngeal nerve** can be damaged during **thyroidectomy** and **oesophagectomy** (Christou and Mathonnet, 2013; Sato et al., 2016). These various laryngeal injuries have implications for phonation and respiration. Carcinomas of the larynx, pharynx, and nasal and oral cavities are also managed by otolaryngologists and maxillofacial surgeons. The National Cancer Institute in the United States estimated that in 2015 there were 45,780 new cases of oral cavity and pharynx cancer and 13,560 new cases of laryngeal cancer. SLT students must have knowledge of the epidemiology and aetiology of oropharyngeal and laryngeal carcinomas and an understanding of how these disorders are assessed and treated by otolaryngologists and maxillofacial surgeons. An advanced laryngeal tumour, for example, may necessitate not only a laryngectomy, but also surgical removal of all or part of the tongue (glossectomy), pharynx (**pharyngectomy**) and oesophagus (oesophagectomy). An adult with **oral cancer** may require surgical removal of part of the mandible (**mandibulectomy**) alongside glossectomy. Each of these surgical procedures has significant implications for speech and swallowing function. Individuals who undergo them must be managed pre- and post-operatively by specialist SLTs.

KEY POINTS: ENT Medicine

- As well as knowledge of the normal anatomy and physiology of the ear, larynx, pharynx and oral and nasal cavities, SLT students must be introduced to congenital, developmental and acquired pathologies of these structures.
- Congenital anomalies of the ear include unilateral and bilateral atresia of the external auditory meatus and microtia. The association of atresia with various syndromes (e.g. Treacher Collins syndrome) and its effect on hearing must be understood by SLT students.
- SLT students must also understand the embryological basis of congenital ear anomalies that cause sensorineural hearing loss. For example, cochlear aplasia and hypoplasia involve no development (aplasia) or malformation of the cochlea in the inner ear.
- Pathologies of the ear can also have their onset in adulthood. Cholesteatoma may develop in the middle ear and cause conductive hearing loss that is unilateral and progressive in nature. Noise exposure is a significant cause of sensorineural hearing loss in adults. It results in poor speech understanding against background noise, recruitment and tinnitus.
- SLT students must have knowledge of the symptoms and effects on voice production of congenital laryngeal abnormalities such as laryngomalacia, vocal fold paralysis and subglottic stenosis. Laryngeal abnormalities may also have their onset in childhood. For example, vocal nodules are related to hyperfunction of the larynx in children.
- The structure and function of the larynx, pharynx and oral and nasal cavities can be compromised by injuries and pathologies in adulthood. Laryngeal trauma may be caused by sports injuries, road traffic accidents and assaults. Carcinomas of these structures demand combined management by otolaryngologists, maxillofacial surgeons and SLTs.

3.6 Audiology

As well as knowledge of the normal and abnormal structure and function of the ear, SLTs must understand how hearing and hearing loss are assessed and treated by audiologists. The RCSLT guidelines for pre-registration courses require SLT students to have an understanding of the following areas of audiology:

- Typical lifespan changes in hearing
- Conductive and sensorineural hearing loss
- Current approaches to assessment of hearing and balance in children and adults
- Current audiological approaches to management of developmental and acquired hearing loss, including the role of hearing aids, cochlear implants, counselling and other approaches
- Impact of hearing loss on communication

(2010: 39)

The peripheral and central auditory systems undergo considerable changes across the human lifespan. Although peripheral auditory function appears to mature by the end of the first few post-natal months, developmental changes of function in the central auditory system continue for several years (Moore, 2002). There is evidence, for example, that some areas of the brain activated by sound stimulation have a maturational course that extends into adolescence, and that the maturation of certain auditory processing skills (e.g. speech recognition in noise) also has a prolonged time course (Ponton et al., 2000). These developmental changes are related to axon myelination and maturation of synaptic mechanisms. Typical maturation of hearing occurs in many, but not all, individuals who receive the services of audiologists. SLT students must be aware of client groups in which there is atypical auditory maturation. For example, there is evidence that **central auditory processing** is hyperactive in individuals with Williams syndrome (Zarchi et al., 2015). Such processing displays delayed or diverse maturation in individuals with this syndrome.

Age-related deterioration of hearing is also a concern of audiologists and SLTs. Age-related hearing loss (**presbycusis**) is characterized by high-frequency-dominated hearing loss, reduced speech understanding, slowed central processing of acoustic information, and impaired sound localization (Roth, 2015). The disorder is highly prevalent, with 30% of men and 20% of women exhibiting a hearing loss of 30 dB HL or more by 70 years of age (Roth et al., 2011). Pure tone audiometry has been used to confirm the presence of presbycusis in the age group 40 to 49 years (Arvin et al., 2013). Interestingly, this same study showed that 16% of 20- to 29-year-olds and 50% of 30- to 39-year-olds also exhibited significant high-frequency hearing loss. There are specific histopathological features and audiometric patterns in different forms of presbycusis.

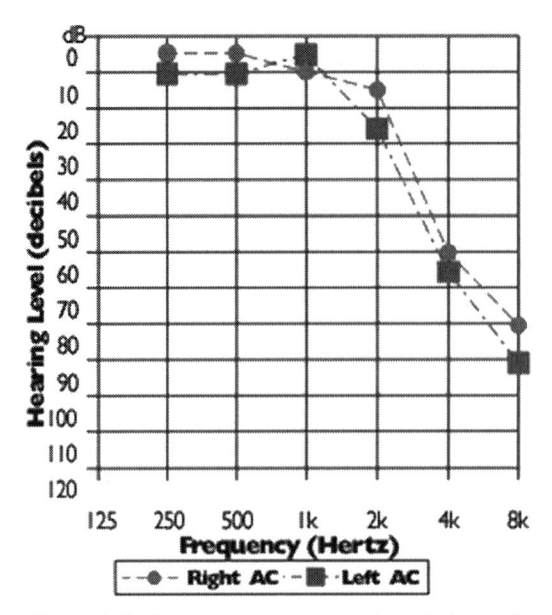

Figure 3.4 *Audiogram in sensory presbycusis (reproduced with kind permission of the International Hearing Society from: P. E. Connelly PhD, CCCA 'Presbycusis – A Look into the Aging Inner Ear')*

In sensory presbycusis, there is a loss of hair cells at the beginning of the basal end of the cochlea. Audiometrically, there may be normal hearing. There may also be a mild hearing loss in the lower frequencies with a sharp drop beginning at 1000 Hz to a severe loss in the higher frequencies (Busis, 2006) (see Figure 3.4). In neural presbycusis, there is a loss of cochlear neurons. The audiogram shows a high-frequency loss with a more gradual curve from low frequency to high frequency. In strial or metabolic presbycusis, there is deterioration of the **stria vascularis**, which is important in inner ear homeostasis, particularly the generation and maintenance of the endocochlear potential. There is a flat or slightly descending pure-tone threshold audiometric pattern. Cochlear conductive presbycusis is characterized by stiffness of the **basilar membrane**. According to Busis (2006: 80), there is a gradually descending pure tone threshold over a range of at least five octaves, with a difference of at least 50 dB between the best and worst thresholds. There is no more than 25 dB difference between any two adjacent frequencies.

Like audiologists, SLT students must have a sound understanding of conductive and sensorineural hearing loss. Knowledge of the general population prevalence of both types of hearing loss has been made possible by universal hearing screening of newborns, at least in developed countries. The prevalence of conductive hearing loss in newborns is 2.97 per 1,000 (Aithal et al., 2012). This type of hearing loss may be caused by ear canal atresia, otitis media, cholesteatoma and congenital malformation of the ossicles. On an audiogram,

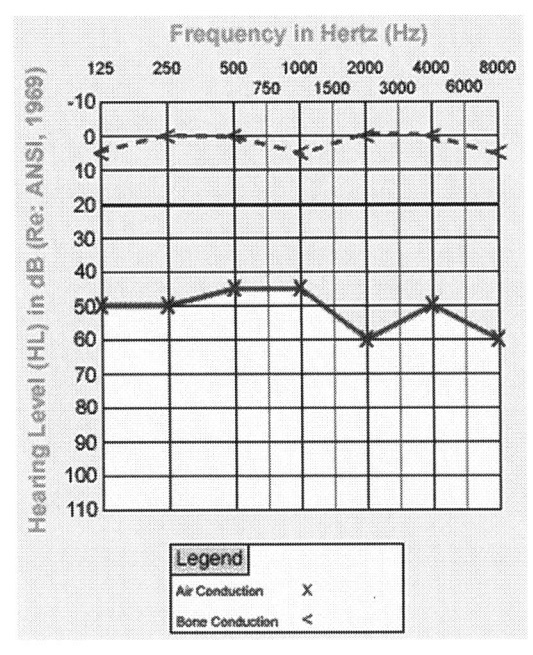

Figure 3.5 *Audiogram in conductive hearing loss (reproduced with kind permission of the Occupational Safety and Health Administration, Washington, DC, USA)*

conductive hearing loss appears as a difference of at least 10 dB between bone conduction responses, which must be in the range of normal, and air conduction responses (see Figure 3.5). Bone conduction responses are obtained during pure tone audiometry by placing a bone conduction oscillator on the mastoid bone. From this position the oscillator stimulates the inner ear directly, thus bypassing the conductive part of the hearing mechanism (i.e. outer and middle ear). The prevalence of sensorineural hearing loss in newborns is 0.36% (Arslan et al., 2013). This type of hearing loss may be caused by congenital infections (e.g. cytomegalovirus), genetic factors and malformations of the cochlea (e.g. cochlear hypoplasia). Sensorineural hearing loss can have many different appearances on an audiogram. **Ménière's disease** is an inner ear condition that typically affects people aged 30 to 60 years. It causes feelings of fullness or pressure in the ear, hearing loss, tinnitus, and recurrent bouts of vertigo (Wright, 2015). There is low-frequency sensorineural hearing loss in Ménière's disease initially in one ear. This appears as a sloping curve from right to left on an audiogram (see Figure 3.6). This audiogram has a quite different appearance from the audiograms for noise-induced hearing loss (Figure 3.3) and presbycusis (Figure 3.4).

Several forms of audiometry are used to assess hearing in children and adults. A complete audiometric assessment includes tests of mechanical sound transmission (middle ear function), neural sound transmission (cochlear function) and speech discrimination ability (central auditory processing). Pure tone audiometry

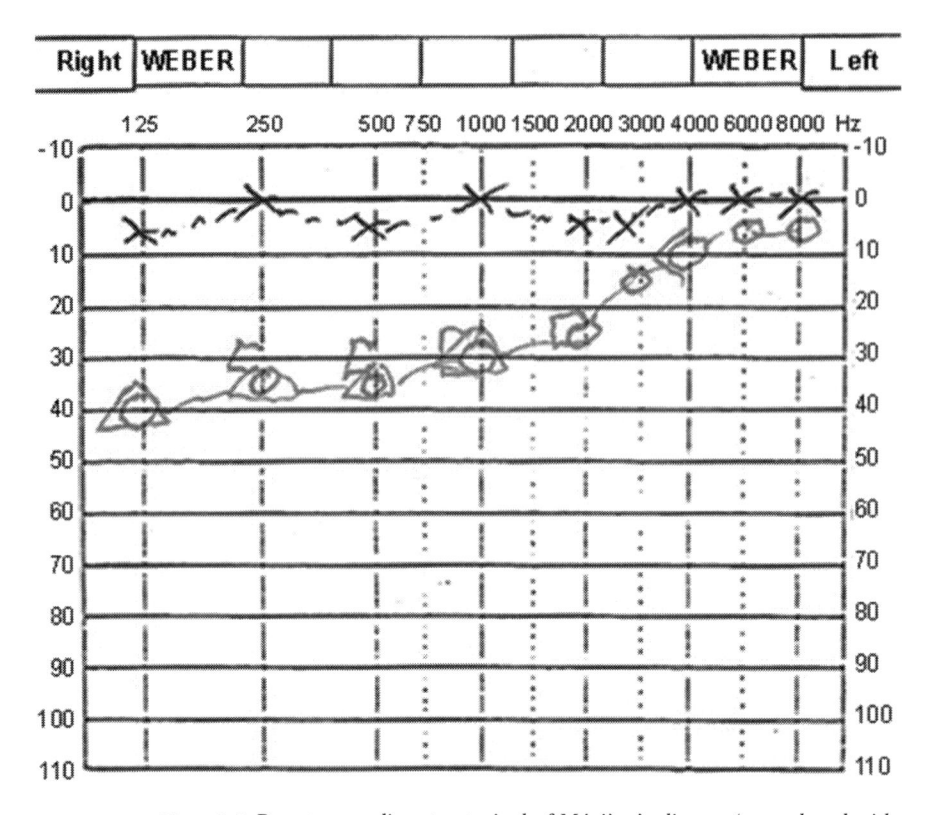

Figure 3.6 *Pure tone audiometry typical of Ménière's disease (reproduced with kind permission of Maurice H. Miller, PhD, Steinhardt School of Education, New York University)*

is the most widely conducted hearing test. The bone conduction form of this test was described above. During air conduction testing, a pure tone is presented to the ear through an earphone. The audiologist measures the lowest intensity in decibels at which this tone is perceived 50% of the time and records this threshold on an audiogram. This procedure is repeated for each ear for specific frequencies between 250 and 8000 Hz. To prevent the participation of the non-test ear, masking noise is sometimes used. During **speech audiometry**, the audiologist tests a person's ability to hear and understand speech. Phonetically balanced, one-syllable words are presented at 25 to 40 dB above the hearing threshold obtained from the pure tone audiogram. The audiologist measures the speech reception threshold, which is the lowest decibel level at which a subject can correctly repeat 50% of these test words. Speech discrimination scores are usually good in conductive hearing loss (if the presentation level is sufficiently loud) and variable in sensorineural hearing loss. Retrocochlear disease (e.g. lesion on the VIIIth nerve) is suspected when there is poor speech discrimination in the presence of little loss for pure tones (Saunders et al., 1990).

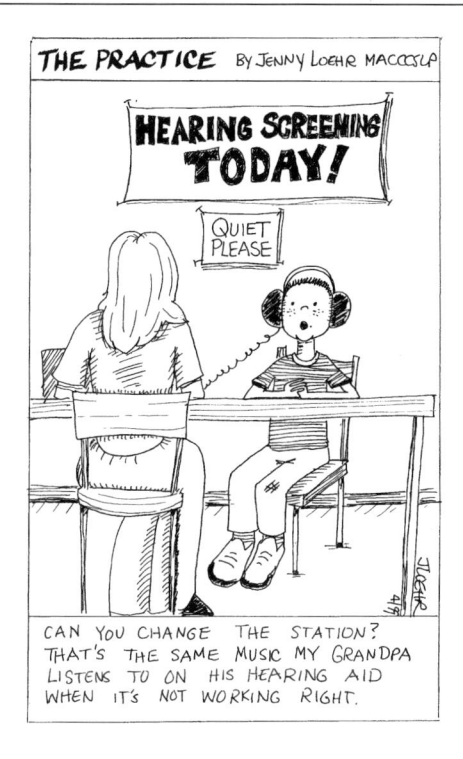

Audiologists also make extensive use of **immittance audiometry** or **impedance audiometry**. Acoustic immittance measures can be used to determine middle ear pressure, mobility of the tympanic membrane, Eustachian tube function, continuity and mobility of the middle ear ossicles, and acoustic reflex thresholds (Northern and Downs, 2002). During **tympanometry**, a hermetic seal is formed by inserting a probe tip into the ear canal. The pressure in the enclosed cavity is varied and the change in sound pressure level of a probe tone is graphed. This shows the movement of the middle ear system as pressure is varied (Saunders et al., 1990). There is maximum compliance of the middle ear system when the pressure in the middle ear cavity is equal to the pressure in the external auditory canal. This compliance is known as static acoustic admittance and is represented by the highest peak of the curve in the normal type A tympanogram shown in Figure 3.7. In otitis media with effusion, there is decreased mobility of the tympanic membrane and a type B tympanogram is obtained. This is a flattened tracing with low static acoustic admittance. Following tympanometry, the contraction of the **stapedius muscle** in response to a loud sound can be measured (**acoustic reflex test**). Reflex thresholds should be seen at 70 to 90 dB above the pure tone thresholds in the normal ear. The contraction of the stapedius muscle should be sustained for at least 10 seconds at 10 to 15 dB above the reflex threshold at 500 and 1000 Hz. Reflex decay, or failure to

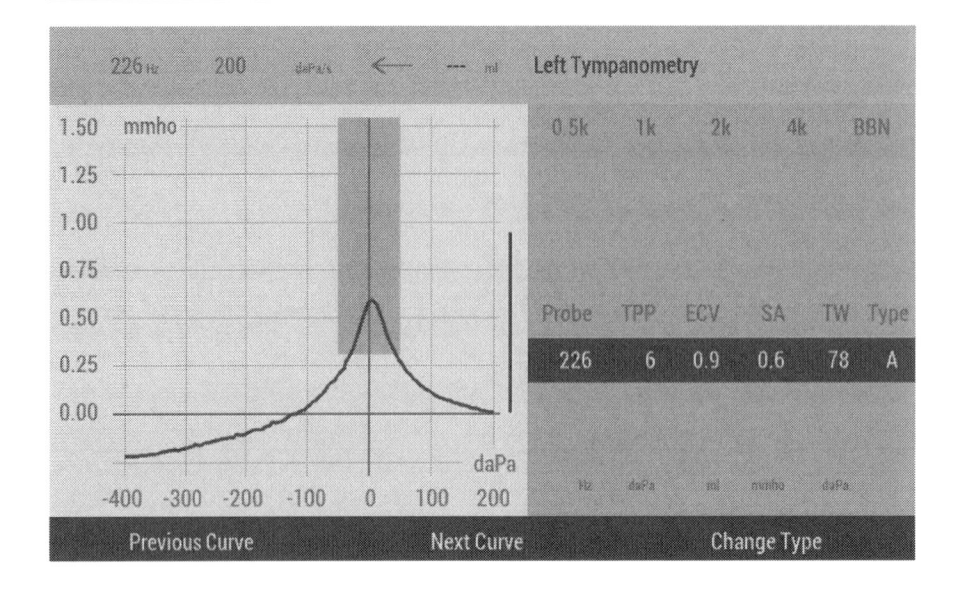

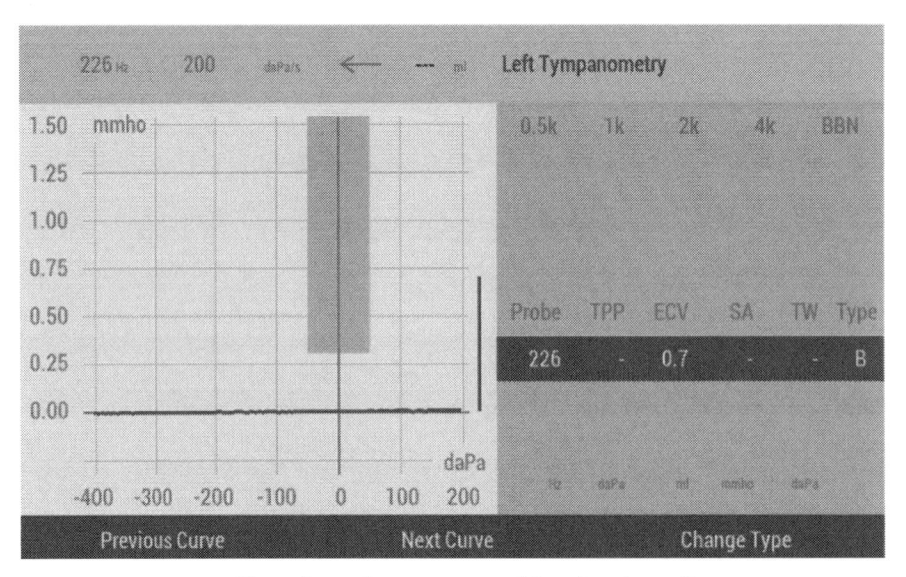

Figure 3.7 *Normal type A tympanogram (above) and type B tympanogram (below) in otitis media with effusion (Data provided by MADSEN Zodiac from GN Otometrics)*

sustain contraction for 10 seconds, is an early sign of retrocochlear disease (Saunders et al., 1990).

Auditory brainstem response (ABR) audiometry measures the electrical activity of the auditory nervous system. Electrodes are placed on the subject's vertex (crown of the head), earlobes and forehead. A series of clicks is delivered

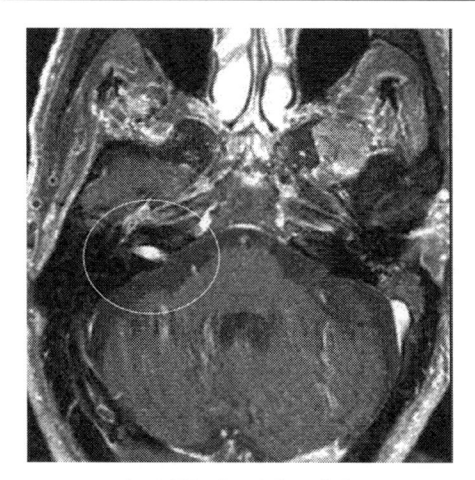

Figure 3.8 *An MRI of a right-sided acoustic neuroma (Image provided courtesy of Dr John Rutka and reprinted with permission from the* Canadian Hearing Report *1:4 (2014))*

through ear phones. A computer calculates the time-locked responses for the first 10 milliseconds after sound stimulation. A display of five waves is generated at predictable latencies (Saunders et al., 1990). These waves represent the auditory nerve response (waves I and II), the lower pons response (wave III), and the upper pons response (waves IV and V). In healthy subjects, the travel time from wave I to wave V is 4.00 milliseconds. There is suspicion of an acoustic tumour (**acoustic neuroma**) when travel time is delayed by 0.5 milliseconds (Ackley, 2014) (see Figure 3.8).

The results of audiometry inform the management of children and adults with hearing loss. Aural rehabilitation may be achieved through the use of amplification devices (e.g. hearing aids) and electronic prosthetic devices (e.g. cochlear implants). All hearing aids share certain basic electronic components including a microphone that detects sound, amplifier circuitry that amplifies sound, a receiver that delivers amplified sound into the ear canal, and batteries that power these electronic parts. However, hearing aids vary in how they are worn. Some are worn behind the ear, with clear tubing connecting the aid to an earpiece. The mini behind-the-ear aid (or on-the-ear aid) is smaller, with a thin, almost invisible tube connecting the aid to the ear canal. In-the-ear hearing aids are contained in a shell that sits in the outer part of the ear. These aids are larger than hearing aids which fit partly or completely into the ear canal. Hearing aids may be analogue or digital. The difference between analog and digital hearing aids is that in a digital hearing aid, the audio signal is converted to a sequence of discrete samples, which are processed digitally, and then converted back to an analogue signal. Hearing aids can also have optional features which assist communication in different situations (e.g. a 'T-coil' setting which facilitates better hearing on the telephone).

Cochlear implants are increasingly being used in the rehabilitation of children and adults with hearing loss. A cochlear implant consists of two parts. There is an external portion (a sound processor) and an implanted portion (an internal receiver-stimulator). The sound processor contains a magnet and a microphone. Associated with the magnet is a radiofrequency coil which connects to the implanted portion. An active electrode that is placed into the **scala tympani** of the cochlea through a **cochleostomy** is stimulated by the coil (Grisel and Samy, 2010: 55). These different components of a cochlear implant are shown in Figure 3.9. The Food and Drug Administration (2015) has estimated that as of December 2012, there were approximately 96,000 individuals in the United States who had received a cochlear implant. Some 58,000 of these individuals were aged 18 years and older, while 38,000 were individuals who were 17 years and younger. As clinical experience with implant technology has grown, the candidacy criteria for implantation have changed, with the result that more people than ever before are now eligible for this procedure. Despite this, there is still widespread under-utilization of implant technology. In the UK, for example, Raine (2013) reported that between 2006 and 2011, only 74% of eligible children aged 0–3 years and 5% of eligible adults actually received a cochlear implant.

GROUP EXERCISE: Cochlear Implantation and the Deaf Community

Cochlear implantation has generated considerable controversy in the Deaf community, with many deaf individuals rejecting the technology for cultural and political reasons. The following extract is taken from an article entitled 'Why Not All Deaf People Want to Be Cured' which was published in the British newspaper *The Telegraph* on 13 September 2012. It describes the experiences of two people, one who received implants and one who did not. In a group, discuss the issues that the article raises.

> Increasingly deaf from the age of four, Rebekah Moore, a 29-year-old from South Derbyshire, had an implant fitted eight years ago. She sends me an email listing some of the things she'd never heard before her operation: 'Birds, footsteps, zips, water running, wind in the trees, paper rustling, kettles boiling, keys jangling. I had an apple and I was astonished at how noisy it was.'
>
> It takes time for patients to get used to an implant and Rebekah had regular appointments to retune her device and gradually increase the parameters of her hearing. 'Each session would be followed by a period of readjustment as I got used to more sounds and more clarity,' she writes. 'Each time I couldn't quite believe it could get any better but it did.'
>
> But not everybody who's deaf is so keen to join the 'hearing world'. Sara Kendall, profoundly deaf from birth, lives with her deaf mother and deaf boyfriend in Nottingham, and feels she has nothing to gain from an implant. 'I was offered cochlear implants when I was younger but my parents refused and I'm very happy with that because I've seen some cochlear users admit that they feel they don't belong.'
>
> What many hearing people might not realise is the strong community that exists in the silent world. In fact, it's more than a community. Deaf people (with a

capital D) see themselves more as an ethnic minority, with their own (sign) language, schools and proud history. The National Association of the Deaf was created by deaf people to advocate for deaf rights in 1880. The Deaf don't see deafness as a disability but a cultural identity (motto: different but not deficient). It's a world so warm and welcoming, many wouldn't want to become hearing, even given the choice.

'I don't feel upset that I can't be in the hearing world completely, because I'm content where I am,' says Sara.

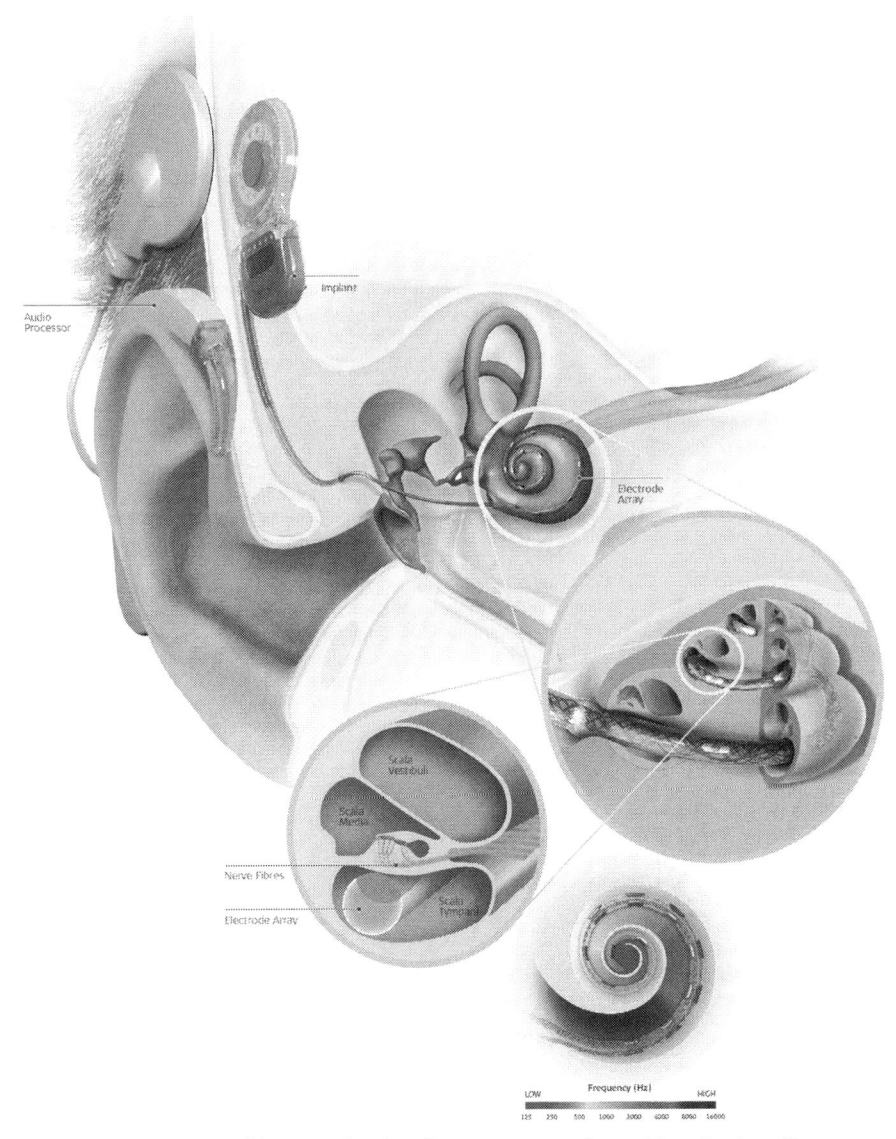

Figure 3.9 *Diagram showing the components of a cochlear implant (Image provided courtesy of MED-EL)*

Audiologists and speech and language therapists must have a sound understanding of the impact of hearing loss on communication. For children, this impact includes delayed speech and language skills, with implications also for social functioning and behaviour. Netten et al. (2015) examined the receptive and expressive language skills of 85 early identified deaf and hard-of-hearing preschool children aged 30–66 months. Language scores revealed that 47% of these children scored one SD or more below the mean on receptive language, while 57% and 56% scored one standard deviation or more below the mean on word and sentence development, respectively. The mean length of utterance of 19 (22%) of the children was one standard deviation or more below the mean. The parents of deaf and hard-of-hearing children reported lower social functioning and more behavioural problems compared to normative scores from hearing children. There is evidence that these communicative and other consequences of hearing loss can be mitigated by early amplification. Attaway et al. (2015) found that children aged 3 to 6 years with conductive hearing loss due to atresia exhibited fewer delays in speech and language development when they received amplification before 1 year of age. For adults, there are also implications of hearing loss for occupational functioning, mental health and quality of life (Tyrrell et al., 2015; Vannson et al., 2015).

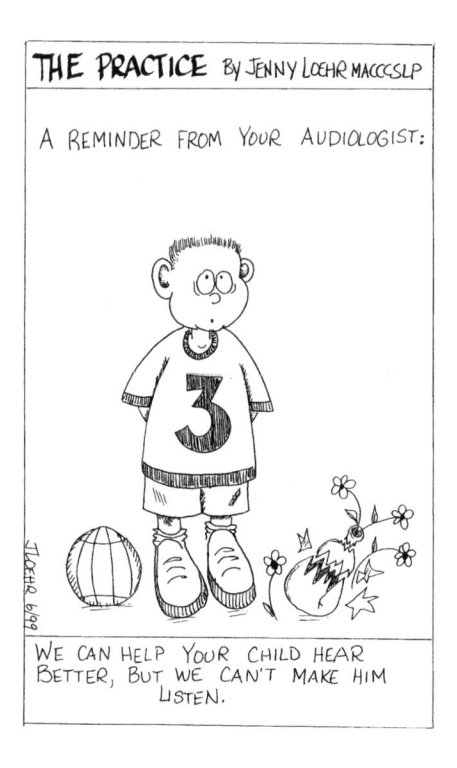

THE PRACTICE By Jenny Loehr MAcCCSLP

A REMINDER FROM YOUR AUDIOLOGIST:

WE CAN HELP YOUR CHILD HEAR BETTER, BUT WE CAN'T MAKE HIM LISTEN.

> **KEY POINTS: Audiology**
>
> - SLT students must have knowledge of developmental changes in peripheral and central auditory function as well as age-related deterioration of hearing in conditions such as presbycusis.
> - Many children and adults in SLT have conductive and/or sensorineural hearing loss. SLT students must appreciate the prevalence, causes and audiometric patterns of these different forms of hearing loss.
> - A comprehensive evaluation of hearing can involve a range of tests including pure tone audiometry, speech audiometry, immittance (impedance) audiometry and auditory brainstem response (ABR) audiometry. SLT students must have an understanding of the technical features of these tests, the specific purposes they serve and how to interpret their results.
> - Aural rehabilitation involves the use of hearing aids for the most part but increasingly cochlear implantation as well. Several different types of hearing aid are available, with the selection of aid dependent on a client's amplification needs. With changes in candidacy criteria, more children and adults than ever before are eligible for cochlear implantation. SLT students must be aware of different methods of aural rehabilitation.
> - Hearing loss has a significant adverse impact on speech and language development in children. Other consequences of hearing loss include reduced social and occupational functioning, behavioural problems, poor quality of life, and mental health difficulties.

3.7 Psychiatry

Psychiatry is the medical discipline that is concerned with the assessment, diagnosis and treatment of children and adults with mental health conditions. It is to be expected that SLTs will encounter a significant number of clients in their clinics with these conditions. This is because mental health problems have a high prevalence in all countries around the world (Kessler et al., 2009), and SLT caseloads will naturally reflect these large figures. But there is an even more specific reason why SLTs need to have an understanding of psychiatry. Communication impairments are a presenting feature of many psychiatric disorders including schizophrenia and bipolar disorder. Knowledge of the communication features of these disorders thus forms an integral part of their clinical characterization. The importance of psychiatry to the work of SLTs is recognized in the RCSLT guidelines for pre-registration SLT courses in the UK. The guidelines state that SLT students must have an understanding of the following:

- Classification of psychiatric conditions
- Current approaches to assessment and intervention in psychiatry

(2010: 39)

An internationally recognized classification system that has assumed increasing prominence in SLT is the *Diagnostic and Statistical Manual of Mental Disorders* (DSM).[1] Published by the American Psychiatric Association and now in its fifth edition, DSM-5 contains diagnostic criteria and detailed text descriptions of most of the disorders which SLTs encounter in clinics. Although it is not within the professional remit of SLTs to diagnose conditions such as schizophrenia and bipolar disorder, therapists must be aware of the criteria that psychiatrists and others use to make these diagnoses. For example, a diagnosis of schizophrenia in DSM-5 is made on the basis of six criteria, the first of which requires that an individual display two or more of the following: (1) delusions; (2) hallucinations; (3) **disorganized speech**; (4) grossly disorganized or catatonic behaviour; and (5) negative symptoms. Two of these behaviours – disorganized speech and a negative symptom known as **alogia** or **poverty of speech** – involve linguistic features which SLTs and psychiatrists must be able to identify.

In disorganized speech, or **formal thought disorder**, individuals with schizophrenia display **derailment**, tangentiality, and incoherence. All three linguistic features are amply illustrated by the following extract from Thomas (1997: 41), which has been produced as part of a doctor–patient interview. The client with schizophrenia displays derailment early on when he asks a question about the doctor's tie. Moreover, he never returns to his original topic, which is an account of where he lives. Several tangential utterances are produced, including the remark about the weather in San Diego and the questions about the conch shell on the doctor's desk and scuba diving. The language is incoherent notwithstanding the use of one type of cohesion (namely, anaphoric reference) between two of the utterances ('where did you get that tie? It looks like ...'). The impression of incoherence stems in large part from the lack of any logical connections between individual utterances, several of which appear to be little more than randomly generated thoughts.

> Then I left San Francisco and moved to ... where did you get that tie? It looks like it's left over from the 1950s. I like the warm weather in San Diego. Is that a conch shell on your desk? Have you ever gone scuba diving?

Alogia, or poverty of speech, is also identifiable on the basis of linguistic features. Clients with schizophrenia who display alogia produce substantially reduced verbal output. Utterances may be single words or turns of a few words even when a more extended conversational turn is appropriate or is directly encouraged. The latter is the case in the following exchange between a doctor (DR) and a 53-year-old male patient (PQ) with schizophrenia who was studied by Clegg et al. (2007). Although the entire exchange is not reproduced below, PQ's much reduced output is evident in a mean length of utterance (MLU) of 3.4 compared to an MLU of 9.4 for the doctor. Lengthy pauses at the end of each of PQ's turns arise because the doctor is trying to delay speaking in an effort to encourage PQ to continue his response. With one exception in the final turn, the doctor's strategy does not succeed in encouraging PQ to continue speaking:

DR: I gather the medication has been causing excess salivation, has it been happening a lot?
PQ: Bit of salivation occasionally (pause of 6 seconds).
DR: When does this happen?
PQ: Possibly at night (pause of 8 seconds).
DR: What have you enjoyed doing this week on the ward PQ?
PQ: Possibly relaxation (pause of 2 seconds).
DR: What do you feel you benefit from by doing the relaxation sessions?
PQ: To relax, get a bit uptight (pause of 5 seconds).
DR: Do you feel uptight all the time?
PQ: Occasionally (pause of 3 seconds).
DR: Do you feel less anxious now than when you first came?
PQ: About the same (pause of 3 seconds).
DR: Can you tell me a bit more? Are you feeling less anxious than you were?
PQ: Could be a bit better ... (pause of 3 seconds) slightly ... (pause 4 seconds) possibly.

Anomalies such as disorganized speech and alogia in schizophrenia are just two of a number of linguistic features that are central to the diagnosis of mental health conditions in classification systems such as DSM-5. Other examples of the role played by linguistic features in the **nosology** and diagnosis of psychiatric disorders include the use of conversational anomalies to identify symptoms of inattention and hyperactivity-impulsivity in the neurodevelopmental disorder ADHD. In this way, the feature 'often does not seem to listen when spoken to directly' is a symptom of inattention in ADHD, while behaviours such as 'often talks excessively' and 'often blurts out an answer before a question has been completed' are symptoms of hyperactivity-impulsivity. The presence of language impairments and symptoms in many of the conditions which psychiatrists assess and treat guarantees a central role for psychiatry in the clinical education of SLT students. For further discussion of the role of language – and pragmatic aspects of language in particular – in the diagnostic criteria of a number of psychiatric disorders, the reader is referred to Cummings (2012).

SLTs must also be aware of the different approaches that psychiatrists use to assess clients with mental health conditions. These approaches include the use of interviews to establish a client's history and prior and current levels of functioning. Screening tools and rating scales are used extensively in psychiatry. Some of these tools and scales are administered by clinicians, while others are completed by parents and teachers. Many have been developed to assist clinicians in arriving at a specific diagnosis, e.g. the *Autism Diagnostic Observation Schedule –Second Edition* (ADOS-2; Lord et al., 2012) is a standardized instrument that is used for the diagnosis of autism. As well as assessment, SLT students must be aware of approaches to intervention in psychiatry. Interventions include **cognitive behavioural therapy**, pharmacotherapy and **psychotherapy**. Psychotherapy is often used in the management of clients with **psychogenic**

dysphonia (Sudhir et al., 2009). Pharmacotherapy has particular relevance for SLTs, as several drugs used in the treatment of mental health conditions can have adverse consequences for motor speech production. Olanzipine long-acting injection for the treatment of schizophrenia is associated with a cluster of symptoms termed post-injection delirium/sedation syndrome (PDSS). In a study of 338 cases of PDSS, dysarthria was reported to occur in 54% of patients (Bushe et al., 2015).

KEY POINTS: Psychiatry

- Mental health conditions have high prevalence rates worldwide and are commonly found in clients who are assessed and treated by SLTs.
- SLTs must be familiar with the classification of psychiatric disorders in internationally recognized systems such as DSM-5.
- Many mental health conditions (e.g. schizophrenia) have specific linguistic disturbances among their symptoms. SLTs must be aware of these disturbances and understand how they relate to the diagnosis of mental health conditions.
- Psychiatrists use a range of approaches and techniques to assess clients with mental health conditions. These include the use of interviews, screening tools and rating scales. Instruments vary in terms of their administration, diagnostic purposes and the chronological ages of clients assessed by them.
- A range of interventions are used to treat clients with mental health conditions. Several have direct relevance to SLT, such as the use of psychotherapy in the management of clients with voice disorders. Some drugs (e.g. olanzapine in the treatment of schizophrenia) can cause side effects such as dysarthria.

3.8 Other Medical Disciplines

The medical disciplines examined above are not exhaustive of the branches of medicine that have relevance to SLT. The RCSLT guidelines for pre-registration SLT courses in the UK state that SLT students must have knowledge of **oncology** and **palliative care**, **gerontology**, **paediatrics**, **orthodontics** and **maxillofacial surgery**. To this list could be added infectious diseases, gastroenterology and endocrinology. In this final section, just three of these disciplines will be examined: gerontology and geriatrics; gastroenterology; and endocrinology. Their selection does not diminish the significance of the other disciplines but is merely an indication of limitations of space. Readers can obtain information on these other medical disciplines in the suggestions for further reading at the end of the chapter.

Gerontology is the study of ageing and older adults. It is a multidisciplinary area that incorporates biology, psychology and sociology. A related discipline, geriatrics, is the study of the medical conditions and diseases associated with old age. Both gerontology and geriatrics are relevant to SLT. It is important for SLTs to understand how typical ageing impacts on communication skills. This is often overlooked in research and clinical practice where the emphasis has traditionally been on the study of how communication is disrupted in clients with conditions such as dementia. However, there is now clear evidence of significant communication impairment and communication-related reduction in quality of life in the normal elderly population. Golub et al. (2006) reported the prevalence of dysphonia in a geriatric population to be 20%. Moreover, more than 50% of elderly individuals with voice problems incurred significant quality-of-life impairment as a result of their dysphonia. A range of cognitive skills that are important for communication are also in decline in normally ageing individuals. In a study of 106 adults aged 50–90 years, Charlton et al. (2009) reported that **theory of mind** (ToM) ability declined with increasing age. SLTs must understand the language and cognitive changes that are part of the normal ageing process if they are to adapt their methods of working with older people in mind. Also, end-of-life care raises important communication issues for older people, particularly in relation to the older person's perceived competence to communicate decisions and wishes. SLTs have an important role to play as advocates for older clients at the end of their lives.

Gastroenterology is the medical discipline concerned with disorders and conditions of the gastrointestinal (or digestive) tract. This includes the oesophagus, stomach, small and large intestines (colon), pancreas and liver. At first sight, it might appear that gastroenterology has limited relevance to SLT. However, as the role of SLT has expanded into dysphagia management and knowledge of the aetiology of voice disorders has developed, SLTs are increasingly working alongside gastroenterologists in the assessment and treatment of clients. Oesophageal dysphagia may be caused by a range of organic conditions including **achalasia** (the lower oesophageal muscle does not relax sufficiently to let food enter the stomach), oesophageal stricture (a narrowed oesophagus traps large pieces of food) and tumours. When oesophageal tumours arise in advanced malignancies related to **laryngeal cancers** and oral cancers, an oesophagectomy may be performed alongside a laryngectomy and a glossectomy. Individually, these surgical procedures can have a significant impact on swallowing anatomy and physiology. When combined, the implications for swallowing are particularly critical. SLTs must have a sound understanding of the structure and function of the upper digestive tract in order to understand these implications. Regardless of the cause of oesophageal dysphagia, SLTs must work in close collaboration with gastroenterologists in order to ensure safe and effective oral and **non-oral feeding** for clients.

SLTs must also work closely with gastroenterologists in the management of clients with dysphonia. There is increasing recognition of the role of gastroesophageal reflux disease (GERD) in the development of dysphonias. Martins et al. (2016) reported gastroesophageal symptoms in 535 (26.5%) of 2,019 patients with dysphonia. In adults aged 19–60 years, **acid laryngitis** (12.5%) was the second largest aetiology of dysphonia behind functional dysphonia (20.5%). GERD is also implicated in the aetiology of laryngeal carcinomas, although tobacco is still the principal aetiological factor (Gale et al., 2016). Proton pump inhibitors, which suppress gastric acid secretion, are the most potent drugs available for the management of GERD. SLTs must understand how the medical treatment of GERD by gastroenterologists contributes to the overall management of clients with dysphonia. A combined intervention based on SLT and proton pump inhibitors can result in good voice outcomes for clients. Beech et al. (2013) reported improvements in subjective voice measurements in a study of 74 patients who received twice daily proton pump inhibitors and speech therapy. SLTs should be aware of the role of GERD in the **pathogenesis** of voice disorders and undertake referral to gastroenterology whenever GERD is suspected.

CASE STUDY: Medical and Scientific Disciplines in Action

This case study is designed to make you think about some of the medical and scientific disciplines that are part of the knowledge base of SLTs. Read the case study carefully. Then, individually or in a group, answer the questions that follow it.

> An SLT works in a voice clinic of a large, regional hospital. She receives a referral from an otolaryngologist in the clinic. The client is a 55-year-old woman with dysphonia. The woman describes to the SLT the long-running nature of her vocal problems. She reported making multiple visits to her general practitioner before a referral to otolaryngology was made. Her vocal complaints include a chronic cough, a sore throat and throat clearing, hoarseness and a sensation of a lump in the throat (globus). A laryngological examination revealed inflammation of the laryngeal mucosa but no lesions. The vibratory pattern of the vocal folds was disrupted. There was abrupt adduction of the folds during the abductory phase of the cycle. The client reported reduced self-esteem and anxiety as a result of her voice disorder. These difficulties had adversely affected her occupational performance and had caused social withdrawal.
>
> After examining the client, the SLT and otolaryngologist agree that the vocal picture is a complex one that involves possibly two vocal pathologies. One is dysphonia related to the presence of acid reflux disease. For further investigation of gastroesophageal reflux disease (GERD), the client is referred to gastroenterology. The other vocal pathology that is consistent with the observed abnormalities of vocal fold adduction and abduction is spasmodic dysphonia. The SLT is also concerned about the psychosocial impact of the client's voice disorder and the extent to which psychiatric factors may be perpetuating the client's voice disorder. She recommends a psychiatric evaluation of the client. The SLT also suspects that the client's chronic cough and throat clearing are contributing to her voice disorder. She institutes vocal hygiene and education as a means of raising awareness of the damaging effects of these behaviours.

Questions

(1) The SLT must have knowledge of at least four medical disciplines in order to engage fully with the client's overall management. Name these four disciplines.
(2) The client is a 55-year-old woman. Which scientific study tells us that this client fits the age and gender profile of the adult with dysphonia?
(3) The otolaryngologist in this case is attempting to establish the causes of the client's dysphonia and diagnoses GERD-related dysphonia and spasmodic dysphonia subject to further evaluation. What scientific discipline studies the causes or origins of medical conditions?
(4) The client is referred to gastroenterology for further evaluation. Which laryngological finding might be explained by a diagnosis of GERD by a gastroenterologist?
(5) Which two of the four disciplines identified in response to (1) play a role in the management of clients with vocal fold paralysis?

Endocrinology is the medical discipline that studies the endocrine system and its various disorders. SLTs must understand the effects of hormones and hormonal imbalances on vocal fold function and vocal quality. These effects include lowered speaking fundamental frequency in the menopause (D'haeseleer et al., 2013) and increased **jitter** in women with premenstrual syndrome (Chae et al., 2001). The oral contraceptive pill also has implications for vocal quality. Although, historically, contraception has been believed to affect the voice negatively, a review of more recent studies using low-dose oral contraceptive pills showed that they stabilize the voice (Rodney and Sataloff, 2016). An understanding of hormonal influences on the voice is also important for the SLT management of transgender clients. Long-term androgen therapy can result in an acceptable male voice in female-to-male transsexual persons. However, pitch-lowering difficulties can occur in approximately 10% of cases and is related in part to diminished androgen sensitivity (Cosyns et al., 2014). A wide range of oestrogens can be used to induce feminization in male-to-female transsexuals. However, their effect on the voice is not as significant as that experienced by female-to-male transsexuals who receive androgen therapy. As these various cases illustrate, endocrinology has considerable links to the work of SLT. Accordingly, SLT students must be introduced to endocrinology as part of their clinical education.

KEY POINTS: Other Medical Disciplines

- Several other medical disciplines are relevant to SLT. These include oncology and palliative care, paediatrics, geriatrics, orthodontics and maxillofacial surgery.
- SLTs must be aware of communication and cognitive changes that occur as part of normal ageing. These changes are one aspect of the study of ageing

- and older adults in gerontology. Geriatrics is the study of medical conditions associated with old age (e.g. dementia). It is also relevant to SLT.
- SLTs must have a sound working knowledge of the anatomy and physiology of the upper digestive tract, and gastroenterology in general, in order to assess and treat clients with dysphagia and dysphonia. Gastroesophageal reflux disease (GERD) is implicated in the aetiology of voice disorders and laryngeal carcinomas.
- The study of the endocrine system and its disorders in endocrinology is a further important medical discipline for SLTs. Therapists must understand hormonal influences on vocal function and vocal quality during the menopause and in women who take the oral contraceptive pill and who experience premenstrual syndrome. Also, the effect of androgen and oestrogen therapies on the voice in transsexual clients is a vital part of the SLT's medical knowledge.

WEBSITE: Medical and Scientific Disciplines

After reading the chapter, visit the website and test your knowledge of medical and scientific disciplines by answering the short-answer questions for this topic.

Suggestions for Further Reading

Seikel, J. A., Drumright, D. G. and King, D. W. 2016. *Anatomy & physiology for speech, language and hearing*, 5th edn, Clifton Park, NY: Cengage Learning.

This accessible, well-illustrated textbook examines the anatomy and physiology of respiration, phonation, articulation, resonation and hearing. It also addresses neuroanatomy and neurophysiology as well as mastication and deglutition. There is also a detailed glossary of terms.

Welling, D. R. and Ukstins, C. A. 2015. *Fundamentals of audiology for the speech-language pathologist*, Burlington, MA: Jones & Bartlett Learning.

This is a complete treatment of all aspects of audiology for speech-language pathologists. There are accessible chapters on sound and hearing; audiometric equipment; pure tone audiometry and masking; speech audiometry; otoscopy and the middle ear test battery; interpretation of audiometric results; hearing aids and hearing assistance technology for children and adults; understanding auditory development and the child with hearing loss; hearing issues in the early intervention years; audiology services in the school system; aural (re)habilitation; and diagnosis and treatment of (central) auditory processing disorders.

Golper, L. A. C. 2010. *Medical speech-language pathology: a desk reference*, 3rd edn, Clifton Park, NY: Delmar Cengage Learning.

This volume is written for speech-language pathologists who work in medically allied settings. As such, it addresses a range of medical disciplines including medical genetics, oncology, infectious diseases and geriatrics.

QUESTIONS: Medical and Scientific Disciplines

(1) For each statement in Part A, indicate if it relates to the *prevalence* or the *incidence* of a communication disorder. For each statement in Part B, indicate if the aetiology of the communication disorder is *infectious*, *neurological* or *genetic* in nature.

Part A:
(a) It is estimated that there are more than 350,000 people in the UK who have aphasia.
(b) It is estimated that approximately 480,000 people aged 65 or older will develop Alzheimer's disease in the USA in 2017.
(c) Eadie et al. (2015) reported that 3.4% of an Australian cohort of 4-year-old children exhibit speech disorder.
(d) Taylor et al. (2013) reported that 1.2/1000 boys and 0.2/1000 girls were newly diagnosed with autism each year between 2004 and 2010.
(e) It is estimated that approximately 1% of the population has developmental stuttering.

Part B:
(a) Children with congenital cytomegalovirus infection exhibit language disorder.
(b) Children with fragile X syndrome exhibit language disorder.
(c) Adults who sustain a cerebrovascular accident may develop aphasia.
(d) Adults with Williams syndrome exhibit language problems.
(e) Children with cleft palate have conductive hearing loss related to otitis media.

(2) Each of the following statements describes an aspect of impaired anatomy or physiology that is of relevance to SLTs. For each statement, indicate if the impairment relates to the anatomy or physiology of the structures described.
(a) A child with a repaired palatal cleft develops hypernasal speech related to the presence of a large fistula.
(b) An adult with motor neurone disease exhibits speech production problems related to poor respiratory function.
(c) An adult with total glossectomy can articulate bilabial plosives but not alveolar and velar plosives.
(d) An elderly woman develops hypernasal speech related to stroke-induced velopharyngeal incompetence.
(e) A professional voice user presents with hoarseness related to the presence of vocal nodules.
(f) An adult with a large nasal polyp exhibits hyponasal speech.
(g) A child has conductive hearing loss that is related to complete atresia of the ear canal.

(h) A child with hypernasal speech exhibits normal palatal excursion during velopharyngeal closure and an excessively capacious pharynx.
(i) An adult with dysphonia displays frequent, abrupt abduction of the vocal folds during phonation.
(j) An adult with Parkinson's disease displays reduced vocal loudness related to an inability to generate subglottal pressure for speech production.

(3) The following statements describe communication and swallowing disorders in children and adults with a range of neurological impairments. For each statement, indicate if the neurological impairment is *developmental* or *acquired* in nature. Also, indicate if the child or adult has a *progressive* or *non-progressive* neurological impairment.
  (a) Molly is 8 years old. She was born with spastic quadriplegia cerebral palsy. She has severe dysarthria and language disorder.
  (b) Bill is 55 years old and has multiple sclerosis. He has ataxic-spastic dysarthria and dysphagia.
  (c) John is 30 years old. He has a speech disorder following TBI caused by a motorbike accident.
  (d) Sally is 5 years old and was born with cerebellar agenesis. She is attending SLT because of a speech disorder.
  (e) Anne is 60 years old. She has aphasia and dysarthria following a left-hemisphere cerebrovascular accident.
  (f) Jack is 4 years old and has Möbius syndrome. An SLT diagnoses dysarthria related to impairment of a number of cranial nerves.
  (g) Michael is 40 years old. He developed meningitis as a young adult which caused sensorineural hearing loss.
  (h) Tom is 65 years old and is in recovery from laryngeal cancer. He has iatrogenic dysarthria related to nerve damage that occurred during laryngectomy.
  (i) Mike is 25 years old. He sustained a penetrating head injury in a violent assault. He has mildly dysarthric speech.
  (j) Sam is 15 years old and has Duchenne muscular dystrophy. He is receiving SLT for the treatment of unintelligible speech and swallowing problems.

(4) The following statements relate to aspects of otolaryngology that have relevance to SLTs. For each statement, indicate if it is *true* or *false*:
  (a) Children who exhibit hyperfunction of the larynx are at risk of vocal nodules.
  (b) Expiratory stridor is a feature of laryngomalacia.
  (c) Unilateral vocal fold paralysis necessitates a tracheotomy.
  (d) Hearing loss in cholesteatoma is unilateral and progressive.
  (e) Malformation of the ossicles can occur alongside atresia.
  (f) Stereocilia of cochlear hair cells are damaged in noise-induced hearing loss.
  (g) There is no development of the cochlea in cochlear hypoplasia.
  (h) Trauma to the laryngeal framework is most often caused by surgery.
  (i) The superior laryngeal nerve may be damaged during thyroidectomy.
  (j) A client with advanced oral cancer may require a mandibulectomy as well as a glossectomy.

(5) Part A: Each of the following statements describes a pattern on an audiogram. Relate each of these descriptions to a particular hearing disorder.
  (a) a sloping curve from right to left on an audiogram
  (b) a notch at 4 kHz with better hearing at higher and lower frequencies
  (c) a sharp drop beginning at 1000 Hz and continuing into the higher frequencies
  (d) normal bone conduction responses with air conduction responses at least 10 dB lower

  Part B: Which type of audiometry would an audiologist use to assess each of the following?
  (a) middle ear pressure
  (b) bone conduction hearing
  (c) contraction of stapedius muscle
  (d) speech understanding

(6) SLTs and psychiatrists are jointly involved in the management of a range of clients. Among the clients listed below, identify those where a close working relationship between SLT and psychiatry may be expected to occur:
  (a) children with specific language impairment
  (b) adults with fluent aphasia
  (c) adolescents and adults with gender dysphoria
  (d) children with developmental apraxia of speech
  (e) adults with developmental stuttering
  (f) adults with conversion aphonia
  (g) children with developmental dysarthria
  (h) children with conductive hearing loss
  (i) adults with Huntington's disease
  (j) children with vocal nodules

(7) SLTs must have knowledge of medical disciplines such an endocrinology, oncology and paediatrics in order to assess and treat clients with communication and swallowing disorders. Match each of the disciplines listed below to one of the statements in (a) to (j):

  oncology – palliative care – geronotology – paediatrics – orthodontics – maxillofacial surgery – infectious diseases – geriatrics – gastroenterology – endocrinology

  (a) A man with herpes simplex encephalitis presents with semantic impairments.
  (b) An SLT discusses options for alternative communication with a man with motor neurone disease as part of his end-of-life care.
  (c) An SLT is asked to write a report on a child's communication development as part of a wider assessment of developmental progress to date.
  (d) A professional singer reports to an SLT that her vocal quality fluctuates according to her menstrual cycle.
  (e) A man with dysphonia complains of heartburn and other gastroesophageal symptoms during an assessment by a voice therapist.
  (f) An SLT receives a referral from an otolaryngologist about a 60-year-old man with an advanced squamous cell carcinoma of the larynx.

(g) An SLT is asked by the manager of a local residential home to devise a communication stimulation programme for its healthy elderly residents.
(h) An SLT delivers a lecture to nurses and doctors on the linguistic and communication features of a range of dementias.
(i) An SLT is asked to assess the speech of a child with Pierre Robin syndrome who has received surgery for correction of micrognathia.
(j) An SLT is asked to assess the speech of a child with cleft palate who has received treatment for the eruption of teeth in the middle of the palate.

4 Psychological Disciplines

4.1 SLT and Psychology

A wide range of psychological disciplines informs the work of speech and language therapists. The psychological knowledge base of SLTs includes aspects of the following disciplines: developmental psychology; educational psychology; cognitive psychology; neuropsychology; and clinical psychology. The broad relevance of psychology to SLT is recognized by the bodies that oversee the clinical education of SLT students in the UK. In its standards of proficiency for speech and language therapists, the Health & Care Professions Council (2013) states that therapists must 'understand psychology as relevant to lifespan development and change, normal and impaired communication, and psychological and social wellbeing' (12). In its benchmark statement for speech and language therapy, the Quality Assurance Agency for Higher Education (2001: 10) requires therapists to have knowledge of the following aspects of psychology:

- The impact of communicative need on the psychological and social well-being of the person and his/her relationships.
- The relevant aspects of psychology (cognitive, neuropsychology, social, health, developmental, clinical, learning theory) and the application of such knowledge to normal and impaired communication.

The psychological content of the SLT curriculum is most explicitly articulated by the Royal College of Speech and Language Therapists (2010) in its guidelines for pre-registration SLT courses in the UK. The guidelines require SLT students to have an appreciation of theoretical frameworks in psychology, psychological development and change, neuropsychology, and applications of psychology. Some consideration of the guidelines for each of these areas provides a useful orientation to the following discussion. To this end, they are listed in full below. SLT students are expected to have an understanding of:

Theoretical frameworks in psychology

- Models of psychological development across the lifespan: social, cognitive
- Theoretical models of cognition and neuropsychology
- Psychological processes: motivation, perception, attention, memory

- Learning theories
- Human information processing

Psychological development and change

- Biological and socio-cultural influences on psychological development
- Social and individual psychology
- Individual differences: intelligence, personality and temperament
- Development and change in non-verbal communication across the lifespan
- Play
- Psychological issues in key life transitions: adolescence, parenting, mid-life challenges and retirement

Neuropsychology

- Cognitive neuropsychology
- Atypical psychological processing

Applications of psychology

- Current psychological approaches to assessment and intervention (educational, clinical, health)
- Counselling
- Health psychology
- Forensic psychology

(RCSLT, 2010: 32–3)

Clearly, psychology has relevance to SLT across a number of areas. It is not possible to address all these areas in a single chapter. But it is possible to distil key themes and disciplines from the above guidelines. One such theme is developmental aspects of psychology. **Developmental psychology** is a core element of the SLT curriculum. Among the issues addressed in developmental psychology, students are introduced to Jean Piaget's theory of cognitive development in infants and children. According to **Piaget**, children's intellectual development proceeds through a series of stages. The first of these stages, which occurs between birth and 2 years, is the sensorimotor period. During this stage, infants learn through sensory and motor interactions with their physical environment. The final stage is the formal operational stage. This stage begins around 12 years of age and is when hypothetical-deductive thinking is established for the first time. Piaget's work is included as standard in developmental psychology courses for SLT students. However, there are many other aspects of psychological development across the lifespan that are equally relevant but less often addressed in these courses. One such aspect is the maturation and deterioration of theory of mind (ToM) skills across the lifespan. ToM is the ability to attribute mental states such as beliefs, knowledge and intentions to one's own mind and to the minds of others. The attribution of mental states to others allows us to predict their behaviour and is a key cognitive skill for language and communication. When ToM is impaired, as is the case in a range of clinical populations including autism spectrum disorder, the use and understanding of language are disrupted (Cummings, 2013, 2014b). ToM will be examined in section 4.2 along with other aspects of developmental psychology that are of relevance to SLT.

Related to developmental psychology and also contained in the RCSLT guidelines is educational psychology. Educational psychology is the application of knowledge about learning and motivation, development, and measurement and statistics to both school- and community-based educational settings. Many children who are assessed and treated by SLTs have statements of special educational needs (SEN). These statements provide a wide-ranging assessment of a child's abilities and needs and include recommendations about the additional support services that a child should receive. (There is similar provision for children in the USA under the Individuals with Disabilities Education Act (IDEA) which was signed into law in 2004.) In developing SEN statements, local education authorities receive reports from a range of medical, health and educational professionals. An educational psychologist is one of these professionals. Using their knowledge of child development, play, learning and behaviour, educational psychologists are uniquely placed to assess a child's intellectual functioning and potential for learning as part of the 'statementing' process. A range of psychometric tests such as the *Wechsler Intelligence Scale for Children – Fifth Edition* (WISC-V; Wechsler, 2014) are used for this purpose. Educational psychologists are also trained to assess children who have suspected dyslexia, **dyscalculia** and **dyspraxia** either in isolation or alongside general learning difficulties. SLTs must have an understanding of these different dimensions of the work of educational psychologists. For this reason, educational psychology will be examined further in section 4.3.

Cognitive aspects of psychology are also extensively acknowledged in the RCSLT guidelines. **Cognitive psychology** is the study of human cognition and in particular mental functions such as **attention**, **perception**, memory, language, reasoning and learning. These functions are often impaired in children and adults who are assessed and treated by speech and language therapists. For example, attention is compromised in individuals with attention deficit hyperactivity disorder (ADHD), while **episodic memory** is impaired in adults with **Alzheimer's dementia**. Cognitive psychology is not a unitary discipline but subsumes a number of distinct approaches, each of which employs a different methodology to study human cognition. These approaches include experimental cognitive psychology, cognitive neuropsychology, computational cognitive science and cognitive neuroscience. **Cognitive neuropsychology** is the study of patterns of cognitive impairment shown by brain-damaged patients with a view to increasing our understanding of normal human cognition. One of its theoretical principles is **modularity**, the assumption that the cognitive system consists of many, for the most part independent, modules or processors. Each of these modules is specialized for a given type of processing (e.g. processing of linguistic data). Of all the branches of cognitive psychology, cognitive neuropsychology has had the most profound influence on how SLTs assess and treat clients with language disorders. This influence can be seen in the use of cognitive neuropsychological assessments such as the *Pyramids and Palm Trees Test* (Howard and Patterson, 1992) and *Psycholinguistic Assessments of Language Processing in Aphasia* (PALPA; Kay et al., 1992). In section 4.4, these assessments will be discussed further as part of a wider examination of the contribution of cognitive psychology to SLT.

Neuropsychology is the study of brain–behaviour relationships. Neuropsychologists attempt to explain the way in which the activity of the brain is expressed in observable behaviour. This branch of psychology has two main sub-disciplines: clinical neuropsychology and experimental neuropsychology. Where the clinical neuropsychologist undertakes studies on brain-injured subjects, most often with a view to engaging in rehabilitation of these subjects, experimental neuropsychologists conduct experimental studies on normal subjects. As an area of professional practice, **clinical neuropsychology** has considerable relevance to the work of speech and language therapists. This is because many of the same clients who are evaluated by clinical neuropsychologists are also assessed and treated by SLTs. For example, clinical neuropsychologists assess the cognitive strengths and weaknesses of children and adolescents with developmental disorders such as ADHD and ASD. They can monitor progress in regaining cognitive skills in adults who have acquired brain injury following a stroke or a traumatic brain injury (TBI). Clinical neuropsychologists are also able to determine when cognitive changes in older adults exceed normal ageing and are indicative of **mild cognitive impairment** (MCI), or when MCI has progressed to the point where it has become one of the dementia syndromes. A battery of neuropsychological tests is used to assess clients in areas such as **memory**, attention, processing speed, **reasoning**, judgement, problem-solving, and spatial and language functions. SLTs must be aware of widely used neuropsychological tests and understand their findings in order to assess and treat clients appropriately (e.g. use of the Stroop test (Stroop, 1935) to assess **response inhibition**). Neuropsychology will be examined in more detail in section 4.5.

Clinical neuropsychologists are first and foremost clinical psychologists. Clinical psychology integrates the science of psychology with the prevention, assessment, diagnoses and treatment of a wide range of mental, emotional and behavioural disorders. Increasingly, SLTs and clinical psychologists are working alongside each other in the management of clients with communication and swallowing disorders. Frameworks such as cognitive behavioural therapy are employed to good effect by clinical psychologists and SLTs in the treatment of clients who have psychogenic dysphonia. Indeed, the combined expertise of SLT and clinical psychology is now considered to be a model of best practice for the treatment of these clients (Butcher et al., 2007). Aside from combined interventions, SLTs also work alongside clinical psychologists as part of multidisciplinary teams in a range of settings. This includes community-based mental health teams, acute mental health inpatient services, with clients in the criminal justice system (e.g. prisons, young offender institutions) and with clients who are undergoing **gender reassignment**. Other, less well-known contexts in which SLTs and clinical psychologists work collaboratively are the management of clients with **head and neck cancer** and clients with respiratory and swallowing problems. In each of these cases, SLTs must have an understanding of assessment and treatment methods in clinical psychology and of the ways in which clinical psychology can contribute to the management of clients with communication and swallowing disorders. Clinical psychology will be examined further in section 4.6.

KEY POINTS: SLT and Psychology

- Psychology is a central component of the SLT curriculum. Several branches of psychology are relevant to the work of SLTs and must be part of the clinical education of SLT students for this reason. These branches include developmental psychology, educational psychology, cognitive psychology, neuropsychology and clinical psychology.
- SLT students must have a detailed understanding of normal child development across cognitive, social, motor and linguistic domains in order to assess and treat children with developmental disorders. Early in the SLT curriculum, students are introduced to developmental psychology.
- Educational psychologists assess many of the same children who attend speech and language therapy. SLT students must understand the role of educational psychologists in the assessment of children with special educational needs (SEN). These psychologists assess general intellectual functioning and make diagnoses of conditions such as dyslexia and dyscalculia.
- Cognitive psychology contributes theoretical models of mental functions such as language, attention and memory to SLT. These models have been used to inform SLT assessments of clients with aphasia and other acquired neurological disorders.
- Neuropsychology is the study of brain–behaviour relationships in both brain-injured subjects and subjects with no neurological injury. The sub-discipline of clinical neuropsychology has particular relevance to SLT as it is concerned with the rehabilitation of clients with traumatic and other brain injuries.
- Clinical psychology has many applications to SLT. SLTs and clinical psychologists work together in the treatment of clients with psychogenic voice disorders. SLTs and clinical psychologists are also part of multidisciplinary teams that assess and treat clients who are seeking gender reassignment, or who have mental health conditions, head and neck cancer and swallowing disorders.

4.2 Developmental Psychology

During the human lifespan a range of cognitive, social, motor and emotional abilities emerge, undergo maturation and then deteriorate. The processes by means of which this occurs are of interest to developmental psychologists. They include the attainment of motor milestones during infancy and early childhood, cognitive maturation in children and cognitive deterioration in older adults, and the emergence and development of a range of social skills. Motor milestones are an aspect of child development that has considerable relevance to SLTs. This is because speech production is first and foremost a motor activity. Children who exhibit delays in gross motor milestones such as crawling, sitting without support, and walking unaided often also experience delayed attainment of speech production milestones (see Cobo-Lewis et al., 1996, for an association between delayed hand-banging and canonical babbling in children with Down syndrome). Motor development is also associated with language development (see Iverson, 2010, for a review). For these reasons, SLTs must have a sound understanding of the stages in motor development followed by normally developing children.

Normative values for motor development in children have been investigated in a number of large-scale studies. In a longitudinal study of 816 children aged 4 to 24 months in Ghana, India, Norway, Oman and the USA, the WHO Multicentre Growth Reference Study Group (2006) calculated windows of achievement for six gross motor development milestones. Estimated 1st and 99th percentiles in months for each of these milestones are shown below:

Sitting without support: 3.8, 9.2 months
Standing with assistance: 4.8, 11.4 months
Hands-and-knees crawling: 5.2, 13.5 months
Walking with assistance: 5.9, 13.7 months
Standing alone: 6.9, 16.9 months
Walking alone: 8.2, 17.6 months

These figures show that only 1% of this group of children could sit without support by 3.8 months of age, while 99% of the group could sit without support by 9.2 months of age. During the taking of a case history, SLTs routinely ask parents about the age that their child attained each of these milestones. This is because many children who are referred to speech and language therapy exhibit significant delays in these milestones. Motor milestones are delayed in children with genetic syndromes, cerebral palsy and dyspraxia, and neurodevelopmental disorders. Sharland et al. (1992) reported motor milestone delay in 151 individuals with Noonan syndrome. This cohort of children had a mean age of sitting unsupported of 10 months and walking of 21 months. Hinton et al. (2013) examined 35 males with fragile X syndrome (FXS) and reported that the mean age at which these children first walked was 17.8 months. Several of these children had autism alongside FXS. Motor milestones are also known to be delayed in children with ASD. Liu (2012) examined 26 motor milestones in 44 children with ASDs aged 82–90 months. These children were delayed on all 26 milestones, which included sitting alone, standing with help, crawling, walking with help, standing alone and walking alone.

Delayed motor development may be a child's only developmental difficulty. Often, however, delays in motor development occur alongside delays in cognitive development. To understand delayed cognitive development, SLT students must appreciate the stages that normally developing children pass through on their way to acquiring increasingly sophisticated forms of thinking. In his theory of cognitive development, the Swiss psychologist Jean Piaget attempted to characterize those stages. The concept of equilibration is central to Piaget's theory. Piaget argued that children's cognitive development proceeds by means of adaptation and equilibration. In essence, when children encounter new experiences, they attempt to assimilate them into cognitive structures ('schemes') that they already possess. If assimilation cannot be achieved – a new experience does not accord with existing schemes – a state of cognitive disequilibrium occurs. The only way to resolve this disequilibrium is for the child's cognitive structures to accommodate or adjust and, in so doing, provide a better fit for the new experience. For accommodation to occur, the child must first notice a feature in the environment and then reflect on its significance ('reflective abstraction'). If accommodation is successfully achieved, the child is returned to a state of cognitive equilibrium. 'Equilibration ... is the dynamic process of moving between states of cognitive disequilibrium and equilibrium as we assimilate new experiences and accommodate schemes' (Littlefield Cook and Cook, 2005: 5–8). To the extent that humans continually aim for increasing organization of their psychological structures – another of Piaget's claims – the process of equilibration can continue indefinitely.

At the level of changes to individual schemes just described, equilibration may be thought of as micro-equilibration. However, when larger cognitive structures undergo equilibration ('macro-equilibration'), children begin to exhibit new and more sophisticated ways of thinking. A detailed discussion of the stages through which this is achieved is beyond the scope of this chapter. What follows is a brief overview of these stages. (The interested reader is referred to Littlefield Cook and Cook, 2005, for further discussion.) According to Piaget, infants between birth and 2 years of age can engage only in sensorimotor thought. What infants *know* about the world is entirely mediated by their sensory and motor interactions with it. A child with a toy in his/her hand can derive a range of sensory stimuli from it and can use the toy to undertake actions (e.g. throw it onto the ground). However, because the child at this stage has no representational, symbolic thought and lacks a concept of object permanence, Piaget claims that the child cannot have thoughts about the toy or even know that it exists when it is no longer within his/her grasp. By the end of the sensorimotor stage, young children are less rooted in the sensory and motor interactions that framed their understanding of the world in the early months of life, and are beginning to have thoughts about objects and events without the need for these sensory and motor experiences.

Piaget characterized children's cognitive development between 2 and 7 years of age as preoperational thought. Mental representations develop further during this stage, as is evidenced by children's increasing use of symbols in language, artwork and play. The rapid increase of vocabulary and other language skills that takes place early in this stage is explicable, according to Piaget, only by the development that is occurring in young children's mental representational ability. Also during the preoperational stage, there is emergence of logic based on personal experience (so-called intuitive thought or logic). Intuitive thought is evident in several aspects of preoperational thinking. This includes egocentrism (an inability to take another person's perspective), animism (the idea that inanimate objects have conscious life and feelings) and artificialism (the notion that natural events and objects, such as weather events, are under the control of people or superhuman agents). As children begin to realize that animism and artificialism do not provide satisfactory explanations of events, they start to use a more objective logic. The preoperational tendency for intuitive thought also explains why children fail conservation tasks at this stage. In these tasks the child is first shown two identical containers holding the same amount of liquid. The child acknowledges that the containers hold the same amount. With the child watching, liquid from one of the containers is then poured into a taller, narrower container. When asked again if the containers hold the same amount of liquid, the child responds this time that the taller container holds more liquid. One of the reasons children fail conservation tasks is that they lack an understanding of reversibility – that if the liquid were poured back into its original container, it would be evident that the amount of liquid had not changed. For Piaget, reversibility is a hallmark of cognitive structures that are fully logical. The absence of these structures (Piaget called them 'operations') is why this stage is known as *pre*operational thought.

Between 7 and 11 years, children are in a stage of cognitive development that Piaget called concrete operational thought. Conservation tasks, which are problematic for younger children, are easily understood by children with concrete operational thinking. This is because they exhibit decentred thinking, in which they are able to consider multiple aspects of a problem (that the width as well as the height of the container needs to be considered in conservation tasks). Children's thinking also exhibits reversibility, and they are able to focus on the transformation that occurs in conservation tasks – that simply pouring liquid from one container to another container does not alter its amount. Thinking at this stage is not rooted in intuitive thought but observes objective rules of logic, and a child's cognitive structures are truly operational. Children in the concrete operational stage also understand class inclusion for the first time, e.g. that poodles and dalmations are both types of dog. So, if shown a picture of three poodles and five dalmations and asked 'Are there more poodles or more dogs?', children are able to respond 'Dogs'. Children are also able to draw transitive inferences. For example, if told that Sam is older than Frank, and Frank is older than Bill, and then asked 'Who is the oldest, Sam or Bill?', children are able to respond 'Sam' because of their understanding of the transitive relationships between Sam, Frank and Bill. Notwithstanding these cognitive achievements, thinking at this stage is limited to concrete objects and situations. Mental operations are still concrete in nature, as the name of this stage indicates.

Piaget's final stage of cognitive development – formal operational thought – begins around 12 years of age and extends into adolescence. A capacity for hypothetico-deductive reasoning develops during this time. Also, thinking is no longer limited to concrete objects and situations but involves abstract concepts. Hypothetico-deductive reasoning finds children able for the first time to pose hypotheses about problems and set about systematic testing of those hypotheses. As hypothesis generation and testing suggest, hypothetico-deductive reasoning is a type of formal scientific reasoning. With the development of abstract thinking, adolescents are able to engage in reasoning about concepts such as justice, truth and morality. They are able to participate in complex moral, ethical and social deliberations that involve these concepts. However, adolescents in the formal operational stage still exhibit certain cognitive immaturities, according to Piaget. One such immaturity is adolescent egocentrism, an inability to distinguish between one's own abstract thought and the thinking of others. With further development of hypothetico-deductive reasoning and abstract thinking, and the decline of adolescent egocentrism, mature cognition is finally achieved in young adulthood. Although Piaget believed that further reorganization of cognitive structures continues throughout adulthood, this reorganization does not involve qualitatively different forms of thought.

Piaget's theory of cognitive development is still enormously influential today and is routinely taught to SLT students as part of their introduction to developmental psychology. However, it is not the only approach to children's cognitive development that is relevant to SLT students. In recent years, the role of theory of mind (ToM) in all aspects of language and communication has become increasingly apparent to clinicians and researchers. Although Piaget's studies on perspective taking and egocentrism in children preceded the advent of theory of mind, similarities between ToM and Piaget's earlier work will not escape the reader. ToM is the ability to attribute mental states to one's own mind and to the minds of others with a view to predicting and explaining human behaviour. Mental states include *cognitive* states such as knowledge, belief and desire, and *affective* states such as happiness, fear and disgust. We use ToM to understand how someone is feeling, to establish why an individual acted in a certain way and to imagine how someone will respond to a particular event or set of circumstances. Most importantly, we also use ToM to interpret the utterances of others. When Jack declares *What a delightful child!* in the presence of a disruptive 5-year-old, Mary has little difficulty in establishing the sarcasm of his utterance. This is because Mary has attributed a particular communicative intention to Jack, namely, the intention to be sarcastic. Jack's belief in this case is that the child in question is anything but delightful. Communicative intentions are mental states just like knowledge and beliefs, and their recovery by means of ToM is the basis of all communication. Given the centrality of ToM to communication, some comments are in order about the development of ToM in children and its deterioration in older adults.

The standard test of ToM performed by psychologists is the false belief test (also known as Sally-Anne experiments on account of the names of the two dolls first used in these tests). In a standard false belief test, a story involving two dolls is played out by the tester in front of a child. In one version of the story, Mum enters a room with two bags, each containing balls of wool. She puts one bag in the cupboard and the other bag in the drawer. She then leaves the room. After her departure, John enters the room and proceeds to play with the bags of wool. Before leaving the room, he puts the bags away but, in doing so, mixes them up – the bag that was previously in the cupboard is now in the drawer and the bag that was previously in the drawer is now in the cupboard. Later, Mum is knitting in an adjacent room and needs one of the bags of wool in order to finish the jumper. She calls out to John 'I need one of the bags of wool. It's the bag in the drawer' (Cummings, 2005: 273). It is the child who knows that John will go to the new location of the bag of wool (namely, the cupboard) that can be said to understand that Mum has a false belief about the location of the bag. Such a child passes a test of false belief. He/she is aware that an actor (in this case Mum) can entertain a belief about the location of the bag of wool which is different from his/her own belief.

Normally developing children begin to pass false belief tests at around 4 years of age. However, under certain modifications of these tests, younger children can also pass them. Some of the conditions under which 3-year-olds can pass false belief tests include downplaying the salience of the real state of affairs or making salient the prior mental state of the actor in the scenario (both of which encourage the child to identify the actor's false belief), the child being actively engaged in deceiving the target person, overlearning the key features of the false belief narrative or phrasing the false belief question in certain ways (Wellman and Lagattuta, 2000: 25). Also, the false belief scenario described above is a test of first-order ToM reasoning. First-order ToM is the ability to attribute mental states *about the world* to the mind of another person. When normally developing children are able to establish that Mum in the above scenario has a false belief about the location of the bag of wool, they are attributing to Mum a false belief about the world. However, we also routinely attribute to others mental states *about the thoughts and beliefs of other people*. In order for Mary to establish that Jack is being sarcastic when he utters *What a delightful child!*, Mary must attribute to Jack the belief that the child before them is quite unpleasant (first-order ToM). But she must additionally attribute to Jack the belief that she, Mary, also thinks that the child is quite unpleasant (second-order ToM). Second-order ToM reasoning begins to develop between 6 and 9 years of age. As this example illustrates, it is integral to understanding pragmatic aspects of language such as sarcasm (see Cummings 2013, 2014b, for further discussion).

Psychologists have compared the ToM performance of normally developing children with the ToM performance of children with ASD and children with intellectual disability. In an early study, Baron-Cohen et al. (1985) presented a false belief scenario to three groups of children: 27 normally developing children (mean chronological age 4;5 years), 20 children with autism (mean chronological age 11;11 years) and 14 children with Down syndrome (mean chronological age 10;11 years). Naming, reality and memory questions in the test were passed by all three groups of children. However, while 85% of normally developing children and 86% of children with Down syndrome passed the false belief question, 80% of the children with autism failed this question, a finding that was highly significant. The four children with autism who passed the false belief question had chronological ages from 10;11 to 15;10 years. Clearly, the children with autism had a severe ToM deficit which could not be accounted for by reduced verbal and non-verbal mental ages (the verbal and non-verbal mental ages of the subjects with autism were higher than those of the subjects with Down syndrome in the study). The findings of this study indicate that ToM has a much longer developmental trajectory in children with ASD than in either normally developing children or children with intellectual disability. On average, children with ASD are 10 years of age before they first pass false belief tests.

Like other aspects of cognitive development, ToM development extends into adolescence and adulthood. Dumontheil et al. (2010) examined the development of ToM into adulthood by administering a computerized task to 177 female subjects in each of five age groups: Child I (7.3–9.7 years), Child II (9.8–11.4 years), Adolescent I (11.5–13.9 years), Adolescent II (14.0–17.7 years) and Adults (19.1–27.5 years). The task required participants to use the perspective of a 'director' and move only those objects that the director could see. There was an improvement in the performance of this task between the Child I and Adolescent II age groups. Also, the Adolescent II group made more errors than the Adult group, suggesting that ToM use improves between late adolescence and adulthood. Even in adulthood, ToM skills do not remain static. There is now growing evidence that ToM skills undergo decline with increasing age (Sullivan and Ruffman, 2004; Pardini and Nichelli, 2009). Maylor et al. (2002) examined understanding of ToM stories in young, young-old and old-old age groups (mean ages 19, 67 and 81 years, respectively). The performance of the old-old age group on these stories was significantly worse than the other age groups across all conditions in the study (e.g. memory load present/absent). This age deficit remained significant even after measures of vocabulary, executive functioning and processing speed were taken into account. As with other aspects of cognitive development, ToM development across the lifespan is an area of developmental psychology that has considerable relevance to SLT.

KEY POINTS: Developmental Psychology

- Motor, cognitive, emotional, social and perceptual abilities change across the human lifespan. The processes by means of which these abilities first emerge in infancy, develop during childhood, adolescence and young adulthood and then deteriorate in later life are of interest to developmental psychologists.
- Development of gross motor skills (e.g. walking) and fine motor skills (e.g. writing) in children has considerable relevance to SLT. This is because speech production is also a motor activity. There is evidence of a relationship between delayed motor milestones and delayed speech and language development in children.
- Cognitive development is an essential component of developmental psychology for SLT students. Piaget's theory of cognitive development has widespread currency in SLT curricula. Other aspects of cognitive development such as theory of mind (ToM) are also particularly relevant to SLT students.
- Piaget proposed that children move between states of cognitive disequilibrium and equilibrium in a process known as equilibration. In the transition between these states, children assimilate new experiences into their cognitive structures ('schemes'). When these experiences fail to assimilate, some accommodation or adjustment of schemes is necessary.
- When equilibration occurs across a large number of schemes, children may be seen to exhibit qualitatively different types of thinking. Piaget characterized these types of thinking according to four stages: sensorimotor thought (birth to 2 years), preoperational thought (2 to 7 years), concrete operational thought (7 to 11 years), and formal operational thought (12 years and upwards).
- ToM development has relevance to SLT students. ToM is the ability to attribute cognitive and affective mental states to one's own mind and to the minds of others. ToM allows us to explain and predict the behaviour of other people.
- The standard test of ToM is a false belief test. Normally developing children pass false belief tests around 4 years of age, while children with ASD do not pass these tests until 10 years of age. ToM development extends into adolescence and adulthood. There is evidence of deterioration of ToM skills in older adults.

4.3 Educational Psychology

Educational psychology is a broad area of professional practice that extends well beyond the learning of children in schools. The breadth of this discipline is conveyed in the following description of educational psychology by the American Psychological Association (2016a):

> Educational psychologists apply theories of human development to understand individual learning styles and inform the instructional process. While interaction with teachers and students in school settings is an important part of their work, it isn't the only facet of the job. Learning is a lifelong endeavor. People don't only learn at school, they learn at work, in social situations and even doing simple tasks like household chores or running errands. Psychologists working in this subfield examine how people learn in a variety of settings to identify approaches and strategies to make learning more effective.

Three features of this account are particularly noteworthy. First, educational psychologists must have a sound understanding of human development. Motor, cognitive, social and other aspects of development are not just of concern to developmental psychologists. Knowledge of development informs what it means to learn in different contexts and life stages. Second, while learning is typically associated with formal education and the early years, it is actually a lifelong process. Educational psychologists are interested not only in the learning undertaken by children at school but also in the learning that occurs by adults in the workplace and even by older adults in retirement. Third, educational psychologists study learning with a view to making this process more effective. This might be achieved by changing the instructional methods used in a particular context. Regardless of the specific adjustments adopted, the aim on the part of educational psychologists is to influence the learning process in a positive way.

Although SLTs can work with educational psychologists in any of the aforementioned settings, they are most likely to work in close collaboration with them in schools and colleges. One of the key roles of educational psychologists in these settings is assessment, most often with a view to compiling a statement of a child's special educational needs. When narrowly defined, assessment is usually taken to involve the use of **psychometric tests**. A more holistic assessment of a child's abilities can also involve observation of classroom behaviour, an evaluation of teaching and learning styles and interviews with parents, teachers and pupils. Although educational psychologists have not always welcomed their characterization as IQ testers, psychometric tests are still the mainstay of assessment. Passenger (2014: 23) summarizes the skills that educational psychologists must possess in order to conduct these tests:

> Psychometric testing requires a carefully managed blend of science and art. It demands a keen understanding of the procedures and purposes of the test material; specific interpersonal and observational skills when working one-to-one with pupils who may be young, disaffected, less able, or non-communicative; a sound knowledge of how to analyse and interpret data; and an ability to present this in a way that will be clear to those who may or may not have a full understanding of a pupil's needs (such as other professionals and parents).

SLTs must also understand how psychometric tests are administered, scored and interpreted in order to engage in a meaningful way with the findings of

Full Scale

Verbal Comprehension	Visual Spatial	Fluid Reasoning	Working Memory	Processing Speed
Similarities	Block Design	Matrix Reasoning	Digit Span	Coding
Vocabulary	Visual Puzzles	Figure Weights	Picture Span	Symbol Search
Information		Picture Concepts	Letter–Number Sequencing	Cancellation
Comprehension		Arithmetic		

Primary Index Scales

Verbal Comprehension	Visual Spatial	Fluid Reasoning	Working Memory	Processing Speed
Similarities	Block Design	Matrix Reasoning	Digit Span	Coding
Vocabulary	Visual Puzzles	Figure Weights	Picture Span	Symbol Search

Ancillary Index Scales

Quantitative Reasoning	Auditory Working Memory	Nonverbal	General Ability	Cognitive Proficiency
Figure Weights	Digit Span	Block Design	Similarities	Digit Span
Arithmetic	Letter–Number Sequencing	Visual Puzzles	Vocabulary	Picture Span
		Matrix Reasoning	Block Design	Coding
		Figure Weights	Matrix Reasoning	Symbol Search
		Picture Span	Figure Weights	
		Coding		

Complementary Index Scales

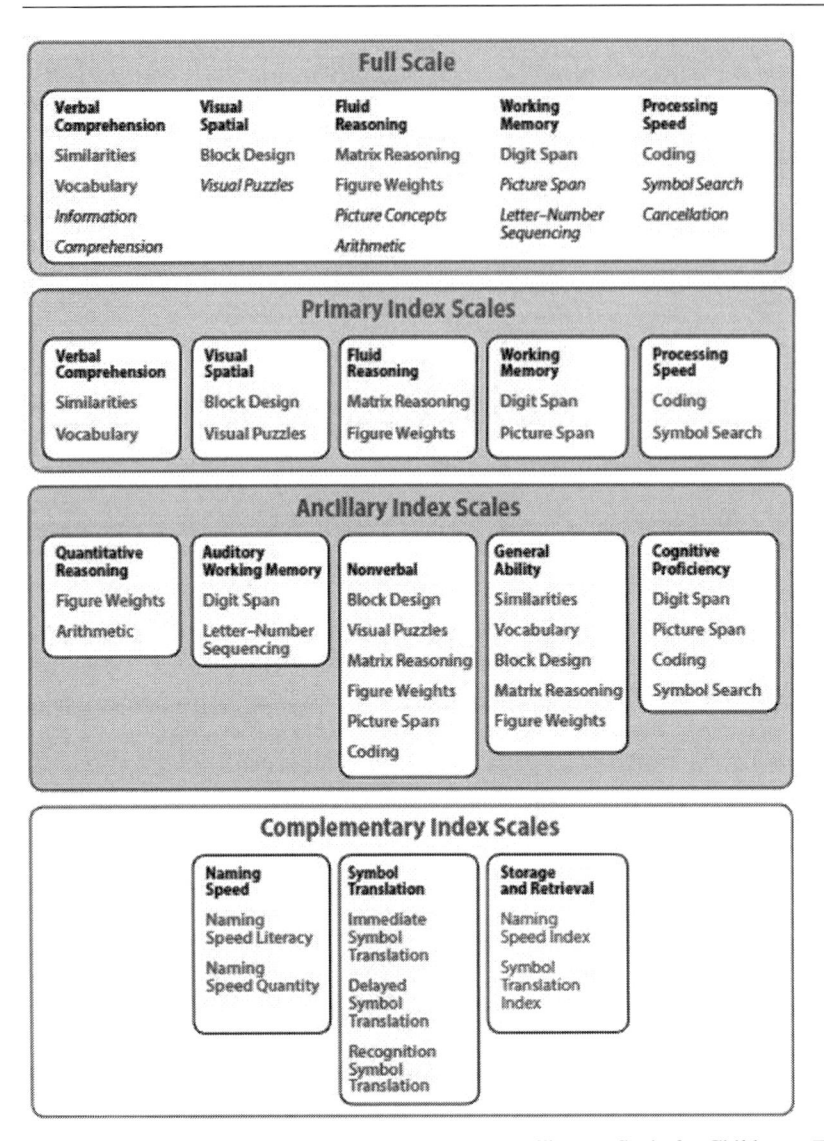

Naming Speed	Symbol Translation	Storage and Retrieval
Naming Speed Literacy	Immediate Symbol Translation	Naming Speed Index
Naming Speed Quantity	Delayed Symbol Translation	Symbol Translation Index
	Recognition Symbol Translation	

Figure 4.1 *The scales of the* Wechsler Intelligence Scale for Children – Fifth Edition *(WISC-V; Wechsler, 2014) (Copyright © 2015 NCS Pearson, Inc. Reproduced with permission. All rights reserved)*

psychological assessment. One widely used standardized intelligence test is the *Wechsler Intelligence Scale for Children – Fifth Edition* (WISC-V; Wechsler, 2014). The WISC-V is a comprehensive assessment of the intellectual abilities of children aged between 6 years and 16 years 11 months. It consists of five primary index scores: Verbal Comprehension Index; Visual-Spatial Index; Fluid Reasoning Index; Working Memory Index; and Processing Speed Index (see Figure 4.1). These five index scores are measured by means of two primary subtests, each of which is shown below. For four of the five index scores, there are also one or more secondary subtests. These subtests are optional and, if administered, can provide additional information regarding a child's performance in a particular domain:

> **Verbal Comprehension Index**
> Primary subtests: Similarities and Vocabulary
> Secondary subtests: Information and Comprehension
>
> **Visual-Spatial Index**
> Primary subtests: Block Design and Visual Puzzles
> No secondary subtests
>
> **Fluid Reasoning Index**
> Primary subtests: Matrix Reasoning and Figure Weights
> Secondary subtests: Picture Concepts and Arithmetic
>
> **Working Memory Index**
> Primary subtests: Digit Span and Picture Span
> Secondary subtest: Letter-Number Sequencing
>
> **Processing Speed Index**
> Primary subtests: Coding and Symbol Search
> Secondary subtest: Cancellation

Full Scale IQ is composed of seven of the ten primary subtests described above: Similarities; Vocabulary; Block Design; Matrix Reasoning; Figure Weights; Digit Span; and Coding. The WISC-V also contains five ancillary measures: General Ability; Cognitive Proficiency; Nonverbal; Quantitative Reasoning; and Auditory Working Memory Indexes. These are optional and permit clinicians to examine hypotheses about a child's WISC-V scores in the context of performance in the classroom, in daily interactions and in everyday demands (Weiss et al., 2015). WISC-V also contains complementary indexes and subtests. These tests are not part of the cognitive abilities assessed by the WISC-V. Rather, they are intended to provide clinicians with more detailed information about those children who are referred with specific learning disorders in reading and mathematics. In total, the core subtests in WISC-V take approximately 60 minutes to complete.

Of course, WISC-V is only one psychometric test, albeit a very prominent one. Other psychometric tests include the *Peabody Picture Vocabulary Test – Fourth Edition* (PPVT-4; Dunn and Dunn, 2007) and the *Stanford-Binet Intelligence Scales – Fifth Edition* (SB-5; Roid, 2003). The PPVT-4 is an individually administered, norm-referenced instrument that is used to assess **receptive vocabulary** in individuals from 2;6 years of age to 90 years and older. The PPVT-4 can be administered by SLTs as well as by psychologists. An examiner reads words aloud. Subjects are required to select from four colour pictures the one that best illustrates a word's meaning. Beyond testing receptive vocabulary, the PPVT-4 may be used as a measure of verbal intelligence. Dunn and Dunn (2007: 1) remark that the PPVT-4 'is useful (perhaps as part of a broader assessment) when evaluating language competence, selecting the level and content of instruction, and measuring learning. In individuals whose primary language is English, vocabulary correlates highly with general verbal ability.'

The SB-5 is the latest in a long succession of Stanford-Binet intelligence tests which were first published in 1916. It assesses intellectual and cognitive abilities in individuals from 2 years of age to 85 years and older. Ten individually administered subtests assess five cognitive factors: Fluid Reasoning; Knowledge; Quantitative; Visual-Spatial; and Working Memory. Each subtest can be administered in 5 minutes. The SB-5 contains an Extended IQ scale that permits the calculation of Full Scale IQ scores that are substantially lower than 40 or higher than 160. An abbreviated test that consists of two subtests – Matrices and Vocabulary – can be used to obtain a Brief IQ score which then determines the starting point for the other subtests. The SB-5 is based on a large normative sample of 4,800 individuals and has been co-normed with and linked to other psychometric tests (e.g. Woodcock-Johnson Tests of Achievement). As part of their clinical education, SLT students must be introduced to the psychometric properties of intelligence tests such as the SB-5 and learn how to interpret the results of these tests.

The role of the educational psychologist does not end with psychometric testing. The results of any psychometric test are useful only to the extent that they can contribute to the diagnosis of a disorder and can assist educational psychologists in identifying a particular intervention. Passenger (2014: 23) states that

> In identifying a particular cognitive profile in those with complex needs, the educational psychologist in today's multi-disciplinary team not only can make a unique contribution to the diagnosis of a range of developmental disorders and syndromes (e.g. Williams syndrome, foetal alcohol syndrome, and Tourette's syndrome) but can also take an active role in identifying the most effective intervention.

One of the developmental disorders that the results of assessment may be used to diagnose is developmental dyslexia. Through their knowledge and training, educational psychologists are ideally placed to advise teachers and classroom assistants on the instructional practices that may be used most effectively with dyslexic students. This knowledge includes specific skills (e.g. automatic word recognition skills) that may be addressed directly in intervention as well as an understanding of how learning may be fostered and hindered by personality features and emotional factors. As well as instituting interventions tailored to individual students with learning disabilities like dyslexia, educational psychologists can also play a key role in establishing whole school programmes that target literacy and other academic areas (e.g. *Success for All* and *Distar*). From assessment and diagnosis to intervention, educational psychologists have a unique understanding of the conditions (including disorders) that compromise learning and how these conditions may best be addressed through instruction. As professionals who work closely with educational psychologists, SLTs must be aware of the remit of this important psychological discipline.

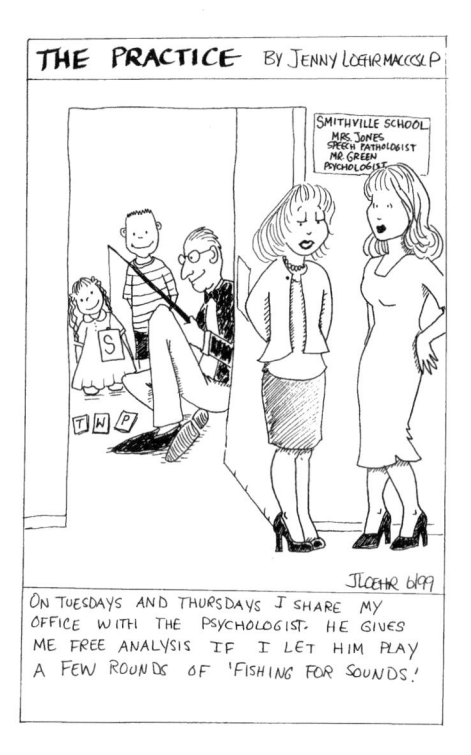

THE PRACTICE By Jenny Loehr MACCSLP

ON TUESDAYS AND THURSDAYS I SHARE MY OFFICE WITH THE PSYCHOLOGIST. HE GIVES ME FREE ANALYSIS IF I LET HIM PLAY A FEW ROUNDS OF 'FISHING FOR SOUNDS!'

GROUP EXERCISE: SLT and Educational Psychology

Perceptions of SLT held by other professionals are seldom examined. SLTs also have attitudes about educational and health professionals that are rarely directly investigated. Yet, knowledge of these perceptions and attitudes is vitally important if the conditions for collaborative practice between educational and health professions are to be realized. One exception is a study by Dunsmuir et al. (2006) that examined the perceptions and attitudes of SLTs and educational psychologists. In this study, the views of SLTs and educational psychologists in two local authorities were sought using a questionnaire. Some of these views are shown below. In a group, discuss these views and their implications for collaborative practice between SLTs and educational psychologists.

What educational psychologists say about SLTs

It seems that SLTs use the results of cognitive assessments to decide whether/how much therapy to offer. This worries me as they see ability as being fixed/static and therefore measurable by a one-off standardised psychometric assessment.

SLTs use non-verbal cognitive scores to compare with their language assessments. They have a narrow view of what we assess – little weight given to other methods.

They make a lot of assumptions about EP assessments, e.g. that a psychological assessment will consist of standardised ability testing – and do not seem familiar with the range of approaches/techniques that we have to offer. Also there is a focus on within child factors – and probably a lack of awareness of broader issues.

What SLTs say about educational psychologists
I think there is a lack of understanding in both professions of each other's role. I find some EPs have little awareness re the specific role of SLT in relation to supporting children's language development. In my experience EPs assume SLTs will work with children with delayed language, and will continue to see them where progress is limited.

Lack of acceptance and respect sometimes of SLTs professional opinion with regards to child's language difficulties.

Lack of understanding that we do not work with all children who have communication difficulties.

KEY POINTS: Educational Psychology

- The branch of psychology that studies human learning across the lifespan. Although most often identified with students and school settings, educational psychology is also concerned with learning by adults in the workplace and the learning of older adults.
- Assessment is a key component of educational psychology. Psychologists administer, score and interpret the results of psychometric tests such as the WISC-V, the SB-5 and the PPVT-4. Tests such as the PPVT-4 may also be administered by SLTs.
- SLTs must have knowledge of the psychometric properties of these tests and understand how to interpret their results. This is because referrals to SLT often include the results of assessments by educational psychologists. Also, educational psychologists are key professionals in the multidisciplinary team that assesses children with special educational needs in compliance with statutory requirements.
- The results of psychometric tests contribute to diagnoses of developmental disorders such as dyslexia, dyscalculia and dyspraxia. Educational psychologists also use the results of assessment to inform the instructional process at both individual and school-wide levels.

4.4 Cognitive Psychology

Cognitive psychology is the branch of psychology that studies mental functions such as perception, attention, reasoning, language, **problem-solving** and memory. A number of different approaches have been taken by cognitive psychologists to explain these functions. One approach that was dominant in the 1960s and 1970s and is still influential today is the use of information-processing models. Although these models vary, they share certain underlying assumptions. One assumption is that the digital computer is a metaphor for how the mind processes information. Linguistic, perceptual and other data enter the mind, are acted upon by processes (algorithms) within it and are converted from one form to another form by means of these processes. Essentially, the mind manipulates symbols in propositions, images and other mental representations in much the same way that a computer manipulates symbols in its internal representations. This computer metaphor extends to the schematic representations that cognitive psychologists use to represent memory, language and other mental functions. Like the computer scientist's flowchart, which represents the processing of information in a number of interlinked stages, information-processing models use 'box-and-arrow' diagrams. Each box contains a specific type of information or data, while each arrow represents the conversion of that information from one form to another form. A typical information-processing model is shown in Figure 4.2. It is the model of language processing that informs the *Psycholinguistic Assessments of Language Processing in Aphasia* (PALPA; Kay et al., 1992), which will be discussed below.

Information-processing models in cognitive psychology subscribe to a number of other assumptions. The boxes in diagrams like the one shown in Figure 4.2 are **cognitive modules**. Modules exhibit a number of properties. The characterization of these properties owes much to the modularity of mind thesis of Jerry Fodor (1983), although different versions of modularity have since been proposed. Fodor enumerates the properties of the mind's input systems or modules as follows: (1) input systems are domain specific; (2) the operation of input systems is mandatory; (3) there is only limited central access to the mental representations that input systems compute; (4) input systems are fast; (5) input systems exhibit **informational encapsulation**; (6) input analysers have 'shallow' outputs; (7) input systems are associated with fixed neural architecture; (8) input systems exhibit characteristic and specific breakdown patterns; and (9) the ontogeny of input systems exhibits a characteristic pace and sequencing. Returning to Figure 4.2, the modules identified as the phonological input lexicon and the orthographic input lexicon are *domain specific* in the sense that they can process only one type of data or information, the spoken and written forms of words, respectively. The operation of these modules is *mandatory* in the sense that as long as their input conditions are satisfied, that is, data of a certain type is available to the modules, the processing of that data occurs automatically. These modules are also *informationally encapsulsated* in the sense that they can provide input to the semantic system, but the semantic system cannot influence the content of these modules.

One further feature of cognitive modules à la Fodor that has particular relevance in the present context is the 'characteristic and specific breakdown patterns' that modules exhibit. When modules are damaged through illness,

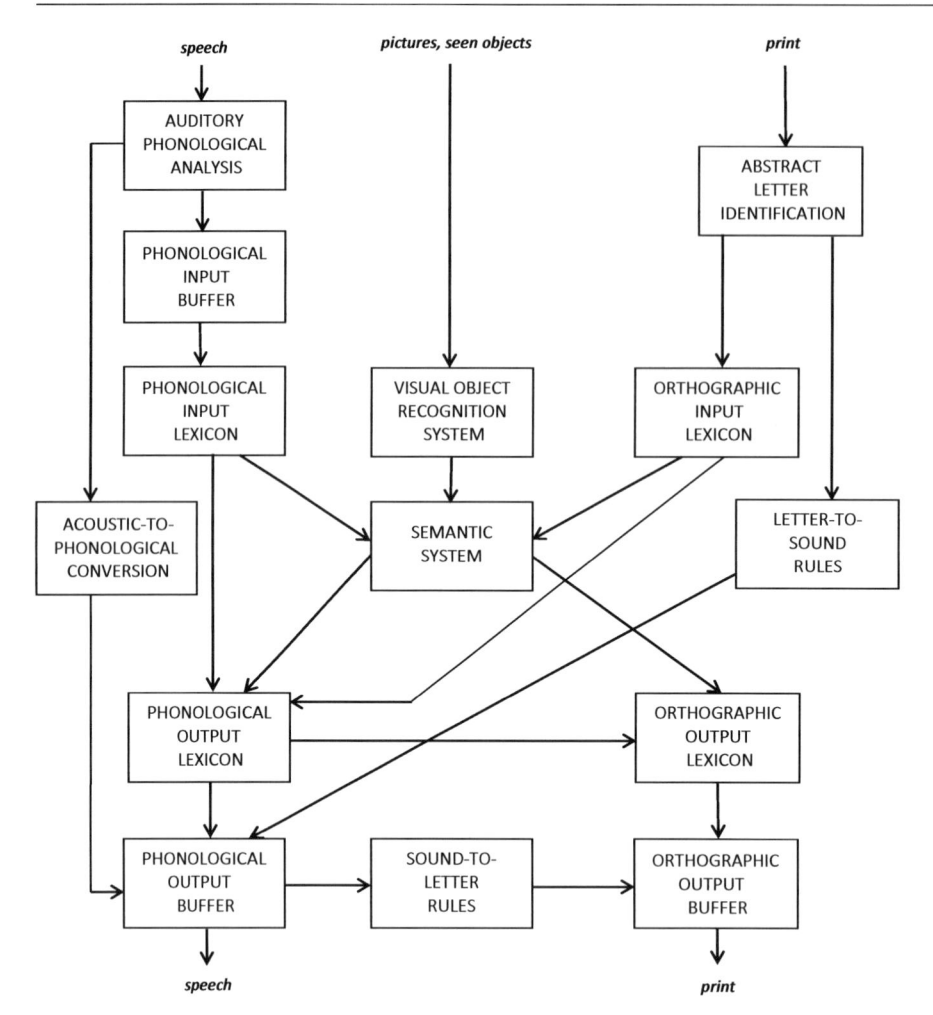

Figure 4.2 *Model of language processing in* Psycholinguistic Assessments of Language Processing in Aphasia *(PALPA; from Kay et al., 1992: 159–80. Reproduced with kind permission of Taylor & Francis Ltd, www.tandfonline.com)*

injury or disease, it is argued that specific impairments arise. For example, an adult who develops aphasia following a stroke and has impairment of the orthographic input lexicon may be unable to read aloud irregular words like *yacht* and *mortgage*. These words are mispronounced if letter-to-sound rules are applied to them and must be accessed in the orthographic input lexicon in order to be read aloud. Also, the vowel sound in the words *hint* (/ɪ/) and *pint* (/aɪ/) would be pronounced the same if the orthographic input lexicon were impaired and reading aloud had to take place via letter-to-sound rules. Such an adult would be unable to complete a lexical decision task because in order to decide if a letter string forms an existing word, the orthographic input lexicon has to be accessed.

In short, quite specific linguistic impairments would arise in the event of damage to the orthographic input lexicon. These same impairments would not occur if another module in Figure 4.2 were damaged. It is the capacity of information-processing models to explain specific linguistic deficits that has made these models attractive to SLTs who assess and treat clients with aphasia. Whitworth et al. (2014: 6) capture the explanatory value of a modular approach in the management of aphasia in the following terms:

> A working assumption is that any of the modules . . . can be lost or damaged as a result of cortical lesions. An individual with aphasia might have damage to one or several modules or the mappings between them. Because of the functional architecture of the brain, some patterns of deficits will be more frequent than others, but because lesions vary both in their precise cortical locations and in the cutting of sub-cortical white matter fibre tracts, identical patterns of deficit in any two people are unlikely. One objective in assessment can be to identify which of the modules and mappings (boxes and arrows) are damaged and which are intact, yielding a concise explanation of the pattern of performance across a range of tasks and materials.

It is the aim of assessments like PALPA (Kay et al., 1992) to establish exactly which modules and mappings (or boxes and arrows) are intact and which are impaired. PALPA contains 60 subtests of language structure in **orthography** and phonology, word and picture semantics, and morphology and syntax. Normative data is available for some subtests. The subtests are arranged in four batteries: auditory processing; reading and spelling; word and picture semantics; and sentence processing. Spoken and written input and output modalities are assessed through the use of tasks that involve lexical decision, matching of items, repetition and picture naming. PALPA is designed to be used as both a clinical assessment and a research tool, although the former use is more common (Bate et al., 2010). Although it is most often used with clients who have stroke-induced aphasia, clinicians also use PALPA to assess clients with a range of other aetiologies including dementia and traumatic brain injury (Bate et al., 2010). To illustrate how this assessment tests specific modules and mappings in the diagram in Figure 4.2, we examine below the processing that is undertaken by subjects as they perform two of the subtests in the word and picture semantics battery in PALPA.

The first subtest is written word–picture matching. In order to match a written word to a picture, a subject must access the semantic system via the orthographic input lexicon (written word) and the visual object recognition system (picture). If either of these routes into the semantic system is impaired, this matching task cannot be performed. For example, the subject who can access the orthographic input lexicon but cannot proceed from there to the semantic system can identify the written forms of the words that he knows. But he cannot access the semantics of these words or engage in matching of them to pictures. The second subtest is spoken word–written word matching. For a subject to match spoken words to

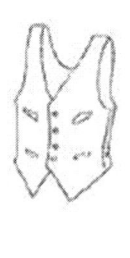

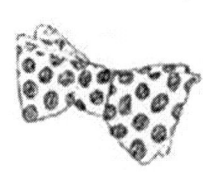

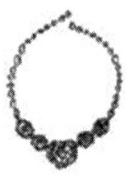

Figure 4.3 *Stimulus pictures from the* Pyramids and Palm Trees Test *(Howard and Patterson, 1992, London: Pearson Education Ltd)*

written words, the semantic system must be accessed via the phonological input lexicon (spoken word) and the orthographic input lexicon (written word). If the mapping between the phonological input lexicon and the semantic system is degraded through illness, injury or disease, then a subject will be able to identify the spoken forms of the words that he knows, but he will not be able to access the semantics of those words. In the absence of this semantic information, he will be unable to match these words to their written counterparts. The PALPA subtests permit specific linguistic impairments to be related directly to degraded modules and pathways within a cognitive model of language processing.

PALPA is not the only assessment based on a modular framework of language processing. The *Pyramids and Palm Trees Test* (Howard and Patterson, 1992) is a cognitive neuropsychological assessment of a subject's ability to access meaning from pictures and words. The subject is presented with a triad of stimuli in the form of spoken words, written words or pictures. One of these stimuli is the reference item (e.g. waistcoat) and the other two are possible choices (e.g. bow tie or necklace) (see Figure 4.3). The subject selects as his response the word or picture that he thinks is most closely associated with the reference stimulus. The word and picture versions of the test contain 52 trials each. There are seven different ways in which the test can be administered. For example, the three test stimuli may all be pictures, or subjects may be required to select a written word for a target picture, or select a picture for a target word, and so on. Using the results of this test, a clinician can locate a subject's semantic impairment in a failure to access semantic and conceptual information in a central, modality-independent semantic system or in a modality-specific deficit in accessing semantics. Like PALPA, the *Pyramids and Palm Trees Test* is used to assess subjects with aphasia. It can also be used to examine subjects with **visual agnosia** and semantic impairment in clients with Alzheimer's disease. Also like PALPA, this test permits clinicians to plan intervention around the specific components – modules and pathways – that are the basis of a subject's semantic impairment. In this way, clinical intervention has a strong theoretical motivation within a cognitive neuropsychological approach to assessment.

> **KEY POINTS: Cognitive Psychology**
> - Cognitive psychology studies mental functions such as attention, reasoning, language, perception, memory and problem-solving.
> - There are a number of different paradigms in cognitive psychology that influence the approach of investigators to these mental functions. One paradigm that has been particularly influential is the information-processing approach.
> - According to the information-processing approach, mental functions such as language and perception are performed by a number of interconnected modules in the mind. These modules and their interconnections are modelled in 'box-and-arrow' diagrams.
> - Modules display a number of properties. On the version of modularity proposed by Jerry Fodor, modules are domain specific, mandatory and exhibit informational encapsulation among other features.
> - On this modular view, specific linguistic impairments can be related to breakdown in one or more modules and/or the interconnections between those modules. For example, the speaker with an impaired orthographic input lexicon cannot engage in written lexical decision tasks (e.g. Is 'splink' a word or a non-word?).
> - SLT assessment has been influenced by the information-processing approach in cognitive psychology. This approach forms the theoretical framework of cognitive neuropsychological assessments such as PALPA and the *Pyramids and Palm Trees Test*. These assessments are used for the most part with clients who have aphasia, although they are also used with clients who have dementia, traumatic brain injury and other neurological disorders.

4.5 Neuropsychology

Neuropsychology can be defined as the study of the relationship between brain structure and behaviour. This branch of psychology is both an academic and a clinical discipline. As an academic discipline, neuropsychology investigates normal brain structure and behaviour and is interested in subjects with organic brain disorders to the extent that they can throw light on normal brain processes. As a clinical discipline, neuropsychology is concerned with the assessment and treatment of individuals with neurological disorders and a range of other conditions. Although SLTs must have an understanding of neuropsychology as both an academic and a clinical discipline, it is clinical neuropsychology that is most directly relevant to the practice of speech and language therapy. In the USA, the National Academy of Neuropsychology (2001) defines clinical neuropsychology in the following terms:

> A clinical neuropsychologist is a professional within the field of psychology with special expertise in the applied science of brain-behavior relationships. Clinical neuropsychologists use this knowledge in the assessment, diagnosis, treatment, and/or rehabilitation of patients across the lifespan with neurological, medical, neurodevelopmental and psychiatric conditions, as well as other cognitive and learning disorders. The clinical neuropsychologist uses psychological, neurological, cognitive, behavioral, and physiological principles, techniques and tests to evaluate patients' neurocognitive, behavioral, and emotional strengths and weaknesses and their relationship to normal and abnormal central nervous system functioning. The clinical neuropsychologist uses this information and information provided by other medical/healthcare providers to identify and diagnose neurobehavioral disorders, and plan and implement intervention strategies.

Among the many disorders that are assessed and treated by clinical neuropsychologists are children and adults with traumatic brain injury (TBI). This population of clients also falls within the remit of SLT on account of the often complex communication disorders that can arise in TBI. (Of course, clients with TBI can also experience swallowing disorders or dysphagia.) In recent years, the communication impairment in TBI has come to be known as a 'cognitive-communication disorder'. This designation reflects the fact that children and adults with TBI often have intact structural language skills and can even pass standardized language tests, but still exhibit significant impairments in everyday communication. These impairments involve pragmatic and discourse aspects of language and are related to the presence of cognitive deficits known as executive function deficits (Cummings, 2009, 2014a). Executive functions are a group of cognitive skills that are integral to the planning, execution and regulation of goal-directed behaviour. These skills include attention, impulse control and self-regulation, initiation of activity, **working memory**, mental flexibility, planning and organization, and selection of efficient problem-solving strategies. Executive functions are typically linked to the brain's frontal cortex, which explains their disruption in clients with TBI and frontal lobe pathology. However, there is now clear evidence that striatal structures also play a role in executive functions (Elliott, 2003: 49). In order to understand the role of executive functions in the cognitive-communication disorders of clients with TBI, SLTs must be aware of how clinical neuropsychologists assess these different functions. Some discussion of this assessment now follows.

SPECIAL TOPIC: Cognitive-Communication Disorder

Many clients who are assessed and treated by SLTs have communication problems in the presence of cognitive deficits. So-called cognitive-communication disorders are found in clients who sustain a traumatic brain injury, in clients with right-hemisphere damage (RHD) and in clients who develop dementia. Communication problems in these clients are most marked in the areas of pragmatics and discourse, although there may also be deficits in other aspects of language.

Penelope Myers undertook the first formal study of communication impairments in adults with RHD. Myers remarked that in a picture description task these adults produced 'irrelevant and often excessive information' and seemed 'to miss the implication of [a] question and to respond in a most literal and concrete way' (Myers, 1979: 38). When attempting to respond to open-ended questions, these patients 'wended their way through a maze of disassociated detail, seemingly incapable of filtering out unnecessary information' (38). The components of a narrative, although available to these patients, could not be assembled into a narrative. There was difficulty 'in extracting critical bits of information, in seeing the relationships among them, and in reaching conclusions or drawing inferences based on those relationships' (39). Although the detail provided by these patients was related to the general topic, its appearance seemed irrelevant because it had not been 'integrated into a whole' (39).

The following data, which is provided by Valeria Abusamra, illustrates many of the features of communication in clients with RHD described by Myers. An examiner (E) is asking an adult (P) with RHD to explain the meaning of a speaker's utterance:

> E: Maryann joyfully looks at her new Ford which is parked in the street.
> P: It's always Ford!
> E: Yes! They're paying us for advertising! So she looks at her new Ford which is parked in the street and says to her husband: 'I love the colour we chose.' What do you think Maryann means by that?
> P: Well, she's very happy to have chosen the car they bought.
> E: Very good. And from the following options, do you think she means to say that she likes the colour they chose or she means she wants her husband to take her for a ride?
> P: For a ride? In theory, one thing has nothing to do with the other. One can be both sitting on the couch watching ... [sic] Plus, besides, plus A doesn't imply B, because it's likely that the idea, instead of coming from the husband, it's her who wants to go for a ride [sic]. Plus, going for a ride doesn't necessarily have to include a car, it could be with other types of rides. Uhm ... it wouldn't be weird if maybe instead of him driving, she drives too.
> E: So which would it be out of the two?
> P: No, the first one, yes. But because there's not one ...
> E: No, maybe one out of the two works best.
> P: A necessary connection ...

Initially, the client displays a correct interpretation of Maryann's utterance: 'she's very happy to have chosen the car they bought'. However, as the exchange unfolds, the client – in Myers' words – wends his way through a maze of disassociated detail,

> seemingly incapable of filtering out unnecessary information. As the client continues to talk, he introduces irrelevant information such as 'sitting on the couch' and uses abstract language like 'plus A doesn't imply B'. The effect of these pragmatic anomalies is to take the client further and further away from the point of the exchange between Maryann and her husband.

From the outset, it should be noted that executive functions are typically examined as part of a wider neuropsychological assessment of clients with TBI. Kosaka (2006) states that a comprehensive neuropsychological assessment of clients with TBI must include the following components: intellect; higher cognitive abilities (executive functioning); attention; memory; visual-spatial abilities; motor and sensory abilities; and emotional status. Historically, neuropsychologists have favoured the use of the fixed battery of tests known as the *Halstead-Reitan Neuropsychological Test Battery* (Reitan and Wolfson, 1993) for this purpose, although other assessments may be used to examine specific aspects of neuropsychological functioning, e.g. the *Wechsler Adult Intelligence Scale – Fourth Edition* (WAIS-IV; Wechsler, 2008) for the assessment of intellect (Kosaka, 2006). The Halstead-Reitan contains ten core subtests, one of which is the Trail Making Test (TMT). The TMT is a measure of executive control (Arbuthnott and Frank, 2000). There are two parts to this test. In Part A, subjects are required to draw lines that sequentially connect 25 encircled numbers distributed on a sheet of paper. The task requirements are similar for Part B, only this time subjects must alternate between circles that contain numbers and letters (e.g. 1, A, 2, B, 3, C, etc.) (see Figure 4.4). These tasks are scored by recording the amount of time in seconds that it takes to complete each exercise. Timed performance which exceeds 39 seconds on Part A and 91 seconds on Part B is indicative of neurological injury (Franzen, 2002).

SLTs who work with neuropsychologists in head trauma rehabilitation units must be familiar with other executive function tests besides the TMT. A neuropsychological assessment also often contains the results of a Stroop test. There are numerous variations of the Stroop test. The *Stroop Colour and Word Test* (Golden, 1978) is the most commonly used tool to assess **selective attention** in individuals with TBI (Ben-David et al., 2011). There are three components to this test. In the first component – the word task – subjects read aloud the names of colour words which appear in black ink. In the second component – the colour task – subjects are required to name the colour of a bar of Xs (XXX) which appears in red, blue or green ink. In the third component – the colour–word task – subjects are shown the names of colours that are printed in conflicting colours (e.g. the word *blue* printed in red ink). They are required to name the colour of the ink rather than the word. A markedly slowed naming response on this latter task for individuals with TBI relative to controls is generally interpreted as reflecting a decrease in selective attention – individuals with TBI are unable to selectively process one visual feature (the colour of the ink) while continuously blocking out the processing of another visual feature (the word form). The slowed naming response may also be explained

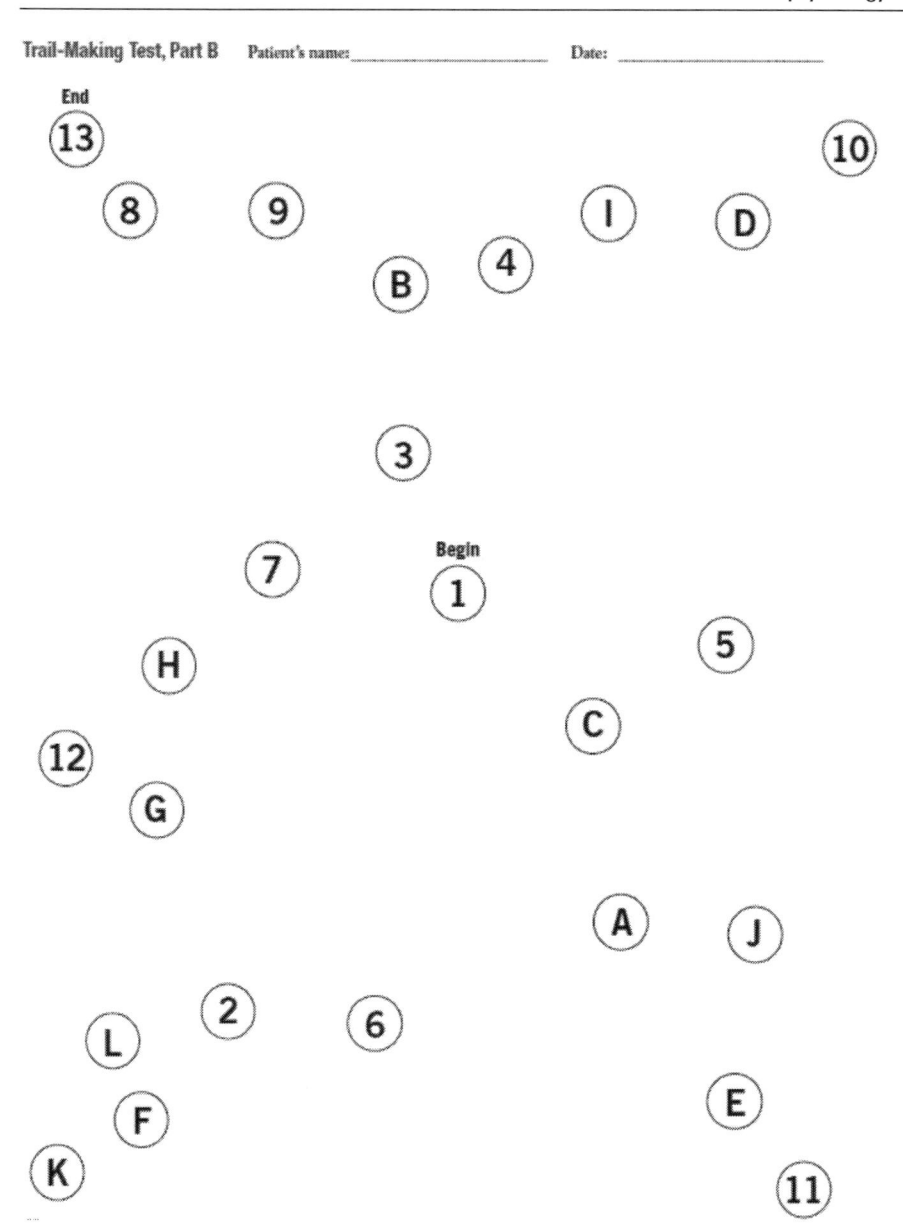

Figure 4.4 *Trail-Making Test, Part B (reproduced with permission of the US Department of Transportation, National Highway Traffic Safety Administration)*

in terms of an inability to inhibit a dominant response – the word form must be inhibited in order to name the colour of the ink that the word is written in. In the original Stroop test, the score is based on the number of words that can be read in a given time limit. On the California Stroop Test, a subtest of the *Delis-Kaplan Executive Function Scale* (Delis ct al., 2001), the time required to correctly read each section is used as the score (Homack and Riccio, 2004).

Neuropsychological assessment has an important role to play in the prediction of recovery in individuals who sustain a stroke or a TBI. But it has an equally important contribution to make to charting cognitive decline in older adults. When cognitive deterioration falls outside normal limits, it may be indicative of mild cognitive impairment (MCI). In more severe cases, the deterioration may be symptomatic of one of a range of dementia syndromes. Neuropsychological assessment is integral to a diagnosis of MCI and the conversion of MCI to dementia: 'Neuropsychological testing can be extremely useful in making the MCI diagnosis and tracking the evolution of cognitive symptoms over time. A comprehensive test battery includes measures of baseline intellectual ability, attention, executive function, memory, language, visuospatial skills, and mood' (Nelson and O'Connor, 2008: 56). Neuropsychological assessment is also relevant to a diagnosis of neurobehavioural disorders such as ADHD, a clinical population in which there is significant impairment of language and communication. The neuropsychological profile of individuals with ADHD is highly variable, with patients displaying deficits in one neuropsychological test or one cognitive domain but not in another (Gualtieri and Johnson, 2005). Notwithstanding this variability, neuropsychological testing makes a vital contribution along with other investigations to the diagnosis of ADHD:

> The 'gold standard' for ADHD diagnosis includes a comprehensive clinical history and examination, rating scales, direct behavioral observations, neuropsychological testing, and objective, comparative analysis of different drug effects. (Gualtieri and Johnson, 2005: 51)

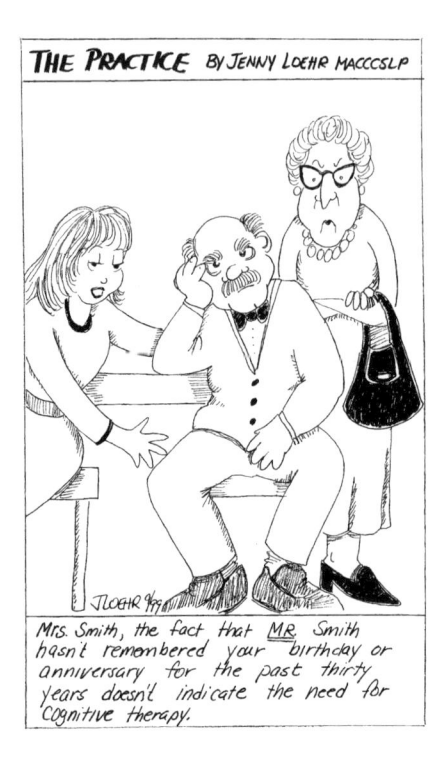

THE PRACTICE BY JENNY LOEHR MACCCSLP

Mrs. Smith, the fact that Mr. Smith hasn't remembered your birthday or anniversary for the past thirty years doesn't indicate the need for cognitive therapy.

SLTs must have a working knowledge of the principles and techniques of neuropsychological assessment in order to assess, diagnose and treat a wide range of clients whose language and communication impairments are related to cognitive deficits.

> **KEY POINTS: Neuropsychology**
> - Neuropsychology is the study of the relationship between brain structure and behaviour. This branch of psychology is both an academic and a clinical discipline. SLTs require knowledge of both dimensions, but work most often in multidisciplinary teams with clinical neuropsychologists.
> - Clinical neuropsychologists assess cognitive skills such as executive functions in children with neurobehavioural and neurodevelopmental disorders (e.g. ADHD and ASD), and in adults with acquired brain injury (e.g. stroke, TBI) or neuropsychiatric disorders (e.g. schizophrenia).
> - Assessment is conducted with a view to predicting recovery from neurological injury and/or to determining the impact of injury on functioning. SLTs must understand the principles and techniques of neuropsychological assessment.
> - Neuropsychological assessment is often conducted through a battery of tests such as the *Halstead-Reitan Neuropsychological Test Battery*. Individual tests may also be used to assess specific cognitive skills (e.g. the *Stroop Colour and Word Test* to assess selective attention).
> - SLTs must understand the significance of neuropsychological findings for a client's language and communication skills. Neuropsychological deficits often manifest in pragmatic and discourse impairments (e.g. in clients with frontal lobe pathology related to TBI).

4.6 Clinical Psychology

There is no standard or widely accepted definition of clinical psychology. Pomerantz (2014: 4) states that '[t]he field has witnessed such tremendous growth in a wide variety of directions that most concise definitions fall short of capturing the field in its entirety'. The American Psychological Association (2016b) defines clinical psychology in the following terms:

> Clinical psychology is the psychological specialty that provides continuing and comprehensive mental and behavioral health care for individuals and families; consultation to agencies and communities; training, education and supervision; and research-based practice. It is a specialty in breadth – one that is broadly inclusive of severe psychopathology – and marked by comprehensiveness and integration of knowledge and skill from a broad array of disciplines within and outside of psychology proper. The scope of clinical psychology encompasses all ages, multiple diversities and varied systems.

As comprehensive as this definition is, it says little about the behavioural and mental health conditions that fall within the remit of clinical psychology. An enumeration of these conditions is given by Plante (2011: 5–6):

> A clinical psychologist might evaluate a child using intellectual and educational tests to determine if the child has a learning disability or an attentional problem that might contribute to poor school performance. Another example includes a psychologist who treats an adult experiencing severe depression following a recent divorce. People experiencing substance and other addictions, hallucinations, compulsive eating, sexual dysfunction, physical abuse, suicidal impulses, and head injuries are a few of the many problem areas that are of interest to clinical psychologists.

Clinical psychologists work closely with SLTs in the management of a range of child and adult clients. This is because **psychopathology** is both a cause and a consequence of many communication disorders. Primary psychiatric disorders such as schizophrenia and bipolar disorder have language disturbances as part of their clinical symptomatology. For example, alogia or poverty of speech is a **negative symptom** in schizophrenia. This linguistic behaviour is evident in the following exchange between a doctor (DR) and a 53-year-old male patient (PQ) with schizophrenia who was studied by Clegg et al. (2007). The exchange occurred during a weekly ward round and was 90 seconds in duration. Only part of it is reproduced below. PQ produces minimal, unelaborated responses to the doctor's questions. The doctor leaves significant pauses at the end of PQ's turns before asking his next question as a means of encouraging PQ to develop his replies. However, this does not occur. The limited responses produced by PQ are reflected in a MLU of 3.4. The doctor's MLU is 9.4:

> DR: So how have you been getting on this week?
> PQ: Okay (pause of 4 seconds).
> DR: I gather the medication has been causing excess salivation, has it been happening a lot?
> PQ: Bit of salivation occasionally (pause of 6 seconds).
> DR: When does this happen?
> PQ: Possibly at night (pause of 8 seconds).
> DR: What have you enjoyed doing this week on the ward PQ?
> PQ: Possibly relaxation (pause of 2 seconds).
> DR: What do you feel you benefit from by doing the relaxation sessions?
> PQ: To relax, get a bit uptight (pause of 5 seconds).
> DR: Do you feel uptight all the time?
> PQ: Occasionally (pause of 3 seconds).
> DR: Do you feel less anxious now than when you first came?
> PQ: About the same (pause of 3 seconds).
> DR: Can you tell me a bit more? Are you feeling less anxious than you were?
> PQ: Could be a bit better ... (pause of 3 seconds) slightly ... (pause 4 seconds) possibly.

Alogia is only one linguistic symptom of schizophrenia. Other linguistic features are anomalies of syntax and semantics (Covington et al., 2005), and pragmatic and discourse deficits (Cummings, 2014a). Pragmatic deficits include impaired comprehension of **figurative language** such as metaphor and idiom and the use of utterances that fail to adhere to Gricean maxims of relevance and quantity. The latter feature is evident in the following extract of language taken from a psychiatric interview with a client with schizophrenia. There is a marked digression after the client's initial response. This failure of relevance is compounded by linguistic impoliteness in the form of a negative remark about the doctor's tie. These combined pragmatic anomalies severely limit the client's effectiveness as a communicator:

> Then I left San Francisco and moved to ... where did you get that tie? It looks like it's left over from the 1950s. I like the warm weather in San Diego. Is that a conch shell on your desk? Have you ever gone scuba diving? (Thomas, 1997: 41)

Psychopathology is the cause of communication impairments in clients with schizophrenia. But psychopathology may also be a consequence of a range of communication disorders. **Depression** and **anxiety** are not uncommon consequences of communication disorders such as aphasia and dysphonia (Martinez and Cassol, 2015; Shehata et al., 2015). Adults with aphasia may experience reduced well-being and quality of life (Cruice et al., 2003; Maggio et al., 2014) as a result of poor adjustment to their disability and its implications for employment, social relationships and other areas of functioning. Significant psychopathology is also reported in children with communication disorders. Children with specific language impairment and stuttering may experience psychological distress and social maladjustment as a result of their communication difficulties (Gunn et al., 2014). Emotional and psychological problems can extend well beyond the developmental period into adolescence and adulthood, and have the potential to compromise functioning in academic, social and occupational domains (but see Bao et al., 2016, who reported a developmentally limited course of psychiatric disorder between late adolescence and young adulthood in children with language disorder). SLTs must be able to identify mental health conditions in their child and adult clients and, where appropriate, undertake referral to a clinical psychologist. Direct management of individuals with these conditions by a clinical psychologist may then occur alongside SLT.

A model of even closer collaborative working between SLTs and clinical psychologists occurs in the management of clients with psychogenic dysphonia. Butcher et al. (2007: 1) define psychogenic dysphonia as a 'dysphonia (impaired or disordered voice) or aphonia (absent voice) where the causative or perpetuating factors are largely psychological or emotional conflict'. These authors further state that a diagnosis of psychogenic dysphonia cannot simply be reached by means of *exclusion* of laryngeal pathology. A diagnosis must also identify the *presence* of psychological factors that play a causative or perpetuating role in the dysphonia. Traumatic and stressful events including sexual assault, bereavement and problematic interpersonal relationships have been reported as significant causes of psychogenic dysphonia (Baker, 2003). An SLT intervention which does not directly address these events is unlikely to be effective. Clinical psychologists have the requisite expertise to identify and analyse conflicts and other psychological traumas that may cause and maintain psychogenic voice disorders. Butcher et al. (2007: 26) also state that 'speech and language therapists can become more skilled and knowledgeable in psychological therapy through joint working with a clinical psychologist'.

One therapeutic approach that has been used successfully with dysphonic clients is cognitive behavioural therapy (CBT). The CBT framework assumes that predisposing and precipitating factors such as stressful life events serve to trigger an initial period of physical symptoms (in this case, vocal symptoms). These symptoms are then maintained by interacting cognitive, behavioural, affective and physiological factors. For example, an adult with voice disorder may experience anxiety or depression (affective factors) or avoid certain speaking situations (behavioural factors) that serve to maintain the dysphonia. CBT focuses on this perpetuating cycle and aims to dismantle the interaction of factors that is hypothesized to perpetuate a client's vocal symptoms (Carding et al., 2013). A recent review of CBT with voice therapy in the management of **functional dysphonia** found that it resulted in an improvement in clients' well-being and distress (Miller et al., 2014). The close interaction between SLT and clinical psychology in the management of clients with psychogenic dysphonia can be illustrated best by means of a case study. Questions relating to this case can be found at the end of the chapter.

CASE STUDY: Woman with Psychogenic Dysphonia

Sudhir et al. (2009) described the case of a 50-year-old married woman ('Ms S') who reported to the authors' hospital with complaints of a hoarse voice and intermittent aphonia which had lasted 5 months. Ms S's vocal symptoms had started abruptly with fluctuations in voice quality. She also reported experiencing low mood, feelings of anxiety and sleeping problems. Ms S had been employed as a teaching assistant at a local school for over 10 years. Her occupational functioning had been affected by her voice problems, as she was unable to take classes. At the time of her referral, Ms S was living with her spouse, two daughters and a son. She reported significant difficulties in her marriage. There were frequent disagreements and anger over the children's futures and the relationship between Ms S and her mother-in-law.

Ms S underwent a laryngeal examination by an **otolaryngologist**, which revealed no organic abnormality. Perceptual and acoustic analyses of Ms S's voice were undertaken. The GRBAS scale (Hirano, 1981) was used to perform a perceptual assessment. This scale assigns ratings of 0 (normal) to 3 (extreme degree of impairment) to a number of parameters: grade (G), roughness (R), breathy (B), asthenia (A) and strained (S). Ms S obtained scores of G_1, R_1, B_0, A_1, S_1 during sustained phonation. On a speech task, her scores were G_3, R_1, B_3, A_3, S_3. Ms S's volitional cough was good. An acoustic analysis was conducted using a speech software system. Sustained phonation of the vowel [a] had a mean habitual frequency of 220 Hz. Ms S's speaking range was from a minimum of 197.53 Hz to a maximum of 266.66 Hz.

Ms S was assessed by a clinical psychologist. The assessment revealed that there were significant interpersonal difficulties between Ms S and her spouse and mother-in-law. Issues concerning communication patterns, decision-making in the marriage, child rearing and Ms S's ability to express her feelings and thoughts about the marriage tended to dominate. Ms S experienced feelings of alienation and distance from her spouse's family whom she perceived to be demanding. The couple did not have a healthy sexual relationship. During joint sessions with her spouse, Ms S was noted to have considerable variation in her voice. This ranged from hoarseness to aphonia, which corresponded with Ms S and her spouse having an argument. The clinical psychologist undertook a number of assessments. Ms S obtained a score of 15 on the Beck's Depression Inventory (Beck et al., 1961), indicating the presence of depression of mild severity. Her responses on the Sentence Completion Test (Sacks and Levy, 1959) revealed significant difficulties in the area of marriage and heterosexual relations. Ms S displayed problems in the approval-rejection domain of the Dysfunctional Attitudes Scale (DAS; Weissman and Beck, 1978). She had difficulty endorsing DAS items on autonomy and endorsed views that others did not like her if they disagreed with her, and that she was worthless if someone she loved did not reciprocate.

Ms S received a programme of therapy which was jointly delivered by a clinical psychologist and speech pathologist. During a three-week period, Ms S received a total of 15 sessions of cognitive behavioural therapy. Dysfunctional assumptions were identified and clarified through Socratic questioning with the aim of cognitively restructuring them. Negative cognitions in the domains of Ms S's children's future and her relationship to her spouse and his family were the focus of sessions. Ms S was encouraged to adopt more neutral alternative interpretations during interactions. During sessions with the couple, tasks and goals were identified which were intended to help improve communication and resolve conflicts about child rearing and sexual interactions.

In each session of voice therapy, Ms S received direct voice therapy and counselling. Direct therapy began with the non-phonatory task of cough, which was immediately followed by sustained production of [a]. From cough and phonation, Ms S progressed to phonation with soft contact. Gradually, phonation was extended to other speech sounds (e.g. [u] and [i]). During counselling the abuse of Ms S's voice in the context of her family problems was subjected to psychotherapeutic examination. Efforts were made to reduce her psychosocial stress. Vocal hygiene and the effects of voice misuse were also addressed. After approximately six 1-hour sessions, Ms S was able to sustain voicing even in the presence of her spouse. By the termination of voice therapy, Ms S had a mean habitual frequency for [a] of 207.79 Hz. Her GRBAS scale scores were zero across all parameters.

> **KEY POINTS: Clinical Psychology**
>
> - Clinical psychologists assess, diagnose and treat a wide range of mental health and behavioural conditions in children and adults. These conditions include anxiety and depression, substance use disorders, sexual and physical abuse, eating disorders, and hallucinations and suicidal ideation.
> - Psychopathology is both a cause and a consequence of communication disorders. Accordingly, SLTs and clinical psychologists work alongside each other in the management of a wide range of children and adults.
> - In primary psychiatric disorders such as schizophrenia, language disturbance is a consequence of psychopathology. Adults with schizophrenia can display alogia (poverty of speech), reduced cohesion and coherence, and impairments of syntax and semantics as a result of their mental health condition.
> - Psychopathology is also a consequence of communication disorders. Individuals with aphasia, dysphonia and stuttering can experience anxiety, depression, reduced well-being and quality of life as a result of their communication impairment.
> - SLTs must understand how clinical psychologists assess and treat a range of conditions in order to work effectively alongside them. Close collaborative working is particularly evident in the management of clients with psychogenic dysphonia where approaches such as cognitive behavioural therapy (CBT) may be used.

> **WEBSITE: Psychological Disciplines**
>
> After reading the chapter, visit the website and test your knowledge of psychological disciplines by answering the short-answer questions for this topic.

Suggestions for Further Reading

Peach, R. K. and Shapiro, L. P. (eds.) 2012. *Cognition and acquired language disorders: an information processing approach*, St Louis, MO: Elsevier Mosby.

This edited volume contains 15 chapters that examine the relationship between cognition, as studied within cognitive psychology, and acquired language disorders. There are also sections on normal language processing from a cognitive psychological perspective and on the clinical management of acquired language disorders.

James, S. and Brumfitt, S. 2016. *Applying psychology for effective speech and language therapy practice*, Guildford: J & R Press Ltd.

Although this chapter examined the main branches of psychology that are relevant to SLT, it could not discuss them all. This volume addresses key ideas in social, health and counselling psychology. It considers how these ideas can be applied in SLT practice with clients of all ages and types of speech, language and communication needs.

Dunsmuir, S., Clifford, V. and Took, S. 2006. 'Collaboration between educational psychologists and speech and language therapists: barriers and opportunities', *Educational Psychology in Practice: Theory, Research and Practice in Educational Psychology* **22**:2, 125–40.

This article examines the collaborative practices of educational psychologists and SLTs. Barriers to collaboration are identified, and ways to overcome them are explored. The views of educational psychologists and SLTs in two local authorities are examined.

QUESTIONS: Psychological Disciplines

(1) Each of the following scenarios describes a situation in which psychologists and SLTs work closely together. Read each scenario and decide what type of psychologist is working with the SLT. The labels you should use are: *developmental psychologist; cognitive neuropsychologist; educational psychologist; clinical neuropsychologist; clinical psychologist.*

  (a) An SLT uses a range of behavioural techniques to treat a 50-year-old woman with dysphonia. Notwithstanding intensive intervention, the woman's dysphonia is not observed to improve. The SLT turns to a psychologist at the hospital to discuss an alternative intervention.

  (b) A 25-year-old man is admitted to a head trauma rehabilitation unit after a number of weeks spent in intensive care. A SLT receives a referral to conduct an assessment of his communication skills. The SLT first reads a report written by a psychologist who has assessed the client and found significant executive function deficits.

  (c) An SLT is part of a multidisciplinary team in a child development clinic at a regional hospital. The therapist has been asked by the team's paediatrician to assess the communication skills of a child with suspected ASD. After assessing the child, the therapist discusses her findings with the team's psychologist.

  (d) As part of a research project, an SLT is working with a psychologist to test a model of lexical access in clients with aphasia. The lexical access deficits of these clients suggest that some revision of the model is required.

  (e) An SLT receives a referral from the local education authority to assess a 5-year-old boy with developmental delay. Among other findings, the psychologist's report indicates that this boy has a verbal IQ of 65 and a performance IQ of 80. His full IQ is 70.

(2) Part A: The following children are assessed and treated by SLTs. In which of these children is the attainment of motor milestones likely to be delayed?

(a) a child with specific language impairment
(b) a child with developmental verbal dyspraxia
(c) a child with foetal alcohol spectrum disorder
(d) a child with developmental stuttering
(e) a child with spastic cerebral palsy
(f) a child with Prader-Willi syndrome

Part B: Children with ToM deficits often display reduced use of mental state language during narrative production. Which words in the following narrative might a child with a ToM deficit have difficulty using? For each word you select, indicate if it is an aspect of *cognitive* ToM or *affective* ToM:

> Sally wanted to visit the zoo. So she got up early one morning and took the bus to the zoo with her friend Paula. When they arrived at the zoo, they discovered it was closed because a gorilla had escaped overnight. Although most other visitors were angry when they heard this news and decided to leave, Sally and Paula were happy to wait for the gates to open. Two hours later, the animal was caught and returned to its enclosure. Visitors were then invited into the zoo. Although many visitors appeared frightened, Sally and Paula decided to head straight to the gorilla enclosure to see the animal that had caused all the panic.

(3) Respond with *true* or *false* to each of the following statements about educational psychologists:
  (a) Educational psychologists are the only professionals who can administer the PPVT-4.
  (b) Educational psychologists assess learning in older adults as well as in children.
  (c) Educational psychologists use their knowledge of learning to inform instructional practices.
  (d) Educational psychologists are part of the multidisciplinary team that assesses children with special educational needs.
  (e) Educational psychologists only conduct psychometric testing of clients.

(4) Each of the following statements describes the function of one of the modules depicted in Figure 4.2. Identify the module in this diagram that is described by each statement:
  (a) This module contains representations of the spoken form of words including metrical information (number of syllables and stress patterns) and segmental information (phonemes and their relative positions).
  (b) This module contains the grapheme sequences that constitute the words of a language and must be accessed in order for irregular words like *debt* and *viscount* to be read aloud correctly.
  (c) This module must be accessed in order to establish that <L, $\mathcal{L}$ and $\mathbb{L}$> are all variants of the same letter.
  (d) This module must be accessed in order for non-words like 'manwag' and 'trimp' to be read aloud correctly.
  (e) This module must be accessed in order to establish that the spoken words *tribe* and *bribe* rhyme while *couch* and *touch* do not rhyme.

(5) Neuropsychological assessment is integral to the management of clients with cognitive-communication disorders. Which of the following statements describes a cognitive-communication disorder in a client?

(a) A 45-year-old man sustains a head injury in a motorbike accident. He displays poor impulse control and self-regulation following his accident. An SLT observes that he is inappropriate in conversation, with several of his remarks judged to be impolite and offensive.
(b) A 5-year-old child with cleft lip and palate and hearing loss is referred to SLT for assessment. His receptive and expressive language skills are delayed. A picture description task reveals poor cohesion and reduced information content.
(c) A 60-year-old man with Alzheimer's dementia displays poor episodic memory. He responds appropriately to greetings and is able to produce 'small talk' in conversation. However, his narrative skills are quite limited and he is unable to relate a significant family event for the SLT.
(d) A 10-year-old boy with specific language impairment has academic problems at school related to his language difficulties. His written language contains many errors of syntax and a limited use of vocabulary.
(e) A 55-year-old woman sustains damage to her right cerebral hemisphere as a result of a stroke. Her structural language skills are intact. However, in conversation she shifts topic abruptly, is tangential in her contributions and displays egocentric discourse.

(6) Examine the case study at the end of section 4.6, and then answer the following questions:
(a) Did Ms S present with any affective disorders that may have caused or served to perpetuate her dysphonia? If yes, what were these disorders?
(b) A laryngeal examination revealed that Ms S had no organic abnormality. Is this sufficient to warrant a diagnosis of psychogenic dysphonia? If not, what else is required for this diagnosis to be made?
(c) Ms S's volitional cough was good. What is the significance of this finding?
(d) Did the results of the clinical psychologist's assessment confirm Ms S's report of her affective state on initial presentation at hospital? Explain your response.
(e) The clinical psychologist embarked on a course of cognitive behavioural therapy with Ms S. Was CBT the only psychological intervention used with this client? Explain your response.

5 Assessment and Diagnosis

5.1 Introduction

Throughout this volume, the discussion of what should be included in the clinical education of SLT students has been guided by the recommendations of the three bodies with responsibility for SLT education in the UK: the Royal College of Speech and Language Therapists (RCSLT), the Quality Assurance Agency for Higher Education (QAA) and the Health & Care Professions Council (HCPC). In earlier chapters, it was described how these bodies require SLT students to have knowledge of a wide range of linguistic, medical, scientific and psychological disciplines. In the same way, these bodies also make specific recommendations about what SLT students and graduates may be expected to know in relation to the assessment and diagnosis of communication and swallowing disorders. In its guidelines for pre-registration SLT courses, the RCSLT states that courses should provide the following:

> Practice in assessment techniques (e.g. standardised and non-standardised tests, informal assessment, oro-facial examination, audiological assessment, conversation analysis).   (2010: 25)

The QAA requires the SLT award holder to be able to

> use published and self-generated assessments, instrumentation and transcription where appropriate to describe, identify, analyse, and evaluate developmental and acquired phonetic, phonological, semantic, syntactic, pragmatic, fluency, voice disorders and swallowing problems.   (2001: 9)

In its standards of proficiency for SLTs, the Health & Care Professions Council states that registrant SLTs must

> be able to administer, record, score and interpret a range of published and self-generated assessment tools to describe and analyse service users' abilities and needs using, where appropriate, phonetic transcription, linguistic analysis, instrumental analysis and psycholinguistic assessment.   (2013: 13)

Of course, assessment is not an end in itself but must lead to a diagnosis of a client's communication or swallowing disorder. Diagnosis is informed to a large extent by the results of assessment. However, it is also guided by the nosology of communication disorders, and classifications of disease and disability in general.

This is formalized in international classification systems such as the *Diagnostic and Statistical Manual of Mental Disorders – Fifth Edition* (DSM-5; American Psychiatric Association, 2013), the *International Classification of Diseases* (ICD-11; WHO, 2018) and the **International Classification of Functioning, Disability and Health** (ICF; WHO, 2001). These systems are regularly updated to reflect current knowledge of the full range of disorders that medical and health professionals encounter in their clinical practice. An understanding of the structure and purpose of these classification systems is an integral part of the clinical competence of today's speech and language therapists.

This chapter will examine assessment and diagnosis within an SLT context. The scope of this area of SLT practice is truly enormous. To facilitate discussion of this expansive aspect of SLT, this section will introduce readers to a number of issues that have general relevance to assessment and diagnosis. Complex clinical decision-making lies at the heart of assessment. To gain some insight into this decision-making, it is necessary to examine the questions that the SLT must address before embarking on assessment. At a minimum, the SLT must provide answers to the following questions:

(1) What aspect(s) of a client's communication skills or swallowing requires evaluation?
(2) How can these skills be best evaluated?
(3) What knowledge, training and clinical expertise are required to evaluate these skills?
(4) What equipment is required to evaluate these skills?
(5) Is the requisite equipment and expertise to assess these skills available in this case?
(6) Are there any circumstances that preclude the use of an assessment in this case?

The answer to (1) may be established at the point of referral. A **paediatrician** may have concerns that a child is displaying developmental delay in a number of areas. A referral may request a wide-ranging assessment of speech, language and communication skills. A referral from a **neurologist** in a head trauma unit may request investigation of a client's receptive language skills with a view to including the client's wishes in decisions about the nature and extent of medical intervention. A referral from a health visitor may simply state parental concerns that a child has 'speech delay'. In this case, an SLT will aim to establish if the child has age-appropriate language as well as speech skills. Aside from referral, the initial meeting with a client provides the SLT with valuable information about the aspects of communication that require evaluation. An informal interaction with the client provides the SLT with an opportunity to assess the intelligibility of speech, the client's ability to comprehend language and construct grammatical utterances, and the client's mastery of conversational dynamics such as turn-taking. This interaction also permits the SLT to establish if social deficits and cognitive impairment may be contributing to a client's communication difficulties. These associated problems may require assessment by other specialists. If a spouse, parent or caregiver attends this initial meeting, they can contribute important information that can help the SLT decide what should be the area of focus in an assessment. For example, the wife of a man with aphasia may remark on **cueing** strategies that help her husband produce words, indicating that **lexical retrieval** is an area that requires examination.

Having established the particular skills that need to be evaluated, the SLT then has to decide how this can best be achieved. In many cases, a formal, standardized test is the most effective method of assessment. An articulation test may be used to assess the speech skills of the child who is referred to SLT with 'speech delay'. One or more tests of receptive and expressive language may also be used to assess this child. A comprehensive language battery may be the most effective way of establishing the linguistic impairments of an adult with aphasia. However, if a client's structural language skills are relatively intact and there is suspicion of a pragmatic impairment, then evaluation is best achieved through the use of informal assessments. These assessments involve the use of techniques such as conversation analysis and discourse analysis, with data taking the form of a recorded conversation between an adult and his spouse or a narrative production task between a child and a parent. For clients with suspected dysphagia, swallowing may be best evaluated using videofluoroscopy. Indeed, videofluoroscopy may be the only definitive way to establish if **silent aspiration** is occurring and to determine if a client is safe to continue **oral feeding**. A perceptual assessment of a client's voice using rating scales is certainly informative. However, in order to understand the specific acoustic features that contribute to the perception of hoarseness or breathiness, the best assessment in this case involves an acoustic analysis of the client's voice. In short, the decision about what constitutes the best assessment of a client's communication skills and swallowing is highly variable and involves the exercise of considerable clinical judgement.

The knowledge, training and clinical expertise that are needed to undertake an assessment of a client's communication skills and swallowing vary considerably. In order to conduct an articulation test in a child with reported speech delay, the SLT must be able to complete a phonetic transcription of the child's single-word productions and connected speech. To establish the presence of simplifying processes in this child's speech, a phonological analysis may also be required. If language delay is suspected, an assessment of expressive and receptive syntax, vocabulary and semantics must also be conducted. A wide range of knowledge, experience and specialist training are needed to make these various linguistic analyses possible. Training in linguistic analysis is an integral part of the curriculum in pre-registration SLT courses (see Chapter 2). All SLT students should be competent to undertake phonetic transcription, for example, upon completion of such a course. However, the assessment of conditions such as dysphagia requires pre- and post-registration knowledge and training (RCSLT, 2014). Many assessments require considerable technical expertise in the use of specialist equipment and the interpretation of results. Nasometry and electropalatography are used to measure, respectively, the acoustic correlate of nasality and tongue-palate contacts during articulation. Both procedures employ equipment (e.g. a nasometer) which must be used safely and competently by the assessing clinician. Specialist knowledge and training are also needed to interpret the results of these instrumental analyses. Where such knowledge and training are not available, onward referral to specialist clinicians and centres is required.

As discussed above, a key component in the clinical decision-making of therapists who are embarking on assessment is knowledge of how best to assess certain skills. However, it is equally important for SLTs to understand when an assessment should not be performed, or at least not performed without modification or in isolation from other assessments. In some cases, this decision may be taken on account of a lack of safety. During **fibreoptic endoscopic evaluation of swallowing** (FEES), compromised breathing may occur in infants if a fibreoptic endoscope is placed in one nostril when a **nasogastric tube** is in position in the other nostril. An alternative method of swallowing assessment may be needed in this case. Alternatively, the feeding tube may need to be removed temporarily to make FEES possible. A further issue of safety arises in patients with a **tracheostomy**. It is physiologically contraindicated to assess swallowing when the cuff of a tracheostomy tube is inflated (see Figure 5.1). This is because a tracheal cannula with an inflated cuff reduces the normal movement of the larynx during swallowing. This can further compromise the patient's swallowing defect.

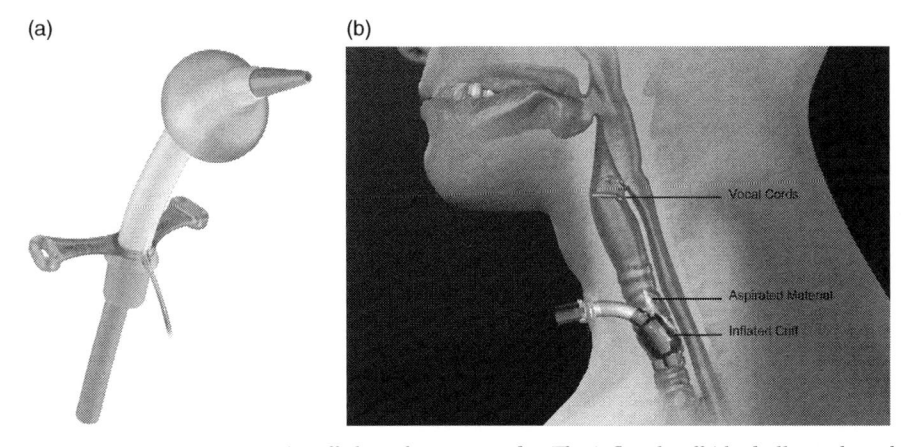

Figure 5.1 *(a) A cuffed tracheostomy tube. The inflated cuff (the balloon-shaped structure) surrounds the body of the tube and fills the tracheal space around it, preventing the leakage of air in a ventilated patient (Permission for use granted by Cook Medical, Bloomington, Indiana). (b) Tracheostomy tube in situ with cuff inflated (Image courtesy of Passy Muir, Inc. Irvine, CA)*

In other cases, an assessment should not be performed, at least not in isolation from other assessments, if there is a lack of evidence to support its clinical validity. Young et al. (2005) found that the *Strong Narrative Assessment Procedure* (SNAP; Strong, 1998) was poor at differentiating pragmatic language disorders in children with autism spectrum disorders when performance was compared to matched controls. The SNAP should, therefore, not be used in isolation to diagnose pragmatic deficits in children with ASD. However, the SNAP can throw light on a child's pragmatic language performance when it is used alongside other assessments such as the *Test of Pragmatic Language* (Phelps-Terasaki and Phelps-Gunn, 2007) and the *Children's Communication Checklist* (Bishop, 2003a). Both of these assessments have been found to be effective in differentiating the pragmatic deficits of children with ASD from pragmatic abilities in other clinical groups (e.g. ADHD) and in normal controls (Geurts et al., 2004; Young et al., 2005).

These introductory remarks highlight the complex clinical decision-making that SLTs must display during assessment and diagnosis. They will be developed further in the sections that follow. In section 5.2, an important distinction between formal and informal assessments is examined. This distinction cannot be straightforwardly captured as the difference between published and unpublished assessments, although most formal assessments are published tests which are available on a commercial basis. The examination of specific types of assessment begins in section 5.3 with a discussion of speech assessments. There is an abundance of published tests available to assess a client's speech. An examination of these tests must necessarily be selective in nature. The same is true of tests of receptive and expressive language, which will be discussed in section 5.4. In section 5.5, assessments of fluency are addressed. A wide range of tools is used to assess speech motor, linguistic, cognitive and affective components of fluency disorders in children and adults. In section 5.6, perceptual, acoustic and physiological techniques used to evaluate voice are considered. The assessment of feeding, swallowing and dysphagia is now a significant area of clinical work for SLTs. The techniques used to assess swallowing function are examined in section 5.7. Finally, the results of assessment are used to inform the diagnosis of disorders. The chapter concludes in section 5.8 with an examination of the major classification and diagnostic systems that are of relevance to SLT. (The use of different types of **audiometry** to assess hearing was discussed in section 3.6 of Chapter 3 and will not be addressed further in this chapter.)

5.2 Formal and Informal Assessment

A distinction of considerable importance in SLT is that between formal and informal assessment. Formal assessments exhibit a range of features that have secured them a significant place in clinical speech and language testing. These assessments are standardized and **norm-referenced**. They are relatively quick and easy to administer. Formal assessments can be used to chart changes in a client's performance over time. These assessments thus have a vital role to play in monitoring progress in therapy. Formal assessments are not without drawbacks, however. They are poor at assessing non-rule-based aspects of language such as pragmatics and discourse. They have poor **ecological validity** in that their tasks do not reflect the use of language in everyday communication. Informal assessments can also lay claim to a range of beneficial features. Through their use of techniques such as conversation analysis, informal assessments provide an in-depth analysis of language skills as used in everyday communication. These assessments thus have greater ecological validity than formal assessments. Informal assessments also give clinicians insight into a large range of language skills rather than one particular skill (e.g. receptive syntax). However, like formal assessments, informal assessments also have their drawbacks. From administration to transcription and analysis, these assessments are labour and time intensive. Findings based on informal assessments can vary with individual assessors and even with the same assessor on different occasions of use of an assessment. These properties and other features of formal and informal assessments can be illustrated through an examination of two scenarios.

Scenario 1 Sally is 5 years old and is referred to SLT by a paediatrician for assessment of her communication skills. Sally was born prematurely and was late to achieve a number of motor milestones. Her mother described her as a late talker and reported that she is moderately unintelligible to people outside of her immediate family. At nursery school, Sally frequently failed to follow instructions which were readily acted upon by her peers. Similar behaviour was observed by Sally's primary school teacher. Her failure to comply with instructions was construed by some teachers and classroom assistants as defiant behaviour. Sally's mother reported that she had many friends at school and at home, and that she enjoyed playing with her older siblings. Sally's hearing is normal. An assessment by an educational psychologist revealed normal performance or non-verbal IQ but reduced verbal IQ. Observation of Sally by an SLT indicated that she has good social communication skills but has evident difficulties with receptive and expressive language. During the first meeting, Sally was able to greet the SLT appropriately, was aware of how to take turns during conversation and contributed a range of speech acts in interactions with her mother and the SLT, albeit with the use of immature grammatical forms. A detailed **case history** indicated that one of Sally's older siblings (a brother) was also a late talker and had attended SLT three years earlier. Problems with speaking and reading were identified in two of Sally's biological uncles.

The scenario described above is familiar to many SLTs. To guide the selection of assessments to be used in this case, the SLT can draw on several sources of information. Observation of Sally in interaction with her mother and the SLT indicates that pragmatic language and social communication skills are appropriate for a child of Sally's age. Because these skills are an area of strength for Sally, informal assessments that examine conversational skills and narrative production and comprehension abilities are not a priority in this case. In order to establish if Sally has a developmental delay, the paediatrician will be interested in comparing Sally's communication skills with those of her same-age peers. Standardized, norm-referenced formal assessments must be used in this case. Sally's poor intelligibility to unfamiliar listeners indicates the need to assess her speech production skills through an articulation test. The *Diagnostic Evaluation of Articulation and Phonology* (DEAP; Dodd et al., 2006) is a standardized, norm-referenced articulation test that can be used with children in the age range 3;0 to 8;11 years. The DEAP also permits a phonological analysis to be conducted, which is important in Sally's case given her unintelligibility.

Further, Sally's inability to follow instructions in class and her use of immature grammatical forms suggest that receptive and expressive language may be areas of weakness that require assessment. A widely used, standardized, norm-referenced assessment of expressive and receptive language is the *Clinical Evaluation of Language Fundamentals – Fifth Edition* (CELF-5; Wiig et al., 2013). Finally, given Sally's delay in achieving certain motor milestones, an assessment of the structure and sensory and motor function of her oral mechanism should be conducted. The DEAP contains an oral motor screen that can be used for this purpose. In conclusion, Sally requires formal assessment of her speech production skills as well as her receptive and expressive language skills. Given Sally's age-appropriate social communication skills, informal assessment is not indicated in this case.

Scenario 2 Mike is 35 years old and is an inpatient in a head trauma unit. He sustained severe frontal lobe damage in a motorbike accident and was in intensive care for three weeks. Mike's neurologist has referred him to SLT for assessment of his communication skills and swallowing. An SLT conducts a **bedside assessment**. In her report, she states that Mike is severely dysarthric. His risk of silent aspiration is assessed to be high, and it is recommended that Mike should be fed non-orally. On account of Mike's severe dysarthria, an assessment of his expressive language skills is difficult to undertake. Mike appears to understand short, grammatically simple utterances. However, his comprehension of longer, more complex utterances is poor. Four months after his accident, Mike is seen in the SLT department of the hospital for the first time as an outpatient. His wife is in attendance. The SLT observes Mike in conversation with his wife. Mike's wife reports considerable communication and cognitive difficulties with him at home. He shifts topics abruptly during conversation and interjects on the turns of his wife. His utterances can be irrelevant and excessively detailed. He frequently makes impolite or inappropriate remarks and is quite often repetitive. Mike's wife reports that his communication difficulties are a source of tension in their relationship and have restricted his activities. His spoken utterances are well structured although he is slow to produce them. Mike appears to rely on contextual cues for comprehension of language during conversation. Mike is now moderately dysarthric. Videofluoroscopic examination of swallowing before discharge from hospital revealed no aspiration and Mike reports no feeding or swallowing problems at home. The SLT wants to begin a new episode of care for Mike with an assessment of his communication skills.

The SLT must decide how best to assess Mike's current communication skills. His dysarthria can be formally assessed by means of the *Frenchay Dysarthria Assessment – Second Edition* (FDA-2; Enderby and Palmer, 2008). This standardized test contains normative data for adults without dysarthria as well as patients with dysarthrias associated with confirmed medical diagnoses. An oral motor and sensory examination is included in the FDA-2. Given Mike's reliance on contextual cues to facilitate comprehension in conversation, formal assessment of his expressive and receptive language skills should also be undertaken. Two widely used, standardized language assessments which may be conducted are the *Western Aphasia Battery – Revised* (WAB-R; Kertesz, 2006) and the *Boston Diagnostic Aphasia Examination – Third Edition* (BDAE-3; Goodglass et al., 2001). The WAB-R was originally normed on just 20 subjects (6 neurologically healthy individuals and 14 subjects with aphasia), although other normative data has been produced since its publication (Milman et al., 2014). The percentiles in the BDAE-3 are based on a sample of individuals with aphasia, while the Boston Naming Test (one component of the BDAE-3) is normed on 210 cognitively intact adults aged 18 to 79 years. All three of these standardized, norm-referenced assessments may be used pre-intervention to establish a baseline for Mike's speech and language skills, and post-intervention to gauge his progress in any therapy that may be implemented.

A comprehensive assessment of Mike's communication skills does not end with the FDA-2, the WAB-R and the BDAE-3. Although Mike can produce well-structured utterances, he does so slowly. This may indicate that cognitive deficits such as slowed information processing are contributing to his language difficulties. Several of Mike's conversational difficulties also suggest the involvement of cognitive deficits. These deficits might necessitate onward referral of Mike to a neuropsychologist for assessment of his cognitive difficulties. There are also standardized tests that SLTs can use to assess cognitive-communication disorders in individuals with traumatic brain injury (TBI) (Turkstra et al., 2005). One standardized, norm-referenced test that can be used for this purpose is the *Repeatable Battery for the Assessment of Neuropsychological Status Update* (RBANS Update; Randolph, 2012), which assesses immediate and delayed memory, attention, language and visuospatial/constructional skills. Mike's communication difficulties are limiting his activity and participation and causing tension in his relationship with his wife. These dimensions can be assessed through the use of the *Functional Assessment of Communication Skills for Adults* (ASHA FACS; Frattali et al., 1995), an assessment of **functional communication** that is consistent with the ICF framework (WHO, 2001). ASHA FACS is one of seven standardized, norm-referenced assessments that met criteria for **validity** and **reliability** in a review of assessments for use with individuals with cognitive-communication disorder following TBI (Turkstra et al., 2005).

Standardized, norm-referenced assessments of Mike's speech, language and cognitive-communication skills provide the SLT with important information thath can be used to plan intervention. However, Mike also displays a range of conversational difficulties that are best evaluated through the use of informal assessments. Conversation analysis can help the SLT investigate Mike's **topic management** and problems with **turn-taking**. Mike exhibits difficulties with **information management** in that his contributions are often irrelevant and excessively detailed. Narrative production tasks can shed light on the nature and extent of these difficulties. Both types of informal assessment may be used to explore Mike's repetitiveness and his use of impolite and inappropriate remarks. It is important to emphasize that 'informal' does not mean 'unstructured'. Specific prompts may be used by the SLT during a conversation with Mike to ensure that a range of topics is addressed or speech acts solicited. Also, checklists and protocols such as the *Pragmatic Protocol* (Prutting and Kirchner, 1987) may be used during the analysis and rating of transcribed conversational data. These techniques ensure that diverse verbal and non-verbal pragmatic skills can be rated for their appropriateness in an exchange. It is also important to emphasize that 'informal' does not mean that only qualitative analyses of data can be undertaken. Quantitative measures including percentage of **correct information units**, correct information units per minute, and words per minute may be used to analyse **narrative discourse**. It emerges that Mike's communication skills are best evaluated through a combination of formal and informal assessments. The advantages and disadvantages of both types of assessment are summarized in Table 5.1.

Table 5.1 *Advantages and disadvantages of formal and informal assessments*

FORMAL ASSESSMENTS	INFORMAL ASSESSMENTS
Advantages: • *standardized:* uniform administration and scoring by different examiners in varied settings reduces influence of tester and context on a client's performance • *norm-referenced:* a client's performance can be compared to the performance of a normative group • *administration:* assessments are relatively quick and easy to perform • *intervention:* assessments permit comparison of pre- and post-intervention skills • *common language:* terms such as test-retest reliability, percentiles and Z scores will be understood by other professionals (e.g. psychologists) **Disadvantages:** • *poor ecological validity:* tasks used in formal assessments do not resemble everyday communication • *discrete skills:* aspects of language which typically interact (e.g. phonology and grammar) are tested in isolation from each other • *formal situation:* clients may become anxious, nervous or reticent if they feel they are being tested • *equipment and stimuli:* test stimuli and equipment may be culturally inappropriate or disadvantage clients from certain social backgrounds • *normative data:* limited normative data may restrict use of tests to clients of certain ages or educational and social backgrounds	**Advantages:** • *language use:* informal assessments can be used to evaluate the use of language (pragmatics) in conversation and other forms of discourse • *good ecological validity:* conversation, storytelling and other forms of discourse closely resemble everyday communication • *compensatory strategies:* SLTs can assess the effectiveness of spontaneous and taught compensatory strategies by clients • *conversation partners:* SLTs can assess the extent to which partners facilitate and hinder communication with the client • *informal situation:* clients are likely to reflect their normal communication styles when they do not feel they are being tested or trying to produce a 'correct' response **Disadvantages:** • *transcription and analysis:* the recording, transcription and analysis of even small amounts of conversation and narrative discourse is time and labour intensive • *non-standardized:* a lack of systematically applied procedures means that a client's performance may not reflect his or her actual abilities • *intervention:* progress in therapy is less easily documented through the use of informal assessments • *normative data:* a lack of normative data makes it difficult to compare a client's performance to peers of similar age, education and social class • *reduced structure:* clients with cognitive deficits may be unable to cope with the reduced structure of informal assessments

KEY POINTS: Formal and Informal Assessment

- SLTs must understand and be able to undertake competently formal and informal assessments. This includes the selection of appropriate tests, the analysis and scoring of data and the interpretation of results.
- Formal assessments are widely used by SLTs. These assessments are standardized, norm-referenced tests that are relatively quick and easy to administer. They can be used to compare performance over time and monitor progress in therapy.
- Formal assessments are most effectively used to test rule-based aspects of language (e.g. phonology, syntax). To assess aspects of pragmatics and discourse, clinicians use informal assessments.
- Informal assessments include techniques such as conversation analysis and discourse analysis. These assessments provide insight into aspects of language that are not readily assessed using formal procedures. Informal assessments are time and labour intensive to conduct, which has limited their widespread use in SLT clinics.
- The selection of which formal and informal assessments to use in a particular case is guided by a range of considerations, including the purpose of referral to SLT, the nature of a client's communication difficulties, and the expertise and equipment available in a clinic.

GROUP EXERCISE: Formal and Informal Assessment

Shipley and McAfee (2009: 254) state that 'informal assessment is an important component of a complete language evaluation. It allows the clinician to assess certain aspects of language more deeply than formal assessment allows, and it provides the opportunity to view a client's functional use of language in natural contexts.' Use this statement as a starting point in your discussion of the respective merits of formal and informal language assessment. Give examples of how each method of assessment has an important role to play in the evaluation of a client's language skills.

5.3 Clinical Assessments: Speech

A speech assessment should be conducted in any client with reduced intelligibility. Problems with intelligibility can arise on account of several disorders. It is the aim of assessment to uncover which of these disorders is responsible for a client's unintelligibility in a particular case. A child or adult may be unintelligible because of a structural defect of the organs of articulation such as the palate (in a child with cleft palate), jaw (in a child with micrognathia) or tongue (in an adult with **glossectomy**). A child or adult with normal speech anatomy may be unintelligible because the programming of motor movements for speech production is impaired (so-called **apraxia of speech**). The programming of movements may occur normally only for a child or adult to have difficulty with the execution of motor movements for speech production (so-called dysarthria). Motor programming and motor execution for speech production may both be intact. Yet, a child may still be unintelligible on account of reduced phonemic contrasts in his or her phonological system. It is the aim of assessment to achieve a comprehensive evaluation of a client's speech skills with a view to conducting a differential diagnosis of these various disorders. A range of procedures can be used by SLTs to assess speech skills. They include an oral mechanism examination, articulation tests, phonological analyses and instrumental techniques. These procedures may be used singly but are more often employed in combination during a speech assessment. Each procedure is examined in turn in this section.

It is important for SLTs to establish if a client has normal anatomy and physiology for speech production. This is achieved through an oral mechanism examination. The structural and functional adequacy of the lips, teeth, tongue, mandible and hard and soft palates for speech production must be determined. Noteworthy structural defects include a **bifid uvula**, a **submucous cleft palate** or palatal **fistulae**, missing teeth or too many teeth, a large tongue (macroglossia), and a small jaw (micrognathia). It is important to record whether structures such as the lips, tongue, mandible and **soft palate** are symmetrical at rest, and to note muscle tone and the presence of any abnormal movements. For example, structures such as the lips and soft palate may deviate to the left or to the right, while the tongue may exhibit fasciculations. To establish the functional adequacy of the articulators, SLTs ask clients to perform movements such as pursing and spreading the lips, protruding and elevating the tongue, and opening and closing the mouth. The symmetry of movement as well as the strength and range of movement should be recorded. The use of a tongue depressor is the most common clinical method for assessing tongue strength. The strength of tongue lateralization can be assessed by having a subject push against a tongue depressor that is placed to the right and left of the lips. An assessment of the movement of the articulators provides SLTs with an opportunity to screen the cranial nerves. For example, the motor function of the hypoglossal nerve (CN XII) can be assessed by examining tongue protrusion (without lip assistance) and tongue tip elevation (without jaw assistance). Other tasks can also be undertaken to assess cranial nerve function. The motor function of the facial nerve (CN VII) can be tested by asking the subject to puff his cheeks and resist the therapist's efforts to push them in.

Abnormalities of symmetry, tone, strength and range of movement, and the presence of abnormal reflexes, may support a diagnosis of dysarthria. In spastic dysarthria, for example, there is increased muscle tone (**hypertonia**), reduced range of movement, weakness, a hyperactive **gag reflex** and pathological oral reflexes (e.g. **suck reflex**). The oral mechanism is only one speech production subsystem. Other systems such as respiration, phonation, resonation and

prosody may also be compromised in dysarthria. For example, the speaker with spastic dysarthria may also exhibit phonatory and prosodic abnormalities such as strained-harsh **voice quality** and reduced variability of pitch (**monopitch**) and loudness (**monoloudness**). An oral mechanism evaluation must not be conducted to the exclusion of an examination of these other speech production subsystems, especially where dysarthria is suspected. If no abnormalities of symmetry, tone, strength and range of movement are identified, an oral mechanism examination can still be revealing in other ways. For example, a client may be unable to protrude and elevate the tongue or round and spread the lips, not on account of any neuromuscular impairment (as in dysarthria) but because of the presence of **oral apraxia**. If apraxia for non-speech oral movements is identified, it raises suspicion of childhood apraxia of speech (CAS) or apraxia of speech (AOS) in adults. CAS and AOS are motor speech disorders in which the speaker has difficulty sequencing muscle movements for volitional production of phonemes and sequences of phonemes. It is with a view to excluding CAS or AOS that most clinicians include a measurement of **diadochokinetic (DDK) rates** (i.e. timed repetition of CV sequences like /pə, tə, kə/) within an oral examination.

A comprehensive oral mechanism examination should be the starting point in an assessment of a client's speech skills. The results of this examination inform the selection of later speech assessments. Where structural defects or neuromuscular impairments are identified, specific instruments may then be used to examine the implications of these anomalies for speech production. In the UK, the *Great Ormond Street Speech Assessment* (GOS.SP.ASS; Sell et al., 1994) is the nationally agreed tool for the assessment and diagnosis of speech difficulties associated with cleft palate (Mildinhall, 2012). The GOS.SP.ASS is a non-standardized assessment that can be used to evaluate phonetic and phonological aspects of speech. The revised assessment (Sell et al., 1999) includes ratings of resonance, **nasal emission**, **nasal turbulence** and **grimace**; the identification of cleft type characteristics such as glottal articulation and developmental speech errors; an assessment of voice, language and the visual appearance of speech (e.g. tight upper lip); and a comprehensive oral examination. Although originally devised as an assessment for the cleft palate population, the GOS.SP.ASS may also be used of individuals who do not have palatal clefts. Shipster et al. (2002) used the GOS.SP.ASS to assess the speech skills of ten children with **Apert syndrome** who were aged from 4;1 to 5;11 years. None of these children had cleft palate.

Where neuromuscular impairment is believed to underlie a client's speech problems, an assessment of dysarthria should be undertaken. Several published assessments are available for this purpose including the FDA-2 (Enderby and Palmer, 2008), mentioned in section 5.2, and the *Dysarthria Examination Battery* (DEB; Drummond, 1993). The FDA-2 contains 11 sections: Reflex; Respiration; Lips; Jaws; Palate; Larynx; Tongue; Intelligibility; Rate; Sensation; and Associated Factors. It may be used to assess dysarthria in children and adults in both research and clinical settings. Eigentler et al. (2012) used the FDA to assess dysarthria in 15 patients with **Friedreich's ataxia**. The FDA sub-item voice (larynx) was most affected in these patients compared to healthy individuals, followed by reflexes, palate, tongue and intelligibility. Lips, jaws and respiration were mildly affected. The DEB contains 15 rating-scale items and 21 quantitative tasks. The battery is organized by speech production subsystems: respiration; phonation; resonation; articulation; and prosody. An assessment of intelligibility is based on listener judgements of single-word and sentence productions. The DEB requires the use of specialist equipment that may not be available in all clinics. For example, an assessment of vital capacity under respiration requires the use of a dry **spirometer**, while speech analysis instrumentation is needed to assess fundamental frequency under phonation.

If an oral mechanism examination reveals a possible apraxic component to a client's speech production difficulties, further investigation of CAS or AOS should be conducted. Although there are several published tests for the assessment of CAS and AOS, only two will be examined in this context: the *Kaufman Speech Praxis Test* (KSPT; Kaufman, 1995) and the *Apraxia Battery for Adults – Second Edition* (ABA-2; Dabul, 2000). The KSPT is a standardized, norm-referenced assessment that can be used to identify CAS in children aged 2;0 to 5;11 years. Items are organized from simple to complex motor speech movements and use meaningful words whenever possible. The assessment is stimulus/response oriented. All items are imitative and can be administered without the need for pictorial stimulation. To illustrate the motor hierarchy used in this assessment, the KSPT scales are shown below along with sample items:

(1) Oral movement (e.g. open mouth)
(2) Simple phonemic/syllabic
  Pure vowels (e.g. /a/ as in *father*)
  Vowel to vowel (e.g. /aI/ as in *high*)
  Simple consonants (e.g. /m/)
  Consonant to vowel (e.g. /pe/ as in *pay*)
  Vowel-consonant-vowel (e.g. /apo/ as in *ah-poe*)
  Repetitive syllables (e.g. *mama*)
  Repetitive syllables with vowel change (e.g. *mommy*)
  Simple bisyllabics with C and V change (e.g. *happy*)
  Simple monosyllabics with assimilation (e.g. *pop*)
  Simple consonants: isolated (/m/); initial (*man*); final (*home*)
(3) Complex phonemic/syllabic
  Complex consonants: isolated (/k/); initial (*cup*); final (*book*)
  Blends: /l/ blends (*clean*); /r/ blends (*green*); /s/ blends (*swing*)
  Front to back / back to front (e.g. *duck*)
  Complex bisyllabics (e.g. *wagon*)
  Polysyllabics (e.g. *banana*)
  Length and complexity (e.g. *soup; sugar; superman*)
(4) Spontaneous length/complexity
  KSPT rating scale

The ABA-2 is a standardized assessment based on normative samples of 40 individuals with apraxia (aged 33–93 years) and 49 individuals with normal speech (aged 30–90 years). The battery consists of six subtests that take around 20 minutes to administer. Subtests include: diadochokinetic rate; increasing word length; **limb apraxia** and oral apraxia; latency time and utterance time for polysyllabic words; repeated trials test; and an inventory of articulation characteristics of apraxia. The inventory includes several features that have diagnostic significance for AOS. Their influence in clinical and research settings is such that they are listed in full below:

(1)   Exhibits phonemic anticipatory errors
(2)   Exhibits phonemic perseverative errors
(3)   Exhibits phonemic transposition errors
(4)   Exhibits phonemic voicing errors
(5)   Exhibits phonemic vowel errors
(6)   Exhibits visible/audible searching
(7)   Exhibits numerous off-target attempts at the word
(8)   Errors are highly inconsistent
(9)   Errors increase as phonemic sequence increases
(10) Exhibits fewer errors with automatic speech than volitional speech
(11) Exhibits marked difficulty initiating speech
(12) Intrudes schwa sound /ə/ between syllables or in consonant clusters
(13) Exhibits abnormal prosodic features
(14) Exhibits awareness of errors and inability to correct them
(15) Exhibits expressive-receptive gap

As well as assessing stroke-induced AOS (Trupe et al., 2013), the ABA-2 can be used to examine AOS in clients with neurodegenerative disorders such as **progressive nonfluent aphasia**, a subtype of **frontotemporal lobar degeneration** (Rohrer et al., 2010).

The assessments examined so far are used to evaluate speech production in clients where motor speech disorders such as dysarthria and apraxia of speech are suspected. Clinicians can also use a range of articulation tests to establish the phonetic inventories of clients who exhibit unintelligible speech but in whom an oral examination raises no suspicion of a motor speech disorder. A widely used, standardized, norm-referenced test of articulation is the *Goldman-Fristoe Test of Articulation – Third Edition* (GFTA-3; Goldman and Fristoe, 2015). The GFTA-3 can be used with individuals in the age range 2;0 to 21;11 years. This test examines 39 consonant sounds and clusters used in Standard American English. Spontaneous and imitative sound production is examined in word-initial, medial and final positions. There are three sections in the GFTA-3. In the sounds-in-words section, examinees respond to picture plates and verbal cues from the examiner with single-word answers. The verbal cue that accompanies the images in Figure 5.2 is 'An apple is a fruit; a carrot is a _____'. Separate images are

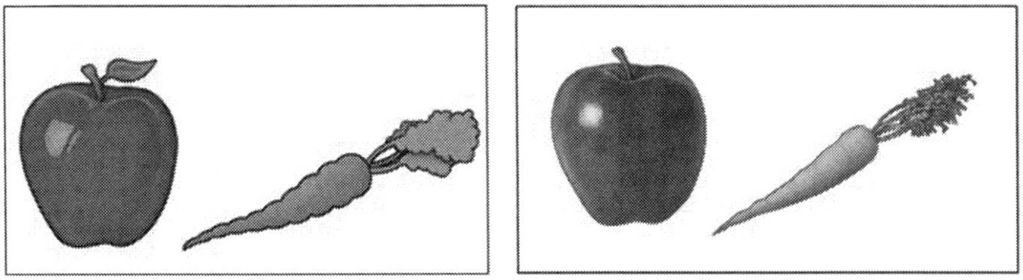

Figure 5.2 *Pictures from the* Goldman-Fristoe Test of Articulation – Third Edition *(GFTA-3; Goldman and Fristoe, 2015) for younger (left) and older (right) examinees (Copyright © 2015 NCS Pearson, Inc. Reproduced with permission. All rights reserved). (A colour version of this image is also available in the plate section.)*

used in the GFTA-3 for younger subjects (2;0 to 6;11 years) and older subjects (7;0 to 21;11 years). In the sounds-in-sentences section, examinees are asked to retell a short story based on a picture cue. This section of the test contains an intelligibility rating. The **stimulability** section measures an individual's ability to correctly produce a previously misarticulated sound after watching and listening to the examiner's production of the sound. The examinee repeats the word or phrase which is modelled by the examiner. Vowels are assessed for the first time in the GFTA-3. It contains dialect-sensitive scoring for a range of American English dialects as well as English which is influenced by another language.

Following assessment of an individual's articulation ability, it is necessary to establish if articulatory errors are related to the presence of phonological processes. There is a wide range of published assessments which can be used for this purpose. One phonological assessment that is used in conjunction with the GFTA-3 is the *Khan-Lewis Phonological Analysis – Third Edition* (KLPA-3; Khan and Lewis, 2015). The KLPA-3 is a norm-referenced analysis of an individual's speech development and phonological process usage. It requires the administration of the 60 target words in the sounds-in-words section of the GFTA-3. The analysis is used to identify the frequency of usage of 12 core and 12 supplemental phonological processes that are grouped into four types of processes (manner; place; reduction; and voicing) as well as other processes used by the individual. The 12 core processes occur frequently in the speech of young children and are considered to be developmental processes, while the supplemental processes occur less frequently and are atypical patterns. Standard scores and percentile ranks by age and sex are available for the core processes. Core and supplemental phonological processes are shown in Table 5.2. As well as using the KLPA-3 to obtain an inventory of consonant phonemes, it can be used to determine if an individual produces vowel alterations.

Finally, SLTs can use a range of instrumental techniques to assess speech production in children and adults. These techniques, which include nasometry,

Table 5.2 *Core and supplemental phonological processes in the* Khan-Lewis Phonological Analysis – Third Edition *(KLPA-3; Khan and Lewis, 2015)*

Core phonological processes	Supplemental phonological processes
Manner:	**Manner:**
Deaffrication	Affrication
Gliding of liquids	Frication
Stopping of fricatives and affricates	Gliding (other)
Stridency deletion	Glottal replacement
Vocalization	Liquidization
	Stopping (other)
Place:	**Place:**
Palatal fronting	Backing to velars or /h/
Velar fronting	
Reduction:	**Reduction:**
Cluster simplification	Deletion of initial consonant
Deletion of final consonant	Deletion of medial consonant
Syllable reduction	
Voicing:	**Voicing:**
Final devoicing	Initial devoicing
Initial voicing	Medial devoicing
	Medial voicing

videofluoroscopy and electropalatography, can be used to assess the effect of structural anomalies (e.g. palatal clefts and fistulae) and neuromuscular deficits (e.g. a paretic or paralysed velum) on speech production. Nasometry is used to measure the acoustic correlate of nasality. The nasometer produces a score which represents the ratio of energy in oral and nasal acoustic sound signals. Nasometry can be used to confirm the perception of **hypernasal resonance** in clients with **velopharyngeal insufficiency** (e.g. children with cleft palate). Videofluoroscopy is a radiographic tool that may be used to assess the movement of the velum and closure of the velopharyngeal port during speech production. (Videofluoroscopy is examined further in section 5.8 in relation to the assessment of swallowing.) Electropalatography is an instrumental technique that can be used to assess lingual involvement in a range of aberrant articulations. This may be maladaptive lingual articulations that children with cleft palate develop as a means of compensating for their compromised speech anatomy. The client wears a palatal plate that contains electrodes. The electrodes record any contact between the tongue and hard and soft palates. As well as an assessment technique, electropalatography is a valuable therapeutic aid on account of its provision of visual feedback to clients. Ultrasound imaging of the tongue is increasingly being used by SLTs, for example, to visualize the tongue in children with speech sound errors (Preston et al., 2017). The use of instrumental techniques may be contraindicated in certain cases. For example, not all subjects can tolerate the artificial palate that must be worn in electropalatography. Instrumental techniques are most often used alongside perceptual measures in a comprehensive speech assessment of clients.

> **KEY POINTS: Clinical Assessments: Speech**
> - Assessment of a client's speech should begin with a comprehensive oral mechanism examination. This examination establishes the structural and functional adequacy of the articulators for speech production.
> - An oral mechanism examination can identify structural anomalies that contribute to a speech disorder (e.g. overbite, fistulae). Anomalies related to cleft palate can be examined further through the use of the *Great Ormond Street Speech Assessment* (GOS.SP.ASS).
> - An oral mechanism examination can identify neuromuscular deficits and raise suspicion of dysarthria. Perceptual assessments such as the *Frenchay Dysarthria Assessment – Second Edition* (FDA-2) can be used to investigate dysarthric speech features. Instrumental techniques may also be used to evaluate dysarthria.
> - Even if an oral mechanism examination does not identify neuromuscular deficits, it may reveal deficits in the volitional production of non-speech, oral movements (oral apraxia). For these clients, assessment of apraxia of speech should be undertaken.
> - SLTs can also undertake articulation testing of clients with no motor speech disorders to establish their phonetic inventories. The *Goldman-Fristoe Test of Articulation – Third Edition* (GFTA-3) is the most widely used test for this purpose.
> - To establish if phonological processes explain a client's speech errors and unintelligibility, SLTs also routinely undertake a phonological analysis. There are many published assessments of phonology. The *Khan-Lewis Phonological Analysis – Third Edition* (KLPA-3) is used in conjunction with the GFTA-3.
> - Alongside perceptual speech assessments, SLTs often use instrumental techniques to assess speech production in children and adults. These techniques are numerous and include nasometry, spirometry, electropalatography and videofluoroscopy.

5.4 Clinical Assessments: Language

The assessment of language involves a combination of formal and informal procedures. Structural levels of language such as phonology, morphology, syntax and semantics are typically assessed through the use of standardized, norm referenced tests and batteries. Some of these tests examine several language levels; others assess only one aspect of language. For example, CELF-5 (Wiig et al., 2013) examines morphology, syntax, semantics and pragmatics, while the *Peabody Picture Vocabulary Test – Fourth Edition* (PPVT-4; Dunn and Dunn, 2007) assesses vocabulary only. Some language assessments examine receptive aspects of language only, such as the *Test for Reception of Grammar – Version 2* (TROG-2; Bishop, 2003b) that assesses the comprehension of **grammar**. Other assessments examine expressive and receptive aspects of language (e.g. CELF-5). Aside from standardized, norm-referenced assessments, language may also be assessed through the use of informal procedures. Informal assessments are particularly suited to the assessment of non-rule-based aspects of language such as pragmatics. Pragmatic language skills such as topic management, use and understanding of a range of speech acts, and the encoding of information in the presuppositions of an utterance are best examined through techniques such as conversation analysis and discourse analysis. Typically, checklists and rating scales may be used alongside these techniques to ensure a comprehensive analysis of a range of pragmatic and discourse features. In this section, each of these approaches to language assessment in SLT will be examined in detail.

Formal procedures tend to dominate the assessment of language in SLT. There are several reasons why this is the case. More often than not, the aim of assessment is to establish if a child's language skills are age-appropriate. This requires that a comparison be made between the child's language skills and those of a normative group of age-matched peers. The use of a norm-referenced assessment of language is the only way to decide if a child has age-appropriate language skills. But there are other reasons why an SLT may decide to assess a child's language skills formally. Increasingly, SLTs are required to demonstrate the efficacy of their interventions to parents, healthcare providers and medical insurance companies. This requires that a comparison be made between pre-intervention and post-intervention language skills, a comparison that can only be achieved if a standardized assessment of language is conducted. Formal assessments of language are also popular among time-pressed SLTs on account of their ease of administration and scoring. Even a small amount of conversation can take several hours to transcribe and analyse, while a formal language assessment can be conducted in 10–20 minutes for smaller assessments (such as TROG-2) or in 30–45 minutes for larger batteries (such as the CELF-5 Core Language Score). For each of these reasons, SLTs may expect to find themselves conducting formal language assessments on a regular basis in clinic. Knowledge of these assessments and experience in conducting them are a vital component of the clinical education of SLT students.

The language battery is a self-contained instrument for the assessment of language at each of its levels (e.g. syntax, semantics) and across all modalities (e.g. speech, reading, and writing). Language batteries are used for the most part either with children or adults and are not restricted to individuals with specific aetiologies or clinical disorders. For example, the CELF-5 can be used to assess clients between 5;0 and 21;11 years who may be at risk of language disorder on account of specific language impairment, intellectual disability, autism spectrum disorder or a range of other conditions. The comprehensive overview of a client's language skills that is possible with a language battery is a large part of the appeal of these assessments to clinicians. The CELF-5, for example, contains 16 stand-alone tests that assess receptive and expressive aspects of all language levels. Each test and its objectives are displayed in Table 5.3. Depending on the objective of an evaluation of a client's language, only some of these tests may be administered. The CELF-5 tests come together to form a Core Language Score and several index scores. The Core Language Score, for example, is based on the following tests: word classes; formulated sentences; recalling sentences; and semantic relationships. Standard scores and test-age equivalents are available for the Core Language Score, the Receptive Language Index, the Expressive Language Index, the Language Content Index and the Language Structure Index. The test's norms are based on a large sample of 2,380 students aged 5–21 years.

A widely used language battery for the assessment of aphasia in adults is the BDAE-3 (Goodglass et al., 2001). The BDAE-3 can be used to diagnose clients with one of the aphasia syndromes. There are three versions of the battery: Standard; Short; and Extended. The assessment can be used with individuals aged 16 years and older and takes 90 minutes to administer (40–60 minutes for the Short Form). The Standard Form contains the following five domains: Conversational and Expository Speech; Auditory Comprehension; Oral Expression; Reading; and Writing. The subtests within these domains are displayed in Table 5.4. Means and standard deviations based on aphasic subjects are provided for these subtests. The Boston Naming Test is a measure of visual confrontation naming. It is incorporated for the first time in BDAE-3 as a subtest in the Oral Expression domain. The Extended Form of the BDAE-3 contains the additional domain Praxis, which has four subtests: natural gestures; conventional gestures; use of pretended objects; and bucco-facial respiratory movements. A separate Spatial-Quantitative Battery examines constructional deficits, **finger agnosia**, **acalculia** and right-left orientation. As well as individual subtest scores, clinicians can calculate three other scores using the BDAE-3. These scores include: the Severity Rating Scale (a rating of the severity of observed speech/language disturbance); the Rating Scale Profile of Speech Characteristics (a rating of observed speech characteristics and of scores in two main language domains); and the Language Competency Index (a composite score of language performance on BDAE-3 subtests).

Batteries like the CELF-5 and the BDAE-3 can be used to reveal areas of language that require more extensive investigation. For example, a child who performs poorly in the sentence comprehension test of the CELF-5 may require further examination of receptive syntax. SLTs can then use more specific assessments to examine the nature and extent of this linguistic impairment. TROG-2 permits the clinician to probe in a detailed way the particular syntactic structures

Table 5.3 *The* Clinical Evaluation of Language Fundamentals – Fifth Edition *(CELF-5; Wiig et al., 2013) tests and their objectives*

Observational rating scale
  Objective: To document a student's ability to manage classroom behaviours and interactions, and to meet school curriculum objectives for following teacher instructions.
  Examples: Statements such as the following are rated as: never or almost never/ sometimes/often/always or almost always
  Has trouble looking at people when talking or listening
  Has trouble understanding facial expressions, gestures or body language

Sentence comprehension
  Objective: To evaluate the student's ability to (a) interpret spoken sentences of increasing length and complexity, and (b) select the pictures that illustrate referential meaning of the sentences.
  Examples: Students are asked to point to one of four pictures corresponding to the following sentences:
  The girl is being pushed by the boy.
  The duck is walking toward the girl.

Linguistic concepts
  Objective: To evaluate the student's ability to interpret spoken directions with basic concepts, which requires logical operations such as inclusion and exclusion, orientation and timing, and identifying mentioned objects from among several pictured choices.
  Examples: The student is shown a selection of pictures and is asked:
  Point to the ball.
  Point to the sun.

Word structure
  Objective: To evaluate the student's ability to (a) apply word structure rules (morphology) to mark inflections, derivations and comparison; and (b) select and use appropriate pronouns to refer to people, objects and possessive relationships.
  Examples: The student is shown pictures as the following sentences are read aloud:
  This boy is standing and this boy is _____ (sitting).
  Here is one book. Here are two _____ (books).

Word classes
  Objective: To evaluate the student's ability to understand relationships between words based on semantic class features, function, or place or time of occurrence.
  Examples: The student is shown a set of three pictures which are named aloud by the examiner. The student is then asked to point to the two pictures that go together:
  <u>cat</u> cow <u>kitten</u>
  <u>marker</u> <u>pencil</u> strawberry

Table 5.3 (*cont.*)

Following directions
   Objective: To evaluate the student's ability to (a) interpret spoken directions of increasing length and complexity; (b) follow the stated order of mention of familiar shapes with varying characteristics such as colour, size or location; and (c) identify from among several choices the pictured objects that were mentioned. These abilities reflect short-term and procedural memory capacities.
   Examples: The student is shown pictures and is asked to:
   Point to the circle and a square.
   Point to the black circle and the white square.

Formulated sentences
   Objective: To evaluate the student's ability to formulate complete, semantically and grammatically correct, spoken sentences of increasing length and complexity (i.e. simple, compound and complex sentences), using given words (e.g. car, if, because) and contextual constraints imposed by illustrations. These abilities reflect the capacity to integrate semantic, syntactic, and pragmatic rules and constraints while using working memory.
   Examples: The student is given the target word 'book' and is shown a picture in which a girl is reading a book.

Recalling sentences
   Objective: To evaluate the student's ability to listen to spoken sentences of increasing length and complexity, and repeat the sentences without changing word meaning and content, word structure (morphology), or sentence structure (syntax). Semantic, morphological, and syntactic competence facilitates immediate recall (short-term memory).
   Examples: The student listens to the following sentences and is asked to repeat them:
   My sister is in the sixth grade.
   Does Mr Gomez teach reading?

Understanding spoken paragraphs
   Objective: To evaluate the student's ability to (a) sustain attention and focus while listening to spoken paragraphs of increasing length and complexity, (b) create meaning from oral narratives and text, (c) answer questions about the content of the information given and (d) use critical thinking strategies for interpreting beyond the given information. The questions probe for understanding of the main idea, memory for facts and details, recall of event sequences, and making inferences and predictions.
   Examples: The student listens to the following paragraph and is then asked questions:
   Andy liked to visit his grandfather who lived on a farm in the country. The last time Andy saw his grandfather, he had promised to send Andy a surprise. Andy was excited because his mom said the surprise would come today. After breakfast, Andy's dad brought a big basket into the kitchen. Andy heard a 'meow' and saw a long furry tail coming from inside the basket.
   Why was Andy excited? (Correct: because the surprise would arrive today)
   What happened after breakfast? (Correct: Andy's father brought a basket/cat into the kitchen)

Table 5.3 (*cont.*)

Word definitions
  Objective: To evaluate the student's ability to analyse words for their meaning features, define words by referring to class relationships and shared meanings, and describe meanings that are unique to the reference or instance.
  Examples: The student is asked to describe the meanings of words in orally presented sentences:
  Mustard: Mom asked 'Would you like mustard on your hamburger?'
  ☐ condiment/something added for taste/put on food
  AND
  ☐ is brown

Sentence assembly
  Objective: To evaluate the student's ability to formulate grammatically acceptable and semantically meaningful sentences by manipulating and transforming given words and word groups.
  Examples: The student is asked to manipulate words and word groups to form sentences:

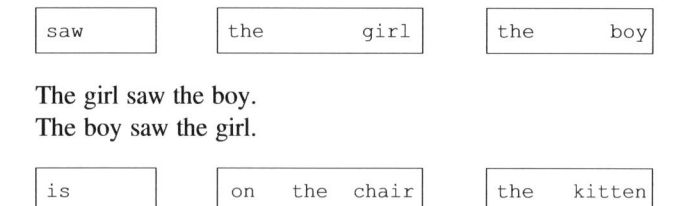

  | saw | the girl | the boy |

  The girl saw the boy.
  The boy saw the girl.

  | is | on the chair | the kitten |

  The kitten is on the chair.
  Is the kitten on the chair?

Semantic relationships
  Objective: To evaluate the student's ability to interpret sentences that (a) make comparisons, (b) identify location or direction, (c) specify time relationships, (d) include serial order or (e) are expressed in passive voice.
  Examples: A student is shown four possible responses and is asked to select the response(s) which complete an orally presented sentence:
  A man is bigger than a
  (a)   house
  (b)   button
  (c)   spoon
  (d)   plane

Reading comprehension
  Objective: To evaluate the student's ability to (a) sustain attention and focus while reading paragraphs of increasing length and complexity, (b) create meaning from narratives and text, (c) answer questions about the content of the information given and (d) use critical thinking strategies for interpreting beyond the information given. The questions probe for understanding of the main idea, memory for facts and details, recall of event sequences, and making inferences and predictions.

Table 5.3 (*cont.*)

> *Examples:* The student is read a short story about a girl called Ying who is apprehensive about starting a new school. Ying meets a new friend called Tia. The student is then asked a series of questions based on the story:
> What is this story about?
> Correct: meeting/making new friends/Ying meeting Tia
> Why do you think Ying was putting on her socks slowly?
> Correct: she was sad/worried/nervous/she didn't want to go to her new school/she wanted to be late

Structured writing
> **Objective:** To evaluate the student's ability to use situational information given by a story title, an introductory sentence, and an incomplete sentence to create and write a thematic, structured narrative of increasing length.
> *Examples:* The student is asked to complete the sentence and write one more sentence on the theme 'Catching the bus':
> Every morning, Eric waits for the bus at the corner. Today it was raining so

---

Pragmatics profile
> **Objective:** To identify verbal and non-verbal pragmatic deficits that may negatively influence social and academic communication.
> *Examples:* The student's pragmatic behaviours are assessed on a scale of 1 (never or almost never) to 4 (always or almost always). The student demonstrates culturally appropriate use of language when:
> (1) making/responding to greetings to/from others
> (2) beginning/ending conversations (face-to-face, phone, etc.)
> (3) observing turn-taking rules in the classroom or in social interactions
> (4) maintaining eye contact/gaze
> (5) introducing appropriate topics of conversation

Pragmatics activities checklist
> **Objective:** To provide the examiner with an opportunity to observe the student's functional communication skills during authentic conversational interactions in order to identify verbal and non-verbal behaviours that may negatively influence social and academic communication.
> *Examples:* After completing three activities with the student (e.g. teach and play a game), each observed behaviour is checked. For example, the student:
> ☐ 1. did not maintain culturally appropriate eye contact with the speaker
> ☐ 2. did not look where speaker pointed
> ☐ 3. did not look at object/person named by speaker

---

that contribute to a client's problems with receptive syntax. Twenty grammatical constructions are tested using a four-picture multiple-choice format that contains lexical and grammatical foils. These constructions range from simple declaratives through to passives and complex embedded clauses. For the grammatical construction postmodified subject, the examinee is asked to point to the picture

Table 5.4 *The domains and subtests in the standard version of the* Boston Diagnostic Aphasia Examination – Third Edition *(BDAE-3; Goodglass et al., 2001)*

BDAE-3 domain	Subtests
Conversational and expository speech	Simple social responses
	Free conversation
	Picture description (Cookie Theft)
Auditory comprehension	Basic word discrimination
	Commands
	Complex ideational material
Oral expression	Non-verbal agility
	Verbal agility
	Automatized sequences
	Recitation
	Melody
	Rhythm
	Single word repetition
	Repetition of sentences
	Responsive naming
	Boston Naming Test
	Screening for naming of special categories (letters, numbers, colours)
Reading	Matching across cases and scripts
	Number matching (three subtasks)
	Picture-word match
	Lexical decision
	Homophone matching
	Free grammatical morphemes
	Basic oral word reading
	Oral reading of sentences with comprehension
	Reading comprehension – sentences and paragraphs
Writing	Mechanics of writing
	Primer word vocabulary
	Regular phonics
	Common irregular forms
	Written picture naming (objects, actions, animals)
	Narrative writing (Cookie Theft)

that corresponds to the sentence 'The elephant pushing the boy is big'. The pictures from which a selection must be made are as follows:

(1)   A little boy pushing a big elephant
(2)   A little elephant pushing a big boy
(3)   A big boy pushing a little elephant
(4)   A big elephant pushing a little boy (correct picture)

The TROG-2 can be used from 4 years upwards and is individually administered in 10 to 20 minutes. It is based on a normative sample of 792 children (aged 4 to 16 years) and 70 adults, stratified by age, gender, geographical distribution and socioeconomic status.

Standardized, norm-referenced assessments of structural aspects of language such as syntax and semantics are routinely conducted in SLT clinics. Less commonly, standardized, norm-referenced tests are used to assess pragmatic aspects of language. One such assessment is the *Test of Pragmatic Language – Second Edition* (TOPL-2; Phelps-Terasaki and Phelps-Gunn, 2007). The TOPL-2 examines six core subcomponents of pragmatics: physical setting; audience; topic; purpose (speech acts); visual-gestural cues; and abstraction (figurative or metaphorical statements). Examinees are shown a series of colour pictures that depict different social contexts. Judgements about each context are probed and scored. For example, in one context, the 'Doctor's Office', a young boy is seen to refuse a doctor who is attempting to give him medicine. The examinee must correctly identify the physical context (the doctor holding the medicine), the purpose (the boy needs to take the medicine) and visual-gestural cues (the boy holding out his arms to reject the medicine) in order to achieve the full mark for this scenario. If any one of these elements is not identified, the mark cannot be awarded. Raw scores, percentiles, standard scores and age equivalents are provided for the TOPL-2. The test is appropriate for individuals aged 6;0 to 18;11 years and is administered in approximately 45–60 minutes. A small number of standardized, norm-referenced assessments of narrative have also been developed. They include the *Renfrew Bus Story* (Cowley and Glasgow, 1994) and the *Test of Narrative Language* (Gillam and Pearson, 2004).

Although pragmatic aspects of language and different types of discourse can be examined in the context of a standardized, norm-referenced test, there is some doubt about the ecological validity of these assessments. It is doubtful, for example, that asking a child to make judgements about a social scenario captured in a picture (as in the TOPL-2) truly reflects the pragmatic and discourse processes that unfold in real time during a conversation or the telling of a story. Informal assessments of language have greater ecological validity than their formal counterparts in the evaluation of non-rule-based aspects of language. A key concern of any informal assessment is the elicitation of a language sample that is broadly representative of the client's skills and of the contexts in which the client is called upon to communicate. For a young child, such a sample may be recorded during play activities with a parent who can use specific prompts to elicit language production. For an adult with stroke-induced aphasia, a naturalistic language sample can be obtained by recording a conversational exchange with a spouse in the setting of the client's home. Extended language samples can be analysed along a number of parameters. Some of these parameters may reflect structural aspects of language. For example, grammatical complexity and lexical semantics may be assessed by measuring a speaker's mean length of utterance and **lexical diversity**, respectively (see Fergadiotis et al., 2013, for an evaluation of four measures used to assess lexical diversity in narrative discourse in people with aphasia).

Other parameters applied to the analysis of language samples reflect pragmatic and discourse features such as topic management, turn-taking, **conversational repair** and **story grammar**. Checklists, pragmatics profiles and rating scales may be used to guide the analysis and ensure comprehensive examination of a range of features. One such instrument is Prutting and Kirchner's (1987) *Pragmatic Protocol*. The Protocol contains 30 pragmatic parameters that are organized according to three categories: (1) verbal aspects (e.g. variety of speech acts); (2) paralinguistic aspects (e.g. vocal quality); and (3) non-verbal aspects (e.g. physical proximity). Assessors judge each parameter as being either appropriate or inappropriate. A parameter is judged to be appropriate if it facilitates the communicative interaction or is neutral. An inappropriate parameter detracts from the communicative interaction and penalizes the individual. A third category of response is used when there is no opportunity to observe a particular parameter.

The *Pragmatic Protocol* has largely been used in research settings. A widely used checklist in clinical settings is the *Children's Communication Checklist – Second Edition* (CCC-2; Bishop, 2003a). The CCC-2 is a 70-item questionnaire that may be used during a semi-structured interview with informants to assess communicative features in general, or to rate language and communication skills following a period of observation of a child. It is suitable for use in children aged 4 to 16 years. The CCC-2 may be completed by a caregiver, speech and language therapist or teacher. Raters respond to a series of statements with one of the following: (a) does not apply, (b) applies somewhat, (c) definitely applies or (d) unable to judge. The checklist contains the following ten scales: (A) speech, (B) syntax, (C) semantics, (D) coherence, (E) inappropriate initiation, (F) stereotyped language, (G) use of context, (H) nonverbal communication, (I) social relations and (J) interests. Standard scores and percentiles are provided for these scales. The checklist contains two composites based on these scales. The General Communication Composite (scales A to H above) is used to identify children who are likely to have clinically significant communication problems. The Social Interaction Deviance Composite (scales A to E and H to J) is used to identify children who may merit further assessment for an autistic spectrum disorder. The CCC-2 can be used in isolation from other measures. Ideally, however, it should be employed alongside other formal and informal techniques within a comprehensive evaluation of language.

SPECIAL TOPIC: Pragmatic Language Impairment

Pragmatics profiles, checklists and rating scales may be used to assess children with suspected pragmatic language impairment (PLI) or social communication disorder (formerly known as semantic-pragmatic disorder). These children present quite differently from most children who are assessed and treated by paediatric speech and language therapists. Their language skills in phonology, morphology and syntax are relatively intact. They also produce fluent, clearly articulated utterances. However, they have marked difficulties in the use of language (pragmatics) and in discourse skills. Some of these difficulties are listed below:

- Fail to observe conversational rules – children with PLI may fail to exchange turns with others, wander off topic, talk excessively or contribute irrelevant utterances
- Difficulty adjusting language to the context or needs of the listener – children with PLI may assume knowledge in their listener which is absent
- Difficulty extracting the gist of a story or the salient points in a conversation
- Literal interpretation of non-literal language like idioms, metaphors and sarcasm
- Difficulty understanding jokes and may be upset by playful teasing
- Unable to draw inferences to establish causal and other links between events in a story
- Lexical choices may be atypical or bizarre

Some of these pragmatic difficulties are evident in the answers given to a series of general knowledge questions by an 8-year-old Swedish girl called Lena who was studied by Sahlén and Nettelbladt (1993):

> E: What do you usually see on the ground when it is autumn?
> L: Mosquitoes and birds and crows.
> E: What season comes after autumn?
> L: Winter and then spring then autumn and then spring ... usually many days are passing.
> E: What is it like in the winter?
> L: (*pause*) You just build a snow man.
> E: Mm ... and in the spring?
> L: At day nursery when was winter then everybody went out and played and she throw snowballs on the wall and it was red.
> E: But look, if I tell you that right now there are already some flowers outside and small, small buds on the trees and so on ...
> L: Flowers ... on the apple trees I think are beautiful to see.
> E: So what season is it when it is like this outside?
> L: (*pause*) Mm ...
> E: Is it winter then?
> L: No ... spring! This is probably not spring (*picks up a pen on the table*). What sort of pen is this?

The first pragmatic anomaly in this exchange occurs when Lena uses 'mosquitoes' to describe what is usually seen on the ground in autumn. Even by the category of all animals, the word 'mosquitoes' is a somewhat atypical choice. Lena disregards the examiner's question about what it is like in the spring. She uses the pronoun 'she' without first establishing a referent for the term. The examiner will not know who

> Lena is referring to at this point. Lena appears not to grasp the significance of the examiner's description of flowers and small buds on the trees. Clearly, the examiner is attempting to cue Lena to say 'spring'. But she responds in an irrelevant way. At the end of the exchange, there is further irrelevance when Lena asks 'What sort of pen is this?'

Finally, language may also be elicited through a range of discourse production tasks. These tasks can take many different forms and include story generation and story retelling, giving directions to a listener or explaining the rules of a game to a hearer (both procedural discourse), and describing a picture to a parent, spouse or therapist. In a review of non-standardized procedures for the assessment of discourse in individuals with traumatic brain injury, narrative production was the most common elicitation task employed for discourse sampling followed by procedural discourse and finally picture description (Coelho et al., 2005). Specific discourse measures have been developed to assist in the analysis of each of these forms of monologic discourse. For narrative production, an SLT may undertake a story grammar analysis in order to establish that all the components of a well-formed story are present and that these components occur in the correct order. For example, in most story grammars a well-formed story consists of a setting, theme, plot and resolution. Characters are introduced during the setting of the story and should not be mentioned for the first time during a story's resolution. Aside from story grammar, there are several other reliable and valid measures of discourse. Some measures relate to structural aspects of language such as number of words and clauses per **T-unit** (a measure of grammatical complexity) and lexical diversity (a measure of lexical semantics). Other measures relate to the amount and accuracy of information or content (e.g. percent correct information units), the number and type of cohesive ties across sentences, and the coherence or thematic unity of discourse.

> **KEY POINTS: Clinical Assessments: Language**
> - Like speech, language can be assessed through the use of formal and informal procedures. Formal procedures are typically standardized, norm-referenced tests. Informal procedures can claim greater ecological validity than formal procedures, and involve recordings and analyses of language in naturalistic contexts.
> - A comprehensive, formal evaluation of expressive and receptive aspects of language is best achieved through the use of a language battery such as the *Clinical Evaluation of Language Fundamentals – Fifth Edition* (CELF-5) and the *Boston Diagnostic Aphasia Examination – Third Edition* (BDAE-3). The subtests in these batteries examine the full range of language levels (e.g. syntax, semantics) and modalities (e.g. speech, writing).

- A language battery can reveal areas of language that require further investigation (e.g. receptive syntax). There are standardized, norm-referenced tests that can be used for this purpose (e.g. *Test for Reception of Grammar – Version 2* (TROG-2)).
- Non-rule-based aspects of language such as pragmatics can be assessed by means of standardized, norm-referenced assessments (e.g. *Test of Pragmatic Language – Second Edition* (TOPL-2)). However, these aspects of language are most often assessed by means of informal procedures.
- Audio- and video-recordings of conversational exchanges can be used to examine a range of pragmatic language skills such as turn-taking, topic management, repair strategies and use of gesture. To ensure a comprehensive analysis of these skills, pragmatic checklists and profiles may be used to guide the analysis.
- Discourse comprehension and production tasks such as responding to questions about a story, explaining the rules of a game to a listener and describing a picture are an effective, informal method of assessing discourse skills. Language elicited by these tasks can undergo story grammar analyses and other discourse measures.

5.5 Clinical Assessments: Fluency

There are two main fluency disorders which SLTs assess and treat: stuttering and cluttering. Wingate (2002: 9) defines stuttering as a speech disorder in which there is 'a unique anomaly in the flow of speech characterized by iterative and/or perseverative speech elements involving word/syllable-initial position'. Iterations involve single phonemes or combinations of phonemes as in iteration of /s/ or /sp/ for *spoke*. Often, one of these phonemes is the schwa vowel as in /spə/ for *spoke*. In perseverations or prolongations, a phoneme is prolonged beyond its normal duration, e.g. /s:::/ for *soap*. Stuttering is most commonly found in its developmental form, with onset generally occurring between 2.5 and 4 years of age. However, there are also acquired forms of the disorder that arise as a result of an acquired brain injury (acquired neurogenic stuttering) or following a traumatic event (acquired psychogenic stuttering). Cluttering often occurs alongside stuttering and may be misdiagnosed as stuttering. The features of this fluency disorder vary with different accounts but include, at a minimum, a perceived rapid and/or irregular rate of speech accompanied by the presence of at least one of the following symptoms: excessive non-stuttering-like dysfluencies (related to thought formulation rather than speech production problems as in stuttering); excessive collapsing or deletion of syllables; and abnormal pauses, syllable stress or speech rhythm. Cluttering can also be developmental or acquired in nature. It has been reported to occur in several syndromes (e.g. Down syndrome) and has been linked to brain damage in adults.

The reader is referred to chapter 8 in Cummings (2014c) and Ward (2006) for further discussion of the features of stuttering and cluttering.

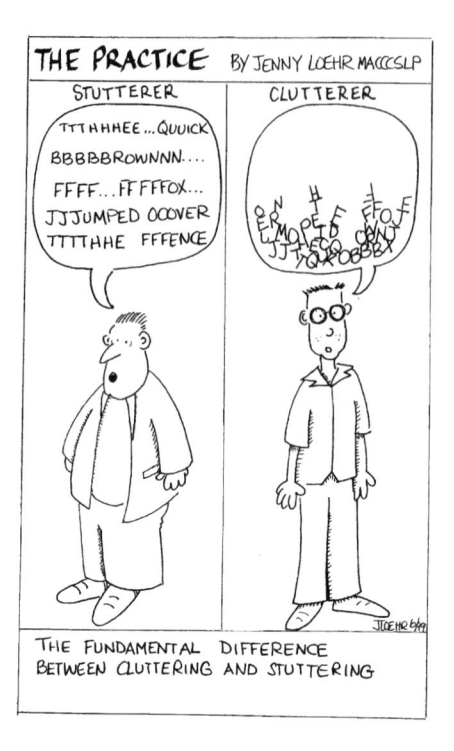

THE PRACTICE BY JENNY LOEHR MACCCSLP

STUTTERER: TTTHHHEE...QUUICK BBBBBROWNNN.... FFFF...FFFFFOX... JJJUMPED OCOVER TTTTHHE FFFENCE

CLUTTERER

THE FUNDAMENTAL DIFFERENCE BETWEEN CLUTTERING AND STUTTERING

Fluency disorders have motoric, linguistic, affective and cognitive dimensions, but before any assessment of these different dimensions is undertaken, SLTs aim to characterize the nature and extent of a client's dysfluency. The most commonly used method of assessing stuttering severity is the stuttering frequency count. This measure is expressed as a percentage of stuttered syllables or words. It is calculated by dividing the total number of stuttered syllables (words) in a speech sample by the total number of syllables (words) spoken, and multiplying the result by 100. Alongside the stuttering frequency count, clinicians often report various measures of speech rate. Expressed as either the number of syllables or words spoken per minute, these measures are calculated by dividing the total number of all syllables spoken (speaking rate) or the total number of non-stuttered syllables spoken (articulatory rate) by the total length of time taken (in seconds), which is then multiplied by 60. Percentage of stuttered syllables is a measure of stuttering frequency alone. A more complete analysis of stuttering is achieved through use of the *Stuttering Severity Instrument – Fourth Edition* (SSI-4; Riley, 2009). The SSI-4 is a norm-referenced assessment that examines the frequency of stuttering alongside stuttering duration, physical concomitants and naturalness of the individual's speech. Stuttering duration is based on the average stutter duration of the three longest stutters in a sample.

Included within physical concomitants are distracting sounds, facial grimaces, head movements and movements of the extremities. The SSI-4 is based on a normative sample of 72 preschool-aged children, 139 school-aged children and 60 adults. It can be administered in 15–20 minutes.

Another norm-referenced assessment of stuttering in children is the *Test of Childhood Stuttering* (TOCS; Gillam et al., 2009). There are three components of the TOCS: the Standardized Speech Fluency Measures; the Observational Rating Scales; and the Supplemental Clinical Assessment. The Standardized Speech Fluency Measures contain four speech fluency tasks: rapid picture naming; modelled sentences; structured conversation; and narration. The latter tasks assess stuttering in a dialogue and monologue context, respectively. In the modelled sentences task, children are shown two pictures side by side that differ in one detail. The examiner produces a sentence about one of the pictures. The examinee is then required to produce other sentences that have the same syntactic structure as the examiner's sentence. This task examines linguistic influences on stuttering, as the child must formulate and produce spoken sentences that vary in syntactic complexity. The Observational Rating Scales contain two scales – the speech fluency rating scale and the dysfluency-related consequences rating scale – which enable the SLT to gather information about stuttering and related behaviours from a range of informants (parents, teachers, etc.). Finally, the Supplementary Clinical Assessment assesses dysfluency-related data in more detail. These assessments include: clinical interviews; comprehensive analysis of dysfluency frequency and types; speech rate analysis; dysfluency duration analysis; repetition length analysis; associated behaviour analysis; stuttering frequency analysis; and speech naturalness analysis. The TOCS is administered in 20–30 minutes to children aged 4 to 12 years.

The cognitions which underlie and reinforce stuttering behaviour are increasingly examined as part of a fluency assessment. The KiddyCAT (Vanryckeghem and Brutten, 2007) is the only assessment of its kind to provide cognitive data about the belief system (or 'attitudes') of preschool children towards their speech. It is a 12-item, binary (i.e. yes or no) response questionnaire which is designed to assess attitudes to communication in children aged 3 to 6 years. Four of the items on the KiddyCAT ask the child to respond to the questions: 'Is it hard for you to say your name?', 'Are words hard for you to say?', 'Do you think that people need to help you talk?' and 'Is talking hard for you?'. A higher score out of 12 suggests that the child has greater negative attitudes towards his or her speech. Preschool children who stutter have been shown to score significantly higher on the KiddyCAT than children who do not stutter regardless of age or gender (Clark et al., 2012).

Negative cognitions about stuttering are also examined in the *Overall Assessment of the Speaker's Experience of Stuttering* (OASES; Yaruss and Quesal, 2010). The OASES is based on the World Health Organization's *International Classification of Functioning, Disability and Health* (2001), and addresses the impact of stuttering on the quality of life of speakers who stutter. There are three different versions of the assessment: School-age (7–12 years); Teenage (13–17 years); and Adult (18 years and above). The OASES contains four sections: General Information; Reactions to Stuttering; Communication in Daily Situations; and Quality of Life. Respondents answer questions that are scored on a 5-point Likert scale, with responses totalled into impact scores and impact ratings. The impact score combines information about (a) the speaker's perceptions about stuttering; (b) the negative affective, behavioural and cognitive reactions that the speaker has to stuttering; (c) the functional communication difficulties a speaker may have in different speaking environments; and (d) the impact of stuttering on the speaker's overall quality of life. The OASES can be completed by speakers in 15 to 20 minutes and takes approximately 5 minutes to score.

Several instruments are now available to assess cluttering in clients. The content of these instruments includes linguistic, cognitive and speech domains and reflects the wide range of problems that contribute to the communicative difficulties of people who clutter. One prominent cluttering checklist is the *Predictive Cluttering Inventory* (PCI; Daly, 2006). The PCI contains 33 descriptive statements that are organized according to four sections: pragmatics; speech-motor; language-cognition; and motor coordination-writing problems (see Figure 5.3). The clinician rates each statement on a scale of 0 (never present) to 6 (always present). The maximum score on the PCI is 198. The higher the client's score on this inventory, the more likely it is that the person is a clutterer. Daly reports that clients with scores of 120 or more are quite rare, and that clients typically present with scores between 80 and 120 (personal communication, 20 June 2016). The former clients are diagnosed 'pure clutterer', while the latter clients are diagnosed 'clutterer-stutterer'. The PCI has not yet been subjected to empirical examination of its validity or reliability. A computer-based assessment of the overall severity of cluttering is the *Cluttering Severity Instrument* (CSI; Bakker and Myers, 2011). The CSI software is available through the website of the International Cluttering Association. Using a speech sample, the clinician completes eight perceptual rating scales of behavioural characteristics that are often considered to be compromised in cluttering. These scales assess: overall intelligibility; speech rate regularity; speech rate; articulation precision; typical dysfluency; language disorganization; discourse management; and use of prosody. After these scales are completed, the CSI software can be used to determine the proportion of the speech sample that reveals the characteristics of cluttered speech as judged by the clinician.

Of course, any assessment of stuttering and cluttering should be conducted alongside a detailed case history of the client. In children, a case history may reveal other biological relatives who stutter. There is an increased incidence of stuttering in families of people who stutter (Kraft and Yairi, 2012). This finding lends support to a genetic aetiology of stuttering. A case history may also reveal delays in achieving motor milestones and/or delays in speech and

INSTRUCTIONS: Please respond to each description section below. Circle the number you believe is most descriptive of this person's cluttering.

	Descriptive Statement	Always	Almost Always	Frequently	Sometimes	Infrequently	Almost Never	Never
	PRAGMATICS							
1.	Lack of effective self-monitoring skills	6	5	4	3	2	1	0
2.	Lack of awareness of own communication errors or problems	6	5	4	3	2	1	0
3.	Compulsive talker; verbose; tangential; word-finding problems	6	5	4	3	2	1	0
4.	Poor planning skills; mis-judges effective use of time	6	5	4	3	2	1	0
5.	Poor social communication skills; inappropriate turn-taking; interruptions	6	5	4	3	2	1	0
6.	Does not recognize or respond to listener's visual or verbal feedback	6	5	4	3	2	1	0
7.	Does not repair or correct communication breakdowns	6	5	4	3	2	1	0
8.	Little or no excessive effort observed during disfluencies	6	5	4	3	2	1	0
9.	Little or no anxiety regarding speaking; unconcerned	6	5	4	3	2	1	0
10.	Speech better under pressure (improves short-term with concentration)	6	5	4	3	2	1	0
	SPEECH-MOTOR							
11.	Articulation errors	6	5	4	3	2	1	0
12.	Irregular speech rate; speaks in spurts or bursts	6	5	4	3	2	1	0
13.	Telescopes or condenses words	6	5	4	3	2	1	0
14.	Rapid rate (tachylalia)	6	5	4	3	2	1	0
15.	Speech rate progressively increases (festinating)	6	5	4	3	2	1	0
16.	Variable prosody; irregular melody or stress pattern	6	5	4	3	2	1	0
17.	Initial loud voice trailing off to unintelligible murmur	6	5	4	3	2	1	0
18.	Lack of pauses between words and phrases	6	5	4	3	2	1	0
19.	Repetition of multi-syllabic words and phrases	6	5	4	3	2	1	0
20.	Co-existence of excessive disfluencies and stuttering	6	5	4	3	2	1	0
	LANGUAGE-COGNITION							
21.	Language is disorganized; confused wording; word-finding problems	6	5	4	3	2	1	0
22.	Poor language formulation; poor story-telling; sequencing problems	6	5	4	3	2	1	0
23.	Disorganized language increases as topic becomes more complex	6	5	4	3	2	1	0
24.	Many revisions; interjections; filler words	6	5	4	3	2	1	0
25.	Seems to verbalize before adequate thought formulation	6	5	4	3	2	1	0
26.	Inappropriate topic introduction, maintenance, or termination	6	5	4	3	2	1	0
27.	Improper linguistic structure; poor grammar; syntax errors	6	5	4	3	2	1	0
28.	Distractible; poor concentration; attention span problems	6	5	4	3	2	1	0
	MOTOR COORDINATION-WRITING PROBLEMS							
29.	Poor motor control for writing (messy)	6	5	4	3	2	1	0
30.	Writing includes omission or transposition of letters, syllables, or words	6	5	4	3	2	1	0
31.	Oral diadochokinetic coordination below expected normed levels	6	5	4	3	2	1	0
32.	Respiratory dysrhythmia; jerky breathing pattern	6	5	4	3	2	1	0
33.	Clumsy and uncoordinated; motor activities accelerated or impulsive	6	5	4	3	2	1	0

TOTAL SCORE:____

COMMENTS:

Figure 5.3 *The* Predictive Cluttering Inventory *(PCI) (reproduced with kind permission of David A. Daly)*

language development in children who stutter. (Choo et al., 2016, reported dissociated development across speech-language, cognitive and motor domains in children who stutter.) In such a case, an SLT evaluation should include a speech-language assessment alongside the specific fluency measures described above. A case history can also be useful in identifying environmental factors that may serve to trigger and maintain stuttering behaviour. For example, it may be reported that a child's dysfluency had sudden onset following the birth of a sibling or a traumatic event such as parental divorce or a family bereavement. In adults with developmental stuttering, a case history may reveal factors that have contributed to the persistence of stuttering or the failure of previous interventions to lead to long-term gains in fluency. A case history can also throw light on **avoidance behaviours** in adults with developmental stuttering. This can include words and sounds that the speaker finds problematic and situations that the speaker may fear. The latter can influence the choice of careers and occupations, the pursuit of interests and hobbies, and the presence and extent of friendships and other social networks. A detailed case history should be viewed as a valuable source of information about all dimensions of a client's dysfluency.

KEY POINTS: Clinical Assessments: Fluency

- There are two main types of fluency disorder: stuttering and cluttering. Fluency can also be compromised in other communication disorders (e.g. aphasia).
- Most cases of stuttering have their onset in childhood (developmental stuttering). However, stuttering can also arise in adults as a result of acquired brain injury (acquired *neurogenic* stuttering) or following a traumatic event (acquired *psychogenic* stuttering). The speech features are iterations and perseverations of phonemes in word- or syllable-initial position.
- Norm-referenced assessments of stuttering such as the *Stuttering Severity Instrument – Fourth Edition* (SSI-4) and *Test of Childhood Stuttering* (TOCS) can be used to examine the frequency and duration of stuttering, linguistic influences on stuttering and the variability of stuttering in dialogue and monologue contexts.
- Cognitive and affective components of stuttering are assessed through instruments such as the KiddyCAT and *Overall Assessment of the Speaker's Experience of Stuttering* (OASES). The OASES is based on the World Health Organization's ICF framework and addresses the impact of stuttering on quality of life.
- Cluttering has both developmental and acquired forms. It can occur in isolation or alongside stuttering. Rate anomalies are a consistent feature of accounts of cluttering. There are other deficits including pragmatic impairments, language deficits (e.g. disorganized language), cognitive problems and articulatory errors.
- Checklists such as the *Predictive Cluttering Inventory* (PCI) permit clinicians to assess the presence and extent of a range of cluttering behaviours. Computer-based assessments (e.g. *Cluttering Severity Instrument*, CSI) are also used to evaluate clients with suspected cluttering.
- Any fluency assessment must include a detailed case history that can reveal biological relatives who stutter and/or clutter, complex avoidance behaviours, and environmental factors that serve to trigger and/or maintain dysfluency.

5.6 Clinical Assessments: Voice

Children and adults with voice disorders must be assessed by SLTs. Voice disorders can arise on account of laryngeal injury or disease. Organic voice disorders may be caused by the presence of vocal nodules and polyps, a malignant laryngeal tumour, or the paralysis of one of the vocal folds. If a comprehensive examination by an otolaryngologist reveals no structural or neurological abnormality of the laryngeal mechanism, a functional voice disorder is diagnosed. Functional dysphonias can be further classified as **hyperfunctional voice disorders** that are related to overuse of the larynx, and **psychogenic dysphonias** that arise on account of psychological factors. The boundaries between these different types of voice disorder are often unclear in practice. This is because organic, psychological and misuse/overuse factors may all play a role in the aetiology of a voice disorder. A client with dysphonia may have laryngeal inflammation which is caused by gastroesophageal reflux disease (GERD). The voice disorder in this case appears to have a clear organic basis. However, the client may engage in excessive coughing and throat clearing, which further exacerbates his dysphonia. This behavioural response to his laryngeal inflammation introduces misuse/overuse factors into the aetiology of his voice disorder. Additionally, the client may experience depression or anxiety related to his dysphonia, especially if there are occupational and social implications of his voice disorder. These psychological factors may also contribute to the client's dysphonia. The complex interplay of these different factors makes it difficult to isolate any one factor as the cause of the voice disorder.

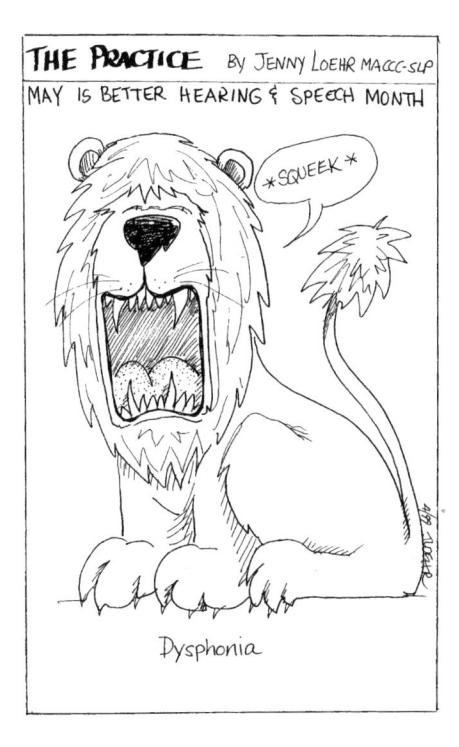

One of the purposes of a voice assessment is to establish the respective contributions of these different factors to a client's voice disorder. This can be achieved through a range of techniques which may be conducted by SLTs and otolaryngologists. Laryngoscopy and **stroboscopy** are important procedures for the visualization of the structures of the larynx and the movement of these structures during phonation. These techniques can be used to detect organic pathologies of the laryngeal mechanism, which may account for a client's voice disorder. A child with persistent **hoarseness**, for example, may be found to have vocal nodules. Perceptual assessments are used to judge the acceptability of a speaker's voice for his or her age and gender (and possibly class and culture). Reduced **vocal intensity** in clients with Parkinson's disease may compromise communication and is a significant perceptual finding that should be investigated during assessment. Also, a client may exhibit deviant vocal quality such as a breathy voice. This perceptual attribute may be explained by an otolaryngological finding, namely, inadequate adduction of the vocal folds during phonation in clients with vocal fold paralysis or bowing (the latter related to presbylarynx). Alongside instrumental and perceptual assessments, SLTs can also use acoustic techniques. These techniques may be used to measure acoustic dimensions of the voice such as fundamental frequency, jitter and **shimmer**. This section will address each of these approaches to the assessment of voice.

For any client who presents with dysphonia, the overriding concern for the assessing clinician is to establish if an organic pathology is responsible for vocal symptoms. To this end, a laryngoscopy is performed by an otolaryngologist.[1] During indirect (mirror) laryngoscopy, an examinee is asked to say 'ee' at a relatively high pitch while the otolaryngologist places a laryngeal mirror against the elevated soft palate. The tongue is wrapped in gauze and is held by the examiner (or where cooperation is achieved it is held by the client). The examiner wears a mirror on his head. Light from an external source is reflected from this head mirror onto the laryngeal mirror, from where it is reflected into the **pharynx** and **larynx**. Some patients are not able to tolerate this procedure. A more appropriate procedure for these patients may be **fibreoptic laryngoscopy** (see Figure 5.4). A flexible endoscope is passed transnasally into a position above the larynx during this procedure. One of the advantages of this technique is that phonation can be observed during connected speech – the presence of the laryngeal mirror in the **oral cavity** prevents visualization of the larynx during connected speech in indirect laryngoscopy. **Strobovideolaryngoscopy** is the most common technique for assessing vocal fold vibration (Heuer et al., 2006). Intermittent flashes of light delivered by means of a rigid or flexible endoscope have the effect of simulating slow motion of the vocal folds during this procedure. This technique allows the otolaryngologist to examine different stages of the vibratory cycle. The effect of even minute lesions of the vocal folds on the mucosal wave can be examined with strobovideolaryngoscopy.

Instrumental techniques are also used in an aerodynamic assessment of voice. In practice, SLTs are less likely to perform aerodynamic assessment than other

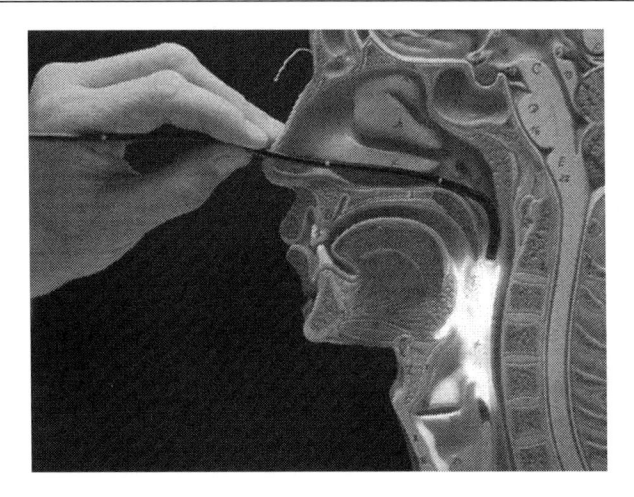

Figure 5.4 *Flexible fibreoptic nasolaryngoscopy (reproduced with permission of James P. Thomas, MD: voicedoctor.net)*

forms of voice evaluation. A study by Behrman (2005) of diagnostic practices among voice therapists revealed that while 81% of respondents were likely to use stroboscopy, only 17% were likely to use aerodynamic measurement. Approximately 42% of respondents indicated that they do not have access to aerodynamic equipment. Where instrumental techniques were used to make aerodynamic measures, these measures included mean airflow, mean subglottal pressure, and glottal efficiency. Airflow measures may be recorded by means of a pneumotachograph. In this technique, a divided air mask may be used to measure oral and nasal airflow separately during speech production. Handheld, battery-operated devices are available that can give real-time estimates of subglottal pressure during speech. Subglottal pressure is one of 22 parameters that are measured by the KayPENTAX Aerophone. Other aerodynamic functions that can be quantified by the Aerophone include laryngeal airway resistance, phonatory flow rate, sound pressure levels and **adduction/abduction** rate of the vocal folds. An instrumental technique that is used to measure patterns of vocal fold approximations (not aerodynamic features) is **electroglottography**. In this technique, an electrode is placed on each side of the **thyroid cartilage** at the level of the vocal folds. Distinct waveforms are generated as the client phonates. These waveforms correspond to clinically judged voice qualities such as hoarseness and **breathiness** (Hegde and Freed, 2011).

Perceptual voice evaluation is a key component of any voice assessment. One instrument used in a perceptual evaluation of voice is the Consensus Auditory-Perceptual Evaluation of Voice (CAPE-V). Ratings on the CAPE-V are based on direct observation of the client's performance in three tasks: sustained production of the vowels /a/ and /i/; production of six sentences designed to elicit various laryngeal behaviours and clinical signs; and the production of at least 20 seconds of natural conversational speech. During these tasks, the clinician assesses the following vocal attributes: (a) overall severity; (b) roughness (perceived irregularity in the voicing source); (c) breathiness (audible air escape in the voice); (d) strain (perception of excessive vocal effort); (e) pitch; and (f) loudness. Each of these attributes is accompanied by a 100-millimetre line that forms a visual analogue scale. The perceived deviance of each attribute from normal is indicated on the line by using a tic. Regions marked as MI (mildly deviant), MO (moderately deviant) and SE (severely deviant) below each line assist clinicians in arriving at their judgements. By physically measuring the distance in millimetres between the tic and the left end of the scale, a score out of a total 100 mm can be assigned to each attribute. A score of 73/100 on 'strain', for example, indicates greater deviancy than a score of 20/100. Each scale is also accompanied by two letters, C ('consistent') and I ('intermittent'), allowing the clinician to indicate, respectively, if an attribute was continuously present or occurred inconsistently across tasks. The clinician may also use two unlabelled scales to rate any additional prominent attributes that are required to describe a given voice. Finally, if a client is aphonic, exhibits tremor or has pitch instability, these and other features may be recorded under 'additional features'.

Another tool for the perceptual evaluation of voice is the GRBAS scale (Hirano, 1981). This perceptual rating system contains five parameters: G (overall grade of hoarseness), R (roughness), B (breathiness), A (asthenic) and S (strained quality). Each parameter is given a rating on a four-point scale between 0 and 3, where '0' indicates non-hoarse or normal, '1' slight, '2' moderate and '3' severe. The GRBAS scale is used extensively in clinical and research settings. It has been used to investigate breathiness in the ageing female voice (Lee et al., 2016), voice function in patients with laryngeal cancer (Bergström et al., 2016) and voice quality in patients with relapsing-remitting multiple sclerosis (Bauer et al., 2015). The GRBAS scale is not fully comprehensive. Unlike the CAPE-V, it does not include parameters for vocal pitch, for example (Freeman and Fawcus, 2000). A high degree of correlation has been observed between the general GRBAS and CAPE-V grades, with similarities in the grades of dysphonia distribution in both scales (Nemr et al., 2012). The GRBAS scale is a reliable method of perceptual assessment that has been shown to correlate with voice-related quality of life (Jones et al., 2006; Karnell et al., 2007).

Increasingly, acoustic measures are used by SLTs to assess voice quality. Technological developments have made computer-assisted voice analysis a reality in many clinics. The *Multi-Dimensional Voice Program* (MDVP; Kay Elemetrics, 1993), in conjunction with the Computerized Speech Lab, is a voice-processing and spectrographic analysis software package that provides an objective, reproducible and non-invasive measure of vocal fold function. The MDVP extracts up to 33 acoustic variables including jitter, shimmer and **noise-to-harmonics ratio**. These variables are compared graphically or numerically to a built-in normative database. This database was originally based on adults. This limited the usefulness of the MDVP in the assessment of paediatric dysphonia.

However, paediatric normative data is now also available (Campisi et al., 2002). The number and range of acoustic parameters included in the MDVP reflects the fact that several acoustic variables are needed to capture an aberration in a client's voice. Gramuglia et al. (2014) identified several acoustic vocal parameters on MDVP which were compromised in children with vocal nodules. The parameters in question were pitch perturbation quotient, amplitude perturbation quotient, noise harmonic ratio and soft phonation index. Other computerized voice analysis systems also exist, e.g. Voice Evaluation Suite. There is evidence that some acoustic variables (e.g. jitter, shimmer, noise-to-harmonics ratio) are not interchangeable between voice analysis systems (Rohrer et al., 2014).

Alongside instrumental, perceptual and acoustic assessments of voice, SLTs now routinely examine the impact of dysphonia on a client's functioning and **quality of life**. Several self-report measures have been developed for this purpose including Voice-Related Quality of Life (V-RQOL; Hogikyan and Sethuraman, 1999) and the Voice Handicap Index (VHI; Jacobson et al., 1997). The V-RQOL is a ten-item outcomes instrument for voice disorders. Clients rate a series of statements using a scale from 1 (none, not a problem) to 5 (problem is as 'bad as it can be'). The ten statements describe aspects of the physical functioning domain (e.g. 'I have trouble speaking loudly or being heard in noisy situations') and the social-emotional domain (e.g. 'I am sometimes anxious or frustrated (because of my voice)'). The VHI is a 30-item questionnaire that is used to quantify the functional, physical and emotional impacts of a voice disorder on an individual's quality of life. Clients give subjective ratings to each item in the questionnaire using a scale from 0 (never) to 4 (always). Statements from the three domains of the VHI include 'People have difficulty understanding me in a noisy room' (functional impact), 'I use a great deal of effort to speak' (physical impact) and 'My voice problem upsets me' (emotional impact). Both self-report measures are reliable and valid and may be used with children as well as adults (Boseley et al., 2006; Zur et al., 2007). The V-RQOL and VHI have also been translated into other languages (Moradi et al., 2013; Sielska-Badurek et al., 2016). The VHI has been adapted for use by singers (Cohen et al., 2007).

KEY POINTS: Clinical Assessments: Voice

- Voice disorders can be classified as organic or functional in nature. An organic voice disorder is caused by a structural anomaly (e.g. vocal polyp) or a neurological abnormality (e.g. Parkinson's disease). Where no organic pathology can be identified, a functional voice disorder is diagnosed.
- Functional voice disorders can be further sub-classified into psychogenic voice disorders (related to stressful or traumatic events) and hyperfunctional voice disorders (related to overuse of the larynx). In practice, most voice disorders have both organic and functional components.

- An evaluation of voice uses a combination of instrumental, perceptual and acoustic techniques. Self-report measures are also used to assess voice-related quality of life.
- Instrumental techniques are wide-ranging in nature and include the use of laryngoscopy and stroboscopy to assess laryngeal structures and function of these structures during phonation. Other instrumental techniques may be used to make aerodynamic measures of the voice (e.g. subglottal pressure). Electroglottography is an instrumental procedure that measures patterns of vocal fold approximations.
- A perceptual evaluation of voice is an essential component of any assessment of dysphonia. Two prominent perceptual assessments are the Consensus Auditory-Perceptual Evaluation of Voice (CAPE-V) and the GRBAS scale. Each of these instruments permits an assessment to be made of the severity of a client's dysphonia according to a number of vocal attributes (e.g. breathiness, strain).
- Acoustic assessments of voice are routinely conducted in well-resourced voice clinics. A widely used computer-assisted voice analysis system is the *Multi-Dimensional Voice Program*. This system can examine 33 acoustic variables including jitter and shimmer.
- Self-report measures are also used in a voice evaluation to establish the impact of dysphonia on a client's quality of life. Two valid, reliable instruments that are used for this purpose are the Voice-Related Quality of Life (V-RQOL) and the Voice Handicap Index (VHI).

5.7 Clinical Assessments: Swallowing

Eating and swallowing are complex volitional and reflexive activities that involve over 30 nerves and muscles. When these activities are disrupted, dysphagia is the result. Dysphagia can arise as a result of structural and functional impairments of the oral cavity, pharynx, larynx or **oesophagus**. The oral cavity is compromised for eating and swallowing in adults with tongue cancer who have a glossectomy and in children with a palatal cleft. Motor disorders such as cerebral palsy can affect the pharyngeal walls, reducing the strength of pharyngeal wall contraction during swallowing. In clients with laryngeal cancer who have a **supraglottic laryngectomy**, reduced elevation of the larynx during swallowing may result in dysphagia. A tumour or stricture of the oesophagus may pose a mechanical obstruction to the passage of the **bolus** from the pharynx into the oesophagus during swallowing. A tumour may compromise only one of the components of swallowing (e.g. oesophagus). Alternatively, in a client with neurological damage as a result of a stroke, the movement of a combination of oral, pharyngeal and oesophageal structures may be compromised. A large range of neurological, infectious, neoplastic and traumatic conditions feature in the aetiology of dysphagia. Dysphagia related to neurological damage (**neurogenic dysphagia**) is most often caused by a cerebrovascular accident or stroke. Viral, bacterial and fungal agents may cause dysphagia. The fungal infection **candida albicans** is the most common cause of infectious **oesophagitis**. Neoplastic conditions such as malignant laryngeal tumours and the surgical procedures that are used to treat them (e.g. laryngectomy) are a significant cause of dysphagia. Finally, among traumatic causes of dysphagia is cervical spine trauma with spinal cord injury.

Only some clients with dysphagia display overt symptoms such as coughing, throat clearing, increased effort during swallowing and repeated swallowing. Clinicians must be aware that 50% of patients who aspirate do not cough or give any external sign of food or liquid entering the airway (Logemann, 2006). Accordingly, it is important to use imaging techniques in an assessment and diagnosis of dysphagia. Techniques such as **videoendoscopy** and videofluoroscopy are essential for visualizing the oral and pharyngeal stages of swallowing and, along with a detailed case history and medical diagnosis, provide SLTs with vital information about the nature and extent of a client's dysphagia. During videoendoscopy – also known as fibreoptic endoscopic examination of swallowing (FEES) – a small, flexible scope is passed through the nose down to the level of the soft palate. Pharyngeal and laryngeal structures can be viewed before and after swallowing but not during swallowing. Videoendoscopy permits clinicians to assess the extent of airway protection, timing of the swallow, the occurrence of spillage before the swallow, the presence of residue after the swallow and ability to clear residue, and the presence of reflux and aspiration (Shipley and McAfee, 2009). There are significant advantages to the use of videoendoscopy. The procedure provides no X-ray exposure to patients. It is also portable, allowing it to be used as a bedside procedure in nursing homes and intensive care units. However, the technique does not allow clinicians to visualize the oral stage of swallowing and critical aspects of the pharyngeal phase of swallowing including laryngeal elevation, tongue-base motion and the upper oesophageal sphincter.

Videofluoroscopy overcomes certain limitations of videoendoscopy. It permits the visualization of all aspects of oropharyngeal swallowing with the exception of vocal fold closure during the pharyngeal phase of swallowing. A videofluoroscopic swallowing study, sometimes referred to as a 'modified barium swallow', uses a contrast agent (usually a barium sulphate preparation), which is swallowed by the patient. Different bolus volumes and viscosities can affect the timing and organization of swallowing and should be examined in consequence. Although protocols for videofluoroscopy vary, the most typical protocol involves presentation of 1, 3, 5 or 10 ml of thin liquids, cup-drinking of thin liquids, straw-drinking of thin liquids, 3 ml of pudding-thick barium and one quarter of a cookie coated with barium pudding to be chewed so that **mastication** can be visualized (Logemann, 2006). Studies are normally conducted with patients in a seated position, although they may be undertaken in a standing position when this is safe and acceptable to the patient. Investigations begin with patients in a lateral view, where aspiration is detected most effectively, and end with an anterior-posterior view to assess swallow symmetry and vocal cord function. Radiographic images are observed on a monitor during the procedure. Some stills are taken and images are simultaneously recorded on videotape or digitally for further analysis. Studies are generally completed in 90 to 120 seconds.

Videofluoroscopy is frequently described as the 'gold standard' in the diagnosis and management of oropharyngeal dysphagia (Belafsky and Kuhn, 2014). However, this procedure is contraindicated in a number of cases. If a patient is medically unstable or is not able to cooperate with the procedure because of cognitive or behavioural reasons, videofluoroscopy should not be performed. Patient pregnancy is a contraindication. Severely obese patients may not be able to fit into the prescribed space limitations that the imaging equipment allows. If a patient is placed nil by mouth for any reason other than oropharyngeal dysphagia (e.g. gastrointestinal tract surgery), videofluoroscopy should not be performed. If a patient has had a previous adverse reaction to the X-ray contrast or if the investigation would not alter the patient's clinical management, then videofluoroscopy is also contraindicated (Newman, 2012).

While a videofluoroscopic swallowing study typically examines the passage of the bolus from the oral cavity to the oesophagus, SLTs must be aware that symptoms reported by some patients may reflect difficulties at the oesophageal stage of swallowing. Oesophageal dysphagia is evaluated and diagnosed by gastroenterologists and radiologists. However, SLTs must understand that oropharyngeal swallowing function is often affected in patients with oesophageal motility disorders and dysphagia. A standard barium swallow may be conducted to evaluate motility and structural abnormalities of the upper gastrointestinal tract, including the stomach and oesophagus. This examination is typically completed by a radiologist and/or a specialist radiographer and does not normally involve SLTs. Gastroenterologists may perform sedated **oesophagoscopy** to evaluate the oesophagus or office-based transnasal oesophagoscopy, which allows the endoscopist to evaluate the oesophagus through to the proximal portion of the stomach (Roe, 2012). Oesophageal dysphagia can result when there is poor propulsion of a bolus along the oesophagus. Motor disorders of the oesophagus are assessed through the use of **manometry**, which can provide clinicians with information on the strength of oesophageal contractions. Where symptoms of reflux are reported by patients, an investigation of gastroesophageal reflux disease (GERD) may be undertaken through the use of oesophageal pH monitoring. (This technique may also be requested by an otolaryngologist as part of an investigation of the role of GERD in a client's voice disorder.) For further discussion of techniques used to investigate oesophageal dysphagia, the reader is referred to Cook (2008).

KEY POINTS: Clinical Assessments: Swallowing

- Structural and functional anomalies may compromise eating and swallowing in children and adults, resulting in dysphagia.
- Tumours of the oral cavity, pharynx, larynx and oesophagus are one of many structural problems that can compromise normal swallowing. Neurological damage resulting from a stroke can compromise the movement or function of these structures. The formation of a bolus of food and its propulsion from the oral cavity into the oesophagus is often compromised by neurological impairment.
- Many disorders are found in the aetiology of dysphagia. They include infectious diseases (e.g. bacterial infections), traumatic events (e.g. neck trauma), neoplastic conditions (e.g. pharyngeal tumours) and neurological disorders (e.g. multiple sclerosis).
- Oropharyngeal dysphagia may be assessed through videoendoscopy and videofluoroscopy. In videoendoscopy, a flexible scope is passed through the nose down to the level of the soft palate. Although this technique has several benefits (e.g. airway protection can be assessed), there is limited visualization of oropharyngeal structures during swallowing.
- Videofluoroscopy is often described as the 'gold standard' in the assessment of oropharyngeal dysphagia. This technique permits the visualization of oropharyngeal swallowing in real time. It is contraindicated in a number of cases (e.g. a patient is uncooperative or medically unstable).
- A diagnosis of oesophageal dysphagia is made by radiologists and gastroenterologists. For their part, SLTs must understand the symptoms of oesophageal dysphagia and the techniques that are used to assess it including standard barium swallow, endoscopy, manometry and pH monitoring.

CASE STUDY: Assessment and Diagnosis

This case study is designed to make you think about some of the issues that are involved in the assessment and diagnosis of clients by SLTs. Read the case study carefully. Then, individually or in a group, answer the questions that follow it.

Bob is 65 years old and was hospitalized following a left-hemisphere CVA. His neurologist referred him to SLT for assessment of his communication skills and swallowing. The SLT conducted a bedside assessment, which was brief on account of Bob's fatigue. This assessment indicated that Bob's motor speech production is intact, as he was able to articulate and sequence speech sounds. He appeared not to have difficulty swallowing liquids and small portions of food, although a final diagnosis of dysphagia awaited a videofluoroscopic examination of swallowing. Bob's main difficulties involved the comprehension and production of language. On a number of occasions, he was unable to point to objects in his immediate environment when asked to do so by the SLT. When the therapist's verbal request was supported by a gestural cue, Bob's response accuracy improved. He also had difficulty naming certain objects, although phonemic cues facilitated naming in several instances.

A comprehensive assessment of Bob's language was undertaken a week later when he was better rested and his performance was less compromised by fatigue. Formal and informal assessments were used. Several subtests from the auditory comprehension and oral expression domains of the *Boston Diagnostic Aphasia Examination* (BDAE) were used. The SLT also engaged Bob in a picture description task and in conversation about his family, holidays and interests. Bob exhibited difficulties across all tasks. His performance on formal assessment tasks was particularly compromised. Bob appeared to use context extensively to facilitate his comprehension of language. For example, he understood syntactic constructions in conversation which he failed to comprehend during the BDAE. The SLT concluded assessment after 45 minutes when Bob's concentration was impaired on account of fatigue. Further, more detailed language assessment was planned for later sessions.

Questions

(1) Why is a diagnosis of dysarthria and apraxia of speech not warranted in Bob's case?
(2) Which tasks provide the SLT with an opportunity to assess Bob's monological and dialogical discourse skills?
(3) Why is Bob's performance on formal assessment tasks so compromised?
(4) Bob's naming improved when the therapist used phonemic cues. Give an example of the use of this type of cue. What other type of cue is used by SLTs to facilitate naming?
(5) To definitively exclude a diagnosis of dysphagia, Bob must undergo a videofluoroscopic examination of swallowing. Explain why this is the case.

5.8 Diagnostic and Classification Systems

The purpose of any assessment is to help clinicians arrive at a diagnosis of a client's communication and/or swallowing disorder. For diagnosis to take place, however, clinicians must agree on the significance of assessment results. That significance can be captured in the form of questions which are unique to the particular communication disorder under consideration. For example, what role do rate anomalies have in a diagnosis of cluttering? What weight should be given to language test scores in a diagnosis of specific language impairment? Should **lexical stress** serve as a diagnostic marker for childhood apraxia of speech, as Shriberg et al. (2003) have argued? The clinical debates that ensue from each of these questions may not always result in a consensus regarding the criteria that should be used to diagnose a communication disorder. But when they do, these criteria may be formalized within a diagnostic system such as the *Diagnostic and Statistical Manual of Mental Disorders – Fifth Edition* (DSM-5; American Psychiatric Association, 2013) and the *International Classification of Diseases – Eleventh Edition* (ICD-11; WHO, 2018). In recent years, both of these international classification systems have given increased prominence to the diagnosis of communication disorders. For example, in 2013, social (pragmatic) communication disorder was included for the first time in the fifth edition of DSM. In this section, some remarks are made about the purpose, structure and use of these systems in the diagnosis of communication disorders.

DSM-5 has relevance to the work of SLTs in at least two respects. The first of these concerns the diagnosis of primary communication disorders. One such disorder, social communication disorder, is defined in DSM-5 as a primary deficit in the social use of verbal and non-verbal communication. The pragmatic anomalies that are a significant barrier to effective communication in children and adults with this disorder are described in Criterion A. They include conversational and narrative difficulties as well as problems making appropriate use of language in context. Each of these pragmatic impairments is supported by the findings of clinical studies (see Cummings, 2009, 2014a, for an extensive review of these findings). Criterion B stipulates that the aforementioned impairments must have limitations on a client's functioning in one or more domains. As with many disorders in DSM-5, these domains for social communication disorder are social relationships, academic achievement and occupational performance. The onset of the disorder is captured in Criterion C. Like other developmental communication disorders, social communication disorder has its onset in the developmental period. However, the pragmatic impairments of social communication disorder may first become manifest when a child is exposed to contexts that exceed his or her limited social communication skills. Criterion D stipulates conditions that preclude a diagnosis of social communication disorder. For example, if a child's social communication difficulties are related to impairments of linguistic structure (word structure and grammar), or are a feature of autism spectrum disorder, or are the result of cognitive limitations (intellectual disability), then a diagnosis of social communication disorder is not warranted. These criteria are displayed in full in Table 5.5.

The second respect in which DSM-5 is relevant to the work of SLTs is in the diagnosis of primary neuropsychiatric, neurobehavioural and neurodevelopmental disorders such as schizophrenia, ADHD and autism spectrum disorder. Typically, it is psychiatrists and psychologists (not SLTs) who diagnose these disorders. However, communication impairments are such prominent features of conditions like schizophrenia and ASD that SLTs must be aware of the criteria used by medical and health professionals to diagnose these disorders. To illustrate the communicative character of some of these criteria, consider the first criterion used to diagnose schizophrenia in DSM-5. For a client to be diagnosed with schizophrenia, he or she must satisfy Criterion A below:

Table 5.5 *Diagnostic criteria for social communication disorder in* Diagnostic and Statistical Manual of Mental Disorders – Fifth Edition *(DSM-5; American Psychiatric Association, 2013)*

Criterion A: Persistent difficulties in the social use of verbal and non-verbal communication as manifested by all of the following:
1. Deficits in using communication for social purposes, such as greeting and sharing information, in a manner that is appropriate for the social context.
2. Impairment of the ability to change communication to match context or the needs of a listener, such as speaking differently in a classroom than on a playground, talking differently to a child than to an adult and avoiding use of overly formal language.
3. Difficulties following rules for conversation and storytelling, such as taking turns in conversation, rephrasing when misunderstood and knowing how to use verbal and nonverbal signals to regulate interaction.
4. Difficulties understanding what is not explicitly stated (e.g. making inferences) and non-literal or ambiguous language (e.g. idioms, humour, metaphors, multiple meanings that depend on the context for interpretation).

Criterion B: The deficits result in functional limitations in effective communication, social participation, social relationships, academic achievement or occupational performance, individually or in combination.

Criterion C: The onset of symptoms is in the early developmental period (but deficits may not become fully manifest until social communication demands exceed limited capacities).

Criterion D: The symptoms are not attributable to another medical or neurological condition or to low abilities in the domains of word structure and grammar, and are not better explained by autism spectrum disorder, intellectual disability (intellectual developmental disorder), global developmental delay or another mental disorder.

Criterion A: Two (or more) of the following, each present for a significant portion of time during a one-month period (or less if successfully treated). At least one of these should include (1) to (3):

(1) Delusions
(2) Hallucinations
(3) Disorganized speech
(4) Grossly disorganized or catatonic behaviour
(5) Negative symptoms (i.e. diminished emotional expression or avolition)

Disorganized speech, also known as formal thought disorder, is a linguistic behaviour that is characterized by disjointed, incoherent and tangential language. Clients with schizophrenia who exhibit disorganized speech display poor use of cohesion, contribute irrelevant utterances to conversation and become derailed while speaking (slip off one track onto an obliquely related or an unrelated track). Disorganized speech is a **positive symptom** of schizophrenia. However, a negative symptom of schizophrenia known as alogia or poverty of speech is also a linguistic behaviour. In alogia, clients with schizophrenia make minimal turns in conversation. Responses to open-ended questions are unelaborated and consist of one or two words. Clients with schizophrenia who display alogia do not conform to a conversational expectation to be informative. It emerges that at least some of the criteria used to diagnose primary psychiatric disorders (and neurodevelopmental disorders) in DSM-5 are communicative through and through. It is thus as important for the SLT to understand the communicative character of criteria used to diagnose conditions such as schizophrenia in DSM-5 as it is to understand the communicative behaviours used to diagnose primary communication disorders such as social communication disorder.

Of course, DSM-5 is only one diagnostic system, albeit a very prominent one. Another classification system of relevance to SLTs is the ICD-11. As a classification system of physical health conditions as well as mental and behavioural disorders, ICD-11 is a much larger system than DSM-5. In its 22 chapters, the full range of communication and swallowing disorders assessed and treated by SLTs are assigned alphanumeric codes. The use of these codes permits easy storage, retrieval and analysis of data. The titles of two chapters in ICD-11 and the alphanumeric codes assigned to voice and fluency disorders within those chapters are shown below:

Chapter V: Mental and behavioural disorders
- F98: Other behavioural and emotional disorders with onset usually occurring in childhood and adolescence
- F98.5 Stuttering [stammering]
- F98.6 Cluttering

Chapter XVIII: Symptoms, signs and abnormal clinical and laboratory findings, not elsewhere classified
- R49: Voice disturbances
- R49.0 Dysphonia
- R49.1 Aphonia
- R49.2 Hypernasality and hyponasality
- R49.8 Other and unspecified voice disturbances

A short description of each disorder is followed by exclusions and cross-references to other parts of ICD-11. For example, cluttering is described as 'a rapid rate of speech with breakdown in fluency, but no repetitions or hesitations, of a severity to give rise to diminished speech intelligibility. Speech is erratic and dysrhythmic, with rapid jerky spurts that usually involve faulty phrasing patterns'. Following this description of cluttering are two exclusions along with cross-references: stuttering (F98.5) and **tic disorders** (F95.-).

There are important similarities and differences between ICD-11 and DSM-5. The classification of autism spectrum disorder is a case in point. Both diagnostic systems have moved away from assigning a separate ASD diagnosis to individuals who meet criteria for ASD but who have a known genetic condition such as **Rett syndrome**. These individuals now receive a standard diagnosis of ASD with these conditions designated as associated features (DSM-5) or as separate genetic conditions (ICD-11). However, where DSM-5 assigns individuals who have significant social and communication difficulties but not the repetitive or restricted behaviours of ASD to a new communication disorder category – social (pragmatic) communication disorder – such a designation is not recognized in ICD-11.

As a reference classification, ICD-11 is used to capture information on mortality and morbidity. Additional aspects of health domains, functioning and disability are classified in another World Health Organization framework called the *International Classification of Functioning, Disability and Health* (ICF; WHO, 2001). The ICF has been widely adopted by speech-language pathologists who have used the framework to develop functional goals and collaborative practice. In its *Scope of Practice in Speech-Language Pathology*, ASHA (2016a) directly aligns the domains of SLP service delivery with the ICF framework. In the ICF, functioning is conceived of in terms of a dynamic interaction between a person's health condition, environmental factors and personal factors. Applied to SLT, a health condition may take the form of a stroke that causes aphasia or a communication disorder such as specific language impairment. A health condition can compromise body structure and function. In children with cleft palate, for example, a palatal cleft is an impairment of body structure, and associated velopharyngeal incompetence is an impairment of body function (namely, the function of the velopharyngeal mechanism).

Impairments of body structure and function can have implications for an individual's activities and participation. An individual with stroke-induced aphasia may no longer be able to write letters and emails (an activity limitation). This may restrict his participation in the role of secretary of the local history society. A child with a palatal cleft and velopharyngeal incompetence may have reduced speech intelligibility that restricts his participation in a significant speaking role in a school play. Environmental and personal factors can help or hinder an individual's activities and participation. Speakers with dysarthria, for example, will be assisted by speaking in a quiet room or by spouses who remember to wear a hearing aid (environmental factors). Also, personality traits such as one's level of motivation, demographic factors (e.g. gender) and one's reaction to disability are all personal factors that can influence the impact of a health condition on an individual's activities and participation. For example, depression following a stroke can serve to exacerbate the activity limitations of aphasia (e.g. reduced contribution to conversation) and restricts to a large extent one's

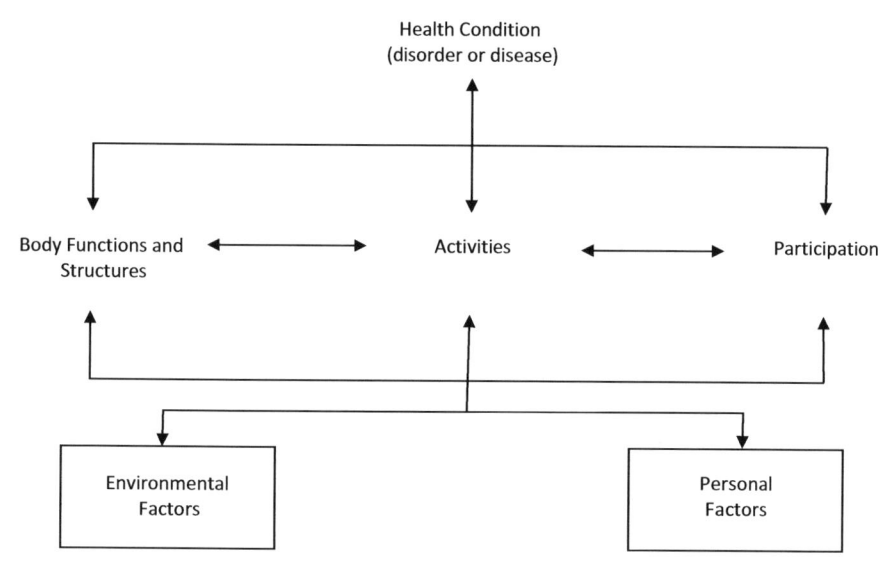

Figure 5.5 *The components of the WHO's* International Classification of Functioning, Disability and Health *(ICF) framework (reproduced with permission of WHO)*

social participation. These various components of the ICF framework are displayed in Figure 5.5.

> **KEY POINTS: Diagnostic and Classification Systems**
>
> - Nosology is the branch of medical science that deals with the classification of diseases. SLTs must be aware of nosology, as it relates to the classification of communication and swallowing disorders.
> - Two international classification systems have relevance to the work of SLTs: the fifth edition of the *Diagnostic and Statistical Manual of Mental Disorders* (DSM-5) and the eleventh edition of the *International Classification of Diseases* (ICD-11).
> - Although the structure and purpose of these systems differ, they both achieve the classification of primary communication disorders such as stuttering and specific language impairment.
> - Many psychiatric and neurodevelopmental disorders have communication impairments as part of their presenting symptoms. These disorders include ASD, schizophrenia and ADHD. SLTs must also be aware of the criteria used to diagnose these disorders and their classification in DSM-5 and ICD-11.
> - ICD-11 is a classification of diseases. Another WHO framework, the *International Classification of Functioning, Disability and Health* (ICF), is a classification of functioning and disability. The ICF is adopted by ASHA in its scope of practice guidelines.

- The ICF framework conceptualizes functioning as an interaction between a health condition, which can cause impairments of body structure and function, and environmental and personal factors. These factors can help or hinder the activity limitations and participation restrictions associated with a health condition.

WEBSITE: Assessment and Diagnosis

After reading the chapter, visit the website and test your knowledge of assessment and diagnosis by answering the short-answer questions for this topic.

Suggestions for Further Reading

Shipley, K. G. and McAfee, J. G. 2016. *Assessment in speech-language pathology: a resource manual*, 5th edn, Boston, MA: Cengage Learning.

This volume examines all aspects of assessment in speech-language pathology. The assessment of speech, language, voice, fluency, hearing and dysphagia is examined in dedicated chapters. There are also chapters on preparatory considerations in assessment (e.g. multicultural considerations); obtaining, interpreting, and reporting assessment information; and assessment of clients with specific conditions (e.g. autism spectrum disorders and neurocognitive disorders).

Kersner, M. and Wright, J. A. (eds.) 2012. *Speech and language therapy: the decision-making process when working with children*, 2nd edn, Abingdon and New York: Routledge.

Part IV in this edited volume contains 13 chapters that examine the assessment of children with communication problems. A wide range of disorders is addressed: specific speech impairment; autism spectrum disorders; specific language impairment; deafness; emotional/behavioural problems; written language difficulties; cleft palate and velopharyngeal anomalies; stammering; learning disabilities; acquired speech and language problems in children; augmentative and alternative communication (AAC); and feeding difficulties. Multicultural issues in assessment are also discussed.

Hegde, M. N. and Freed, D. 2011. *Assessment of communication disorders in adults*, San Diego, CA: Plural Publishing.

The 18 chapters in this volume address all aspects of assessment in adults with communication disorders. The volume is divided into eight parts: foundations of assessment; assessment of motor speech disorders in adults; assessment of aphasia; assessment of right-hemisphere syndrome; assessment of dementia; assessment of traumatic brain injury; assessment of fluency disorders; and assessment of voice.

QUESTIONS: Assessment and Diagnosis

(1) Each of the following statements describes a clinical scenario that involves assessment. For each statement, indicate if a *formal* assessment or an *informal* assessment is required:
  (a) An SLT wants to compare the language skills of a 6-year-old boy to those of his same-age peers for the purpose of an annual team review of the child.
  (b) A 20-year-old man with ASD reports considerable topic management problems to an SLT. The therapist decides to explore his claims that he finds it difficult to change and terminate topics.
  (c) A 45-year-old woman with traumatic brain injury (TBI) reports social withdrawal related to her post-injury conversational difficulties. An SLT decides to examine these difficulties with a view to implementing therapy.
  (d) An SLT conducts an intensive language intervention in a boy with specific language impairment. The therapist wants to compare his post-intervention performance to his pre-intervention language skills.
  (e) A 10-year-old boy with TBI is reported by his teacher to produce narratives that include irrelevant and poorly ordered information. The boy's narratives can also be over-informative. The SLT decides to investigate the teacher's claims.

(2) Part A: The 15 features contained in the inventory of articulation characteristics in Dabul's *Apraxia Battery for Adults – Second Edition* (ABA-2) are listed in full in section 5.3. Match each of the following apraxic speech errors to one of these features:
  (a) pep for 'pet'
  (b) moan for 'man'
  (c) lelo for 'yellow'
  (d) Arifca for 'Africa'
  (e) ben for 'pen'

   Part B: The following single-word productions were recorded in a boy of 4 years of age in response to items in the sounds-in-words section of the *Goldman-Fristoe Test of Articulation – Third Edition* (GFTA-3). Indicate the phonological processes that occur in response to each target word:
  (a) 'swimming' [wɪmɪŋ]
  (b) 'brush' [bʌ]
  (c) 'green' [dɪn]
  (d) 'five' [paɪ]
  (e) 'frog' [pɔ]
  (f) 'ring' [wɪŋ]
  (g) 'car' [tɑ]
  (h) 'wagon' [wædən]
  (i) 'watches' [wɑtɪd]
  (j) 'bath' [bæ]
  (k) 'banana' [nænə]
  (l) 'ball' [bɔ]
  (m) 'spoon' [pun]

(n) 'tree' [ti]
(o) 'jumping' [dʌmpɪŋ]

(3) Imagine you are an SLT who is trying to decide which CELF-5 (*Clinical Evaluation of Language Fundamentals – Fifth Edition*) tests to use to examine language skills in a child who has been referred to your clinic. Each statement below describes a specific language skill that you would like to have information about in relation to the child you are assessing. For each statement, identify the CELF-5 test that should be undertaken to obtain this information:

(a) Ability to comprehend passive voice constructions such as *The car is being followed by the lorry*.
(b) Ability to use inflectional morphemes to form the plural of nouns such as *chair* and *pencil*.
(c) Ability to understand relationships of function between words such as *socks* and *shoes*.
(d) Ability to terminate a topic of conversation in an appropriate way.
(e) Ability to capture the gist of a story and establish the motivations of its main characters.
(f) Ability to interpret the comparative relationships expressed by the sentence *Dan is taller than Jeff, and Lee is taller than both of them*.
(g) Ability to capture the meaning of the word 'little' in the context of the sentence *Dad said, 'There is little left in the box'*.
(h) Ability to arrange the following words and word groups into a sentence: *the runner; the race; to win; going; isn't*.
(i) Ability to engage in repair of conversational breakdown.
(j) Ability to understand the relative clause in the sentence *The girl who has brown hair is holding a doll*.

(4) Respond with *true* or *false* to each of the following statements about the assessment of fluency:

(a) Assessments of stuttering do not include normative data.
(b) Facial grimaces are an avoidance behaviour examined in the *Stuttering Severity Instrument – Fourth Edition* (SSI-4).
(c) The SSI-4 measures the frequency and duration of stuttering.
(d) The *Test of Childhood Stuttering* (TOCS) permits clinicians to examine the influence of syntax on stuttering.
(e) A case history can reveal risk factors for stuttering such as family history.
(f) KiddyCAT examines cognitive aspects of cluttering in preschool children.
(g) Pragmatic anomalies are assessed by the *Predictive Cluttering Inventory*.
(h) OASES examines the impact of cluttering on quality of life.
(i) Pure clutterers are frequently identified on the *Predictive Cluttering Inventory*.
(j) Speech rate is routinely evaluated in an assessment of cluttering.

(5) One of the tasks in the Consensus Auditory-Perceptual Evaluation of Voice (CAPE-V) is the production of the six sentences in (a) to (f) below. These sentences are designed to elicit the various laryngeal behaviours and clinical signs described in (i) to (vi). Match each sentence in (a) to (f) with the description that best characterizes it in (i) to (vi):

(a) The blue spot is on the key again.
(b) How hard did he hit him?

(c) We were away a year ago.
(d) We eat eggs every Easter.
(e) My mama makes lemon jam.
(f) Peter will keep at the peak.
   (i) This sentence elicits hard glottal attack.
   (ii) This sentence is weighted with voiceless plosive sounds.
   (iii) This sentence involves production of every vowel sound in the English language.
   (iv) This sentence incorporates nasal sounds.
   (v) This sentence contains all voiced sounds.
   (vi) This sentence involves easy onset with the /h/.
(6) Which of the following can be established by means of a videofluoroscopic study of swallowing?
   (a) The range of hyoid and laryngeal movement during swallowing.
   (b) Swallowing pressure in the pharynx and cervical oesophagus.
   (c) The presence of post-swallow pharyngeal residue.
   (d) Pressures exerted by lingual peristalsis during the oral phase of swallowing.
   (e) The occurrence of laryngeal penetration or aspiration during swallowing.
(7) Assign each of the following statements to one of these three components of the ICF framework: (1) body structures and functions; (2) activities and participation; and (3) environmental and personal factors.
   (a) A patient with anomic aphasia achieves only 20% accuracy on the Boston Naming Test.
   (b) A child with speech sound disorder displays low motivation during therapy tasks.
   (c) A man with Broca's aphasia following a stroke is unable to return to work as a company director.
   (d) A child with cerebral palsy has weak tongue movements during speech production.
   (e) A client with Parkinson's disease and dysarthria reports difficulties in being understood in noisy environments.
   (f) A woman with voice disorder no longer attends her local amateur drama group.
   (g) An adult with stroke-induced dysarthria exhibits hypernasal speech related to velopharyngeal incompetence.
   (h) A client with TBI is reported to have clinically significant depression and low self-esteem.
   (i) An adult with motor neurone disease displays silent aspiration during swallowing.
   (j) An adult with TBI does not participate in the weekly pub quiz with his friends.

6 Intervention and Outcomes

6.1 Introduction

The results of assessment are used to plan a course of treatment or intervention. If assessment reveals that a client has word-finding difficulties, is unable to construct a coherent narrative and produces weak oral plosives, then an intervention might be expected to address these problems. But this is not always the case. The client who produces weak oral plosives may still be intelligible in all but the most adverse speaking environments. Communication between this client and his work colleagues, family members and friends may not be compromised by this speech difficulty. Indeed, the production of weak oral plosives may have few, if any, implications for the client's social and occupational functioning. Under these circumstances, a clinician may decide not to treat the client's speech difficulty after all but rather to focus on the **word-finding difficulty** that has prevented him from delivering oral presentations in the workplace. What this simple example demonstrates is that intervention is not a process which maps directly onto a client's individual deficits. The planning of intervention must consider a range of concerns only some of which relate to the results of assessment. In this chapter, these concerns are addressed along with the specific techniques that are used by SLTs to treat speech, language, fluency, voice, hearing and swallowing disorders. Of course, any intervention is implemented ultimately with the aim of achieving positive outcomes for a client. Increasingly, researchers are investigating client outcomes in SLT, particularly as a means of demonstrating the effectiveness of interventions. This chapter will also address how outcomes are measured in SLT and what outcomes reveal about intervention in SLT.

Any intervention must satisfy certain minimum requirements. The first, and most important, requirement is that an intervention must not cause harm to clients. Harm can take a number of forms including physical injury or illness (e.g. aspiration in a client with dysphagia) or the presence of psychological or emotional distress. The second requirement is that there must be a demonstrable improvement in a client's communication and/or swallowing skills as a direct result of the intervention. If the improvement in skills would have occurred without the intervention, for example, as a result of developmental maturation in children or spontaneous recovery following a stroke or TBI, the intervention is not effective and should not be implemented. The third requirement is that an intervention must be conducted by an appropriately qualified clinician. An intervention that is normally effective might produce limited gains for a client if it is conducted by a clinician who lacks the knowledge and expertise to implement it appropriately. The fourth requirement is that clients must be convinced that an intervention is a rational approach to the remediation of a communication disorder. If an intervention appears implausible, unrealistic or lacks credibility to a client, then clinicians can expect poor compliance with it. The fifth and final requirement is that an intervention must observe certain temporal parameters. Clients must understand when a course of treatment is to be started and terminated and the frequency of its delivery between these points. An intervention which extends indefinitely becomes a 'way of life' and can foster an unhelpful dependence of the client on the clinician (and possibly vice versa).

Alongside these minimum requirements for an intervention, clinicians must then proceed to set goals for a course of treatment. As described above, goal setting is a complex process that must address a client's impairments without being completely circumscribed by those impairments. Any goal of intervention must be attainable and measurable, and it must represent some improvement in a client's functioning or quality of life. For a client with a neurodegenerative disorder such as motor neurone disease, the restoration of intelligible speech is not an attainable goal. An attainable goal for this client might be the effective use of an alternative communication system. When goals are not measurable, clients and clinicians do not know what it would take to achieve them or even when they have been achieved. While any improvement in the intelligibility of a child with speech sound disorder as a result of intervention is clearly desirable, this becomes a measurable goal only when a percentage level of intelligibility to a specific type of listener (e.g. unfamiliar listener) is specified. Goals must also contribute positively to a client's functioning in one or more domains or result in improvement of a client's quality of life. As described above, the remediation of weak oral plosives is of dubious value as a goal of intervention if this particular speech defect has minimal impact on a client's functioning in social and occupational domains. However, a goal of intervention might be to address a client's mild dysphonia, even before a more significant impairment of language (e.g. word-finding), if there is evidence that the voice disorder is associated with poor self-esteem and reduced quality of life. Goals that are not attainable and measurable, and do not contribute to improvements in functioning and quality of life are unlikely to be met with success in therapy.

The outcomes of intervention are increasingly important in the clinical management of clients. The chief reason for this emphasis on outcomes is economic in nature. Healthcare providers who commission SLT services require evidence that these services are cost-effective. The cost-effectiveness of an intervention is judged in terms of the benefits that clients derive from the intervention. One way to measure these benefits is to examine a client's communication skills and communication-related functioning at the end of intervention and at intervals after the completion of treatment. The measurement of outcomes in SLT is an area of growing research interest. Investigators require answers to two questions: 'What skills should be measured in studies of treatment outcomes?' and 'When should these skills be measured?' In relation to the first question, standardized assessments may permit speech and language skills to be measured in an objective way but may not be a sensitive indicator of the type of communication skills that might constitute a good outcome of treatment for a client (e.g. increased participation in conversation). Improved academic achievement or social and occupational functioning as a result of enhanced communication skills are even less likely to be adequately measured by the assessments normally employed by SLTs. In relation to the second question, research on outcomes should aim to assess skills across a range of time frames. Short-term improvements in speech and language skills or in classroom participation and occupational functioning as a result of intervention are clearly of value to clients. But if therapy gains at 3 months post-intervention are not replicated in positive, longer-term outcomes, then the continued use of a particular intervention may not be warranted.

Even when the type of skills to be assessed and the timing of outcome measurements have been established, SLT researchers must address a number of practical issues. Little research has been conducted into long-term outcomes of children with developmental communication disorders such as specific language impairment. When such research is conducted, it typically involves small numbers of subjects, which limits the conclusions that can be drawn from these studies. For example, in their study of adult psychosocial outcomes of children with specific language impairment (SLI), pragmatic language impairment (PLI) and autism spectrum disorder (ASD), Whitehouse et al. (2009) investigated 19 young adults with a childhood history of SLI, seven with PLI and 11 with high-functioning ASD. Studies of this type are difficult and expensive to conduct. Subjects are often lost to long-term follow-up for reasons such as relocation and change of circumstances. The assessment and monitoring of participants over a 10- or 20-year period is particularly costly and exceeds the resources of most research studies. Even when these practical issues can be overcome, studies of outcomes must address an additional difficulty. A child with SLI may experience poor psychosocial, educational and occupational outcomes as a 25-year-old adult. Such an adult may be in unskilled employment or have no employment, may have few formal qualifications and may report low self-esteem and limited friendships. However, the relationship of impaired language skills to each of these outcomes is unlikely to be a direct, causal one. Even if studies succeed in demonstrating a correlation between language skills and psychosocial outcomes, such correlations must be interpreted with caution.

6.2 Direct and Indirect Approaches to Intervention

SLT intervention can be delivered in many different ways to clients. Traditionally, therapy has taken the form of a one-to-one relationship between a client and an SLT. This traditional method of intervention still remains the most common way in which therapy is delivered to clients. However, as knowledge of communication disorders has increased and technological developments have occurred, this traditional method of intervention now stands alongside a number of other approaches to intervention. It is not uncommon for an intervention to be delivered to a group of clients rather than to a single client, or for more than one therapist to deliver an SLT intervention. Although intervention continues to be delivered for the most part by therapists in schools, hospitals and residential homes, **telerehabilitation** has the potential to deliver interventions in the home or local community via video conferencing and through interactive computer-based therapy activities. Intervention is now as likely to involve spouses, parents and carers as it is clients themselves. In some cases, clients are not treated directly at all, as therapists work only with key individuals in the environment of the client. Therapy tasks may be delivered to a client by a classroom assistant, a spouse or a parent, all of whom work under the guidance of an SLT. Equally common is the use of SLT assistants to administer therapy tasks to clients. What these different methods of delivery all have in common is their positioning on a continuum between direct and indirect intervention. This continuum is shown in Figure 6.1. Each form of intervention it displays will be discussed further in this section.

More often than not, intervention is delivered by an SLT who works directly with an individual client. The client may be accompanied by a spouse, carer or parent, who can play an important supportive role in intervention by completing homework exercises and engaging in monitoring of the client's performance. However, it is the client who is the primary focus of intervention. This direct, one-to-one relationship between the SLT and client is the most effective means of delivering intervention under certain conditions. When clients require intensive practice of specific speech and language targets, individualized intervention is generally recommended. It has long been recognized that children with apraxia of speech require intensive, individualized therapy to improve intelligibility. Campbell (1999) reported that children with apraxia of speech required 81% more individual treatment sessions than children with severe phonological disorder in order to achieve a similar functional outcome. Individualized, direct intervention is warranted under other circumstances. Many clients who are treated by SLTs display cognitive difficulties and behavioural problems. Children with ADHD exhibit **inattention**, **hyperactivity** and **impulsivity**. Not only are these cognitive and behavioural problems difficult for SLTs to manage when other clients are present, but they may also be exacerbated by the presence of these clients. The disorientation of clients with dementia to time and place and

```
          DIRECT                                                    INDIRECT
       INTERVENTION                                               INTERVENTION
    ◄─────────────┬──────────┬──────────────────┬────────────────────────►
                  │          │                  │
                  │    ┌─────┴─────┐     ┌──────┴──────┐
                  │    │ SLT and   │     │ SLT provides│
                  │    │ client in │     │ training    │
                  │    │ one-to-many│    │ and guidance│
                  │    │ relationship│   │ to carers,  │
                  │    │ (e.g. group │   │ classroom   │
                  │    │ therapy with│   │ assistants, │
                  │    │ adults with │   │ etc. who    │
                  │    │ aphasia)    │   │ then        │
                  │    └─────┬─────┘     │ implement   │
                  │          │           │ therapy     │
                  │          │           │ tasks (e.g. │
                  │          │           │ sentence    │
                  │          │           │ production  │
                  │          │           │ exercises   │
                  │          │           │ for child   │
                  │          │           │ with SLI)   │
                  │          │           └──────┬──────┘
```

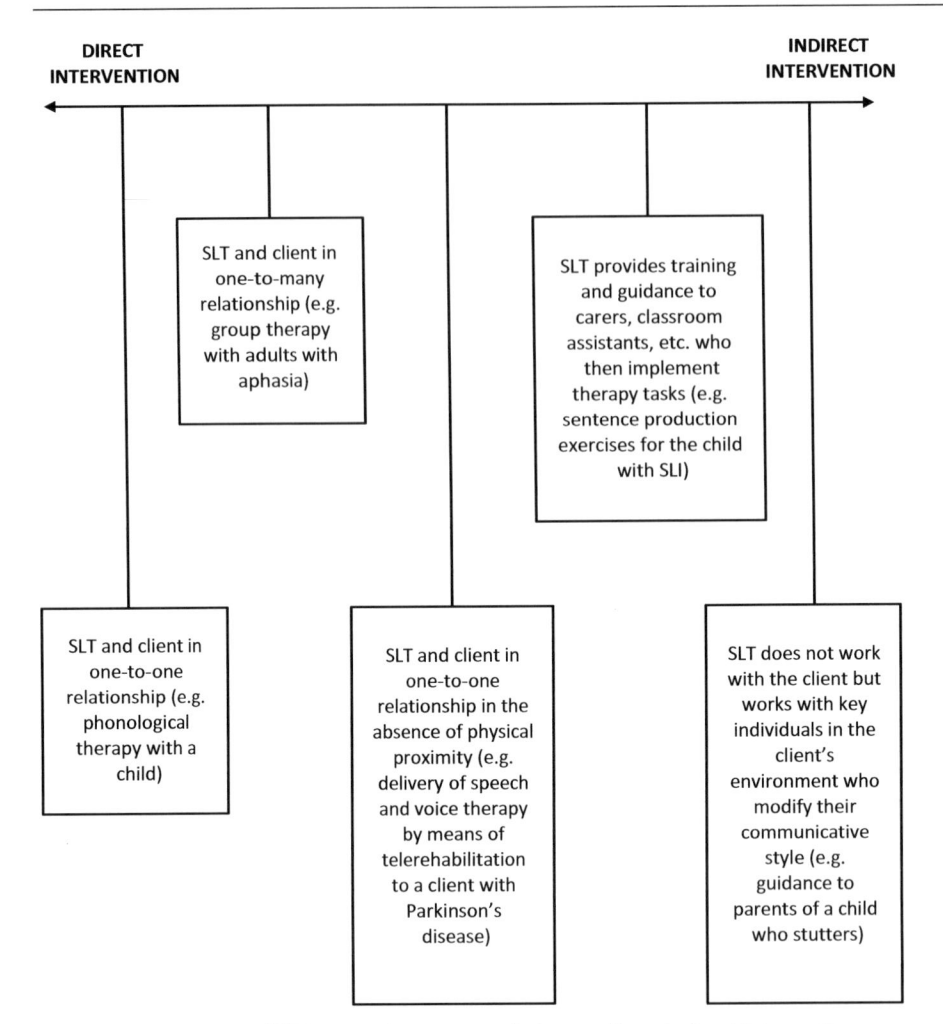

(Figure boxes along the continuum:)

- SLT and client in one-to-one relationship (e.g. phonological therapy with a child)
- SLT and client in one-to-one relationship in the absence of physical proximity (e.g. delivery of speech and voice therapy by means of telerehabilitation to a client with Parkinson's disease)
- SLT does not work with the client but works with key individuals in the client's environment who modify their communicative style (e.g. guidance to parents of a child who stutters)

Figure 6.1 *SLT interventions arranged along a direct-indirect intervention continuum*

symptoms such as delusions and hallucinations in individuals with schizophrenia may be disturbing to other clients. These behaviours and symptoms are most easily managed when clients are treated on an individual basis. For all these reasons, it appears likely that individualized, direct intervention will continue to form the mainstay of SLT intervention.[1]

Direct intervention which is conducted on an individual basis has a considerable body of evidence to support its clinical effectiveness. However, it is also a costly way in which to deliver SLT intervention to clients. With growing pressures on healthcare budgets, there is a strong economic imperative for SLT services to find less expensive, but equally effective ways of delivering intervention to clients. There is evidence that SLT intervention which is delivered to groups of clients is able to address this imperative (Dickson et al., 2009). Group therapy is now used routinely in the treatment of a wide range of client groups including adults with aphasia, children and adults who stutter, and adults with Down syndrome. The benefits of group over individual intervention are considerable. Most everyday communication takes place in conversations involving two or more participants. Group therapy is better able to reflect the dynamics of everyday conversation than an individual intervention in which clients respond to prompts and questions from a therapist. Group therapy also provides clients with an opportunity to practise communication skills in a safe, non-threatening environment before these skills are put into practice in everyday communication. For example, clients who stutter can gain practice in making and receiving telephone calls before progressing to use these skills in real-life situations. Also, group therapy provides clients with much needed psychosocial support. Adults with aphasia can experience depression and reduced quality of life as they struggle to adjust to their disability and its impact on their lives. The opportunity to discuss these concerns with others who are experiencing the same challenges can facilitate adjustment to disability.

In direct individual and group intervention, the SLT and client(s) occupy the same physical setting. The technological developments that have made telerehabilitation possible have changed the therapeutic interface to such an extent that the SLT and client no longer need to be in physical or temporal proximity in order for intervention to take place. Clients and SLTs can be in different geographical areas. Clients can work synchronously (in real time) with a speech-language pathologist or asynchronously (offline) with a stand-in virtual therapist (Cherney and van Vuuren, 2012). In its relatively short history, telerehabilitation has had many applications in SLT, including its use in intensive swallowing therapy during chemoradiotherapy in patients with head and neck cancer (Wall et al., 2017), in intervention with patients with chronic post-stroke aphasia (Choi et al., 2016) and in the treatment of school-age students with speech sound disorders (Grogan-Johnson et al., 2011). Towey (2013) describes the benefits of telerehabilitation in SLT in the following terms:

> Speech telepractice 'costs' people less to get service, in technology expense, and in time spent traveling. Geography or physical limitations are no longer barriers to treatment. For patients who must get services at home, telepractice provides a less instrusive method of service delivery than admitting strangers into the privacy of a home for 'home visits' (Towey, 2013: 106)

Notwithstanding its many clinical applications and reported benefits, telerehabilitation remains an under-utilized resource in SLT. In ASHA's 2015 SLP Health Care Survey, only 2% of survey participants delivered clinical services remotely (i.e. via telepractice) (ASHA, 2015b). Cherney and van Vuuren (2012) reported that regulatory issues including licensure, reimbursement, and threats to privacy and confidentiality hinder the routine implementation of telerehab services into the clinical setting. Perhaps unexpectedly, in a review of telehealth publications in the field of SLT, Keck and Doarn (2014) found that technological adversities were not a cause of discontinuation of teleheath services by practitioners or clients.

Many SLT interventions are delivered indirectly to clients through parents, spouses, carers and SLT assistants. There are many cases where indirect intervention with clients may be implemented to good effect. Some communication disorders (e.g. childhood apraxia of speech) require intensive practice and drills on the part of clients in order for progress to occur. Other communication disorders (e.g. aphasia) display significant improvement when therapy is delivered intensively in the early post-injury period. Still other communication disorders (e.g. speech sound disorder) require intensive intervention before a child enters school. In all these cases, resource limitations mean that SLTs are unable to deliver intervention at the intensity that is required for the client to make progress, and must rely on individuals such as parents and spouses to act as 'proxy' therapists. In this role, parents and spouses may complete homework exercises with the client between weekly sessions, or monitor and provide feedback to the client on aspects of speech and language that are targeted in therapy. In each of these tasks, they are guided by the SLT who is responsible for setting clear parameters for the work that is undertaken by parents and others. It is SLTs who must decide the goals of an intervention and how these goals are to be achieved. Parents and spouses must be provided with materials and instructed in how to use them. They must also receive clear guidance on what constitutes success in a particular task, when and how to reward the client, and when to increase or decrease the difficulty of a task. When appropriately guided, parents, spouses and carers can make a significant contribution to the overall therapeutic input that a client receives. At the same time, they can be kept informed of a client's progress in therapy.

Finally, some SLT interventions involve no direct work with the client at all. Instead, significant others in the client's environment are the sole focus of intervention. This model of intervention is warranted under certain circumstances. First, clients may be too cognitively impaired for SLTs to work with them directly. For example, adults with Alzheimer's dementia may lack the self-awareness and other cognitive skills that are needed to comply with therapy. However, communicative gains may still be possible if conversational partners are instructed in how to modify their communication with these clients. Second, a client's communicative difficulties may originate entirely in behaviours of a conversational partner such as when an adult with aphasia is required to respond to questions to which the partner already knows the answer. Such 'test' questions are a source of frustration for adults with aphasia who may assume a passive role in conversation as a result. Third, many young children experience problems with **fluency**, but only some will go on to become stutterers. When difficulties with fluency first emerge, it is advisable for SLTs to work with parents to achieve environmental adjustments that can facilitate a child's fluency. Simple modifications to parental behaviour and family routine can help a young child achieve fluency in a situation where direct intervention risks adverse consequences.

In each of these scenarios, significant others in the client's environment are the focus of intervention and can become positive agents of change in the client's communication skills. This most indirect method of intervention may need to be replaced by a direct treatment, such as when a child's problems with fluency persist and therapy for stuttering is implemented.

> **KEY POINTS: Direct and Indirect Approaches to Intervention**
> - Most therapeutic encounters in SLT involve a therapist working with one client. Although this has been the traditionally dominant model of SLT intervention, and continues to be the preferred form of intervention for the treatment of certain clients, several other methods of intervention are also routinely used.
> - SLT interventions can be arranged along a continuum from direct to indirect intervention. In a direct intervention, the SLT works with one or more clients without an interface in the form of technology or other people. In an indirect intervention, the SLT works with clients through 'proxy' therapists such as parents and spouses or does not work with clients at all. Between these direct and indirect interventions is telerehabilitation, in which an SLT can work with clients but does so remotely through the use of technology.
> - Direct intervention with an individual or a group may involve phonological therapy with a child or group therapy with adults with aphasia, respectively. There is evidence to support the clinical effectiveness of direct individual and group treatment.
> - Indirect intervention may be undertaken by a classroom assistant who completes language exercises with a child. It may also include advice and training to the parents of a dysfluent child or the conversational partner of an adult with aphasia.
> - The selection of a direct or an indirect intervention is based on a range of factors including costs, training of individuals, needs of the client and purpose of the intervention. Both forms of intervention may be used simultaneously or sequentially, as when an indirect treatment with the parents of a dysfluent child is replaced with a direct treatment as stuttering persists.

6.3 Clinical Interventions: Speech

Speech interventions are a significant aspect of the work of SLTs. The selection of an intervention for a speech disorder is based on several factors including the results of assessment, the medical and communication diagnoses of a client, the severity of a speaker's unintelligibility, personality traits such as motivation, and a client's psychiatric status. In illustration of these factors, consider a scenario in which a speech assessment has revealed limited range and strength of articulatory movements for speech production. For example, tongue movements for the production of oral plosive sounds may be weak, palatal excursion may be insufficient to close the velopharyngeal port and there may be reduced respiratory support for speech. These assessment results are consistent with a communication diagnosis of dysarthria for which a motor speech intervention may be warranted. However, let us also imagine that the client displays moderate unintelligibility and has a medical diagnosis of motor neurone disease. In other words, this client's dysarthria is progressive and will worsen as his underlying neurological disorder deteriorates. A motor speech intervention is less warranted in these circumstances than some form of augmentative and alternative communication (AAC). But an intervention based on AAC is complicated by the fact that the client exhibits depression. Moreover, he has shown little motivation to engage with AAC, preferring instead to make many unsuccessful attempts at spoken communication. In short, a complex interplay of factors must be brought to bear when deciding which form of speech intervention to use in a particular case.

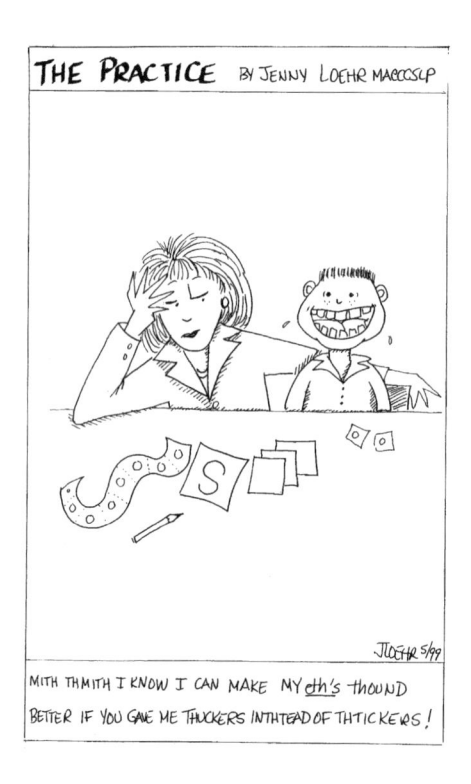

THE PRACTICE BY JENNY LOEHR MA&CCSLP

MITH THMITH I KNOW I CAN MAKE MY *eth's* thOUND BETTER IF YOU GAVE ME THUCKERS INTHTEAD OF THTICKERS!

There are many different speech interventions used with children and adults in clinical practice. In a review of interventions for children with speech, language and communication needs, Law et al. (2012) identified 17 interventions that were specifically relevant for improving a child's speech. These interventions are displayed in Table 6.1. Collectively, they are used to treat children with speech

Table 6.1 *Speech interventions in children*

Intervention	Description
Core Vocabulary Approach (Crosbie et al., 2005)	Designed for use with children who have inconsistent speech disorder (many of their words are produced with inconsistent pronunciations), but there are no signs of developmental verbal dyspraxia
Cued Speech	Designed primarily to help deaf and hearing-impaired speakers to learn English, to help lip reading and to support the development of literacy
Cycles Approach (Hodson and Paden, 1991)	Initially developed for use with children who have speech that is very difficult to understand because of a large number of erroneous speech sounds; used with children who have severe expressive phonological impairments and children who have phonological deviations related to developmental verbal dyspraxia, repaired cleft palate, hearing impairment with and without cochlear implant and learning difficulties
Electropalatography	Used for the assessment and treatment of severe speech disorders related to structural abnormalities of the vocal tract (e.g. cleft palate), developmental speech disorders, developmental neuromotor difficulties (e.g. dyspraxia) and acquired neurological disorders (e.g. dysarthria)
Focused Auditory Stimulation	A component of the Cycles Approach (Hodson and Paden, 1991) to the remediation of very unclear speech; used with children who are young (between 3 and 6 years old) and who cannot make the target sound, or are unwilling or unable to join in with other types of intervention
Gillon Phonological Awareness Training Programme	Based on the work of Gillon (2004), this programme targets phonological awareness, speech production and literacy skills in children aged 5 to 7 years with speech impairment
Lidcombe Program	A behavioural treatment for young children who stutter
Maximal Oppositions	Based on the work of Gierut and colleagues (Gierut, 1992, 2001; Gierut et al., 1987), this intervention subscribes to the idea that

Table 6.1 (*cont.*)

Intervention	Description
	more complex linguistic input promotes greater change in a child's phonological system
Meaningful Minimal Contrast Therapy	One of a number of contrast therapies, the aim of which is to improve speech production in children with phonological impairment
Metaphon (Dean et al., 1990, 1995)	A cognitive-linguistic treatment that aims to increase metalinguistic awareness as a means of improving phonological change and speech sound production
Multiple Opposition Therapy (Williams, 2000, 2005)	A type of contrast therapy that is aimed at children with moderate to severe speech disorder; it is intended specifically for those children who have preferences for particular phonemes such that one phoneme is used as a substitute for multiple targets
Non-Linear Phonological Intervention (Bernhardt, 1992; Berhardt and Stoel-Gammon, 1994; Bernhardt and Stemberger, 1998)	Based on theories of phonology that describe the hierarchical representation of the phonological system from the prosodic phrase down to the individual features of a phoneme; focus of intervention is awareness and production of the phonological form
Non-Speech Oro-Motor Exercises	Targets the sensorimotor functions that underlie speech production; benefits clients whose speech difficulties arise from sensorimotor impairment (e.g. reduced or impaired strength and range of movement)
Nuffield Centre Dyspraxia Programme (Williams and Stephens, 2004)	Designed for children with severe speech disorders and specifically those with difficulties in motor programming and planning
Parents and Children Together (PACT)	Designed for young children aged 3 to 6 years with speech sound difficulties; SLT involves parents and significant others in therapy
Phoneme Factory	Seven computerized activities including sound–symbol matching, rhyming, blending and minimal pair discrimination; designed to increase speech input processing skills leading to changes in the child's phonological system

Table 6.1 (*cont.*)

Intervention	Description
Stimulability Treatment (Miccio and Elbert, 1996)	Designed for young children aged 2 to 4 years who have very small phonetic inventories and are not stimulable for production of many or all absent sounds
Prompts for Restructuring Oral Muscular Phonetic Targets (PROMPT; Hayden, 2006, 2008)*	A sensorimotor, cognitive-linguistic intervention designed for children as young as 2 years who have sensory, motor and phonological impairment affecting speech development

* PROMPT was not included in the 17 speech interventions identified by Law et al. (2012). It is described by the authors as an 'up-and-coming' intervention because it is under development and there is insufficient evidence to judge its value.

sound disorders related to structural anomalies (e.g. cleft palate), neurological impairments and motor programming deficits, or where a speech sound disorder occurs in the absence of an identifiable aetiology. Although space limitations preclude their individual examination, some comments about the features of these interventions are necessary. Some interventions target the sensory and motor substrates of speech production on the assumption that speech will improve by increasing the strength and range of movement of articulators such as the lips and tongue. Typically, these interventions are used to treat children with speech sound disorders that are related to dysarthria. Other speech interventions do not attempt to address neuromuscular weakness of the speech musculature but focus instead on the planning and programming of articulatory movements that are required to produce speech sounds. These interventions are used to treat children with speech sound disorders that are related to apraxia of speech. Still other interventions have the child's phonological system as their therapeutic focus. A wide range of interventions that target the phonological system in children with speech sound disorders have been developed in SLT. Some of these interventions address **phonological awareness** and literacy, while others emphasize stimulability or the use of contrastive therapies. Each of these interventions will be examined further below.

Many childhood-onset disorders including cerebral palsy, Duchenne's muscular dystrophy and traumatic brain injury can compromise the sensory and motor functions that are essential to intelligible speech production. Tongue movements may be weak and limited in range with the result that alveolar plosives are realized as alveolar fricative sounds. Palatal elevation may be insufficient to make contact with the posterior and lateral pharyngeal walls, leading to the production of nasalized vowels and oral plosive sounds. Lip closure for the production of bilabial sounds may be weak, and there may be reduced respiratory support for speech. Each of these anomalies is consistent with the motor speech disorder developmental dysarthria. In Table 6.1, interventions such as PROMPT and Non-Speech Oro-Motor Exercises have the sensory and motor substrates of speech production as their therapeutic focus. PROMPT is a tactile-kinaesthetic approach that uses touch cues to a client's articulators to guide them manually through a targeted word, phrase or sentence. The PROMPT Institute (2016) states that 'the technique develops motor control and the development of proper oral muscular movements, while eliminating unnecessary muscle movements, such as jaw sliding and inadequate lip rounding'. PROMPT therapy may be used with clients who have aphasia, apraxia/dyspraxia, dysarthria, pervasive development disorders, cerebral palsy, acquired brain injuries and autism spectrum disorders.

Non-speech oro-motor exercises (NSOMEs) target non-speech oral movements on the assumption that improvements in these movements can lead to gains in speech production. Ruscello (2008: 380) defines non-speech oro-motor treatments as a 'collection of nonspeech methods and procedures that claim to influence tongue, lip, and jaw resting postures; increase strength; improve muscle tone; facilitate range of motion; and develop muscle control'. The most commonly used NSOMEs include blowing, tongue push-ups, pucker-smile, tongue wags, big smile, tongue-to-nose-to-chin, cheek puffing, blowing kisses and tongue curling. These techniques are widely used in clinical practice. In a nationwide survey of speech-language pathologists, Lof and Watson (2008) reported that 85% of respondents used NSOMEs to address children's speech sound production problems. However, there is little or no evidence to support the clinical effectiveness of these techniques. In a Cochrane **systematic review**, Lee and Gibbon (2015) reported that there is currently no strong evidence to suggest that non-speech oro-motor treatments are an effective treatment or an effective adjunctive treatment for children with developmental speech sound disorders. The issue of **evidence-based practice** will be examined further in section 6.9.

Children with speech sound disorders may display no neuromuscular weakness during speech production and yet still be highly unintelligible on account of a large number of speech errors. For these children, speech production difficulties are related to impairments of motor programming and planning in childhood apraxia of speech (CAS). Several interventions in Table 6.1 can be used to treat the speech errors of children with apraxia of speech. The *Nuffield Centre Dyspraxia Programme – Third Edition* (NDP3; Williams and Stephens, 2004) is the most significant of these interventions. The NDP3 can be used with any child who has a speech disorder. However, it is most suitable for children who have pronounced difficulties producing consonant and vowel sounds and whose speech production is characterized by dyspraxic features such as sequencing difficulties, inconsistency, speech sound omissions and substitutions, and suprasegmental (prosodic) difficulties. The programme starts with pre-speech motor skills and works systematically to connected speech. There is evidence to support the clinical effectiveness of NDP3. Murray et al. (2015) used a randomized controlled trial to compare the NDP3 to the experimental treatment Rapid Syllable Transition. Although both treatments aim to improve motor planning and programming in children with CAS, they differ in the types of stimuli used, principles of motor learning and level of stimulus complexity at the outset of treatment. Treatment was delivered to 26 children aged 4 to 12 years with mild to severe CAS. Large treatment effects, which included significant **generalization** to untreated stimuli, were obtained for both interventions.

Several interventions in Table 6.1 have the phonological system as their therapeutic focus. They include the Cycles Approach, the Gillon Phonological Awareness Training Programme and Maximal Oppositions. Children whose speech disorder is related to a phonological impairment are unintelligible on account of a reduced system of sound contrasts in their phonological system. By increasing these contrasts, children are able to express meanings that cannot be conveyed when they employ one phonetic form to refer to several different words (e.g. the use of [at] to mean *bat*, *cat*, *fat*, *hat* and *mat* in a child with initial consonant deletion). An expansion of sound contrasts can be achieved by working on a child's phonological awareness skills. Phonological awareness refers to an individual's awareness of the sound structure of a spoken word. It is integral to both speech production and literacy development in the Gillon Phonological Awareness Training Programme. On this approach, phonological awareness is developed through direct work on rhyme, phoneme analysis, phoneme identity, phoneme segmentation, phoneme blending and phoneme manipulation. As well as training specific components of phonological awareness, Gillon's intervention links speech to print. Speech gains achieved through phonological awareness training may, therefore, be expected to be matched by gains in literacy. Gillon (2000) demonstrated concurrent gains in phoneme awareness, speech production and early reading skills in children with spoken language impairment and early reading delay who had received an integrated phonological awareness intervention. Another intervention that places central emphasis on phonological awareness is Metaphon (Dean et al., 1990, 1995).

Interventions such as Multiple Opposition Therapy in Table 6.1 are contrast therapies. These therapies focus on production using contrasting word pairs instead of individual sounds. A contrast therapy based on minimal pairs demands least phonological knowledge on the part of the child, as word pairs contain sounds that differ in terms of one **distinctive feature** only. Sounds can differ in terms of voicing (*pin* vs *bin*), place of articulation (*take* vs *cake*), or manner of articulation (*nine* vs *dine*). A contrast therapy that uses maximal pairs demands most phonological knowledge, as sounds differ on all three dimensions simultaneously. For example, the sounds /f/ and /g/ in the word pair *fun* vs *gun* differ in terms of voicing (voiceless vs voiced), place of articulation (labiodental vs velar) and manner of articulation (fricative vs plosive). Other contrast therapies can use many contrasts within a particular phonological error pattern. For example, for the child who exhibits **final consonant deletion**, *pie* can be contrasted with *pipe*, *pine*, *pile* and *pies*. Still other contrast therapies can use multiple oppositions across a phoneme collapse, e.g. where /d/ is used in place of all plosive sounds in *tea*, *pea*, *bee*, *key* and *ghee*. Dodd et al. (2008) compared two interventions that differed in the nature of the word pairs that were contrasted in therapy. One group of children received an intervention that was based on a traditional minimal pair approach. A second group received an intervention that used contrasts that differed across a range of distinctive features. Both interventions produced improvements in speech accuracy and the number of error patterns suppressed. However, there was no difference between the two interventions in terms of the children's progress.

Traditionally, phonological interventions have emphasized teaching early developing, stimulable sounds as a foundation for the acquisition of later developing, more difficult sounds. Stimulability Treatment (Miccio and Elbert, 1996) inverts this traditional approach by giving priority in intervention to the treatment of non-stimulable sounds. Miccio and Elbert undertook stimulability treatment in a girl aged 3;4 years called Stacy. With the exception of the liquids /r/ and /l/, which were not treated and served as controls, Stacy was taught most major consonants at once. Because the goal of intervention was to enhance stimulability, sounds were taught in isolation or in the case of some sounds (e.g. stops or glides) in a CV context. Following treatment, Stacy increased the number of stimulable sounds in her repertoire. More recently, Tyler and Macrae (2010) examined stimulability treatment in a study of 18 children with speech sound disorders. The results confirmed stimulability treatment as an effective method of intervention. Marked relations between stimulability and percentage consonants correct and between stimulability and phonetic inventory size were obtained in these children. However, this approach to intervention is not without criticism. Rvachew and Nowak (2001: 621) stated that 'unless the treatment of unstimulable phonemes boosts the rate of progress for stimulable phonemes beyond that due to maturation, it is difficult to see how the selective treatment of unstimulable phonemes could be the most efficient procedure'.

There is also an extensive range of speech interventions for adults with motor speech disorders such as dysarthria and apraxia of speech. Adults with acquired dysarthria may be treated using one or more of the following interventions: (1) articulation, voice and prosody training; (2) behavioural interventions; (3) the use of sign language as a supplement or alternative to speech; (4) prosthetic devices; (5) assistive communication devices; (6) listener training programmes; and (7) listener advice. An example of the interventions in (1) is the use of the Lee Silverman Voice Treatment to treat speech and voice disorders in adults with Parkinson's disease. An adult with stroke-induced dysarthria may have hypernasal speech related to velopharyngeal incompetence. A **palatal lift** device is an example of a prosthetic intervention in (4) which may be used to achieve adequate velopharyngeal closure for speech production. The interventions in (5) include the use of 'low-tech' aids such as drawing and writing, or communication books, and 'high-tech' aids such as computerized voice output communication devices. These may be used with adults who have progressive dysarthria as a result of neurodegenerative diseases such as motor neurone disease. Interventions in (7) which emphasize listener advice can recommend environmental modifications that improve the **comprehensibility** of adults with dysarthria. Speaking against background noise, in a poorly lit room or to a conversational partner who does not wear a hearing aid can all reduce the comprehensibility of adults with dysarthria. Notwithstanding the widespread use of these different types of intervention, Sellars et al. (2005) concluded in a systematic review that there is limited evidence to support the clinical effectiveness of SLT interventions for adults with dysarthria due to non-progressive brain damage.

SPECIAL TOPIC: Augmentative and Alternative Communication

Spoken language is not a functional means of communication for many children and adults, and must be supplemented or replaced by an augmentative or alternative communication (AAC) system. The clients who can benefit from AAC are wide-ranging in age and medical diagnosis. They include children with cerebral palsy and dysarthria who may be severely unintelligible to all but the most familiar listeners. Progressive dysarthria may compromise speech production in adults with neurological disorders such as multiple sclerosis and motor neurone disease. Children and adults with language disorders may also benefit from AAC. For example, AAC provides adults with progressive non-fluent aphasia with a means of continuing to communicate as verbal expression declines. It can also facilitate communication in children with Landau-Kleffner syndrome, a rare, seizure-related language disorder with onset in childhood.

AAC systems can be broadly classified as aided or unaided. An aided AAC system requires the use of supplemental materials and equipment. This may be a communication board with letters, line drawing symbols or photographs. It may also include the use of picture books, flashcards, texture-based symbols (e.g. Braille), text telephone devices and speech-generating devices. Children with ASD who use the Picture Exchange Communication System to communicate are using an aided AAC system. Unaided AAC systems make no use of materials and equipment and employ non-verbal means of communication. This may be gestures and facial expressions. It can also include manual signs in a formal sign language like British or American Sign Language and Makaton. Adults with aphasia who use gestures in place of words that they cannot produce are using an unaided AAC system.

While the benefits of AAC are clear enough, not every form of AAC is suitable for a client and their communicative partners. Visual field impairments may limit a client's ability to scan letters or symbols on a communication board or a computer screen. Motor impairment may prevent the use of a manual sign system or use of a computer keyboard. Cognitive deficits may limit a client's ability to understand what symbols signify or the use of a complex AAC system that requires considerable learning. Each of these factors affects the selection of an AAC system. Comprehensive assessment of clients is necessary in order to determine which form of AAC is likely to be

> successfully adopted. Assessment should also take place on a regular basis. This is particularly important in the case where a client's medical condition may change (improve or deteriorate) and AAC is no longer required or a different AAC system must be used.

Interventions for acquired apraxia of speech (AOS) generally fall into one of four categories: (1) articulatory-kinematic treatments; (2) rate/rhythm control treatments; (3) intersystemic facilitation/reorganization treatments; and (4) AAC approaches. Articulatory-kinematic treatments focus on improving spatial and temporal aspects of speech production. They employ a combination of repeated motoric practice, modelling-repetition, integral stimulation, and articulatory cueing. In integral stimulation, the client imitates utterances produced by the clinician, with attention focused on both the auditory model and the clinician's face. Rate/rhythm control treatments such as metronomic pacing and metrical pacing improve speech production by manipulating the rate and/or rhythm of speech. An intervention based on intersystemic facilitation/reorganization uses relatively intact systems to facilitate speech production. Iconic gestures such as Amerind (American Indian Sign) and rhythmic gestures such as tapping and fingercounting may be used to facilitate and/or supplement speech. Amerind may also be used as an AAC intervention for AOS along with communication boards/notebooks, spoken computer output and an **electrolarynx** (the latter in the case of **laryngeal apraxia**). In a systematic review of AOS intervention research, Ballard et al. (2015) reported that the weight of evidence supports a strong effect of both articulatory-kinematic and rate/rhythm approaches to AOS treatment.

KEY POINTS: Clinical Interventions: Speech

- Speech interventions may be used to treat children and adults with motor speech disorders (dysarthria and apraxia of speech), speech disorders related to structural anomalies (e.g. cleft palate), and speech disorders for which there is no identifiable aetiology.
- The neuromuscular weakness that gives rise to speech errors in dysarthria may be targeted in non-speech oro-motor exercises. These exercises aim to increase the range and strength of movements for speech production. The effectiveness of these exercises has been questioned.
- Interventions for developmental and acquired apraxia of speech have a different focus: the motor planning and programming of speech production. There is evidence to support the clinical effectiveness of the *Nuffield Centre Dyspraxia Programme* in children and articulatory-kinematic and rate/rhythm approaches to AOS treatment in adults.
- Speech sound disorders in children may also be related to phonological impairments. Phonological interventions are widely used in clinical practice. Some address phonological awareness, literacy and

> stimulability. Contrast therapies are commonly used in the treatment of phonological disorders.
> - Where speech is highly unintelligible and is unlikely to improve, or is unintelligible and is likely to deteriorate, an intervention that has a speech focus may be inappropriate. An AAC intervention may be necessary. Interventions of this type may be 'low tech' (e.g. communication board) or 'high tech' (e.g. computerized voice output communication device).

6.4 Clinical Interventions: Language

An SLT evaluation may reveal that a client's communication difficulties are related to impaired language skills. An extensive range of interventions is available to address these skills. The selection of an appropriate language intervention must be guided by the client's language diagnosis as well as other factors. Children with Down syndrome and children with specific language impairment (SLI) may both omit **auxiliary verbs** (e.g. *He falling down*) and **inflectional suffixes** (e.g. *Sally walk home*) in spoken language. However, the language intervention that works for a child with normal intellectual functioning (SLI) may not be appropriate for a child whose language difficulties are related to intellectual disability (Down syndrome). In the same way, adults with stroke-induced aphasia and adults with Alzheimer's dementia may both display word-finding difficulties. However, while a language intervention may produce gains in a client with a neurological injury (stroke), which may improve or is static, the same gains are unlikely to be achieved in a client whose neurological damage (Alzheimer's disease) is progressive in nature. Having selected an appropriate language intervention, SLTs must consider a range of other factors that are likely to influence the outcome of an intervention. A language intervention that involves twice weekly therapy with no additional stimulation of a client between sessions is unlikely to result in a positive outcome. Yet, this is exactly the situation of child clients who lack parental input, and adults with aphasia who are depressed and display poor compliance with homework exercises. The contribution of personality traits and a client's psychiatric status to the success of an intervention cannot be overestimated.

In a review of interventions for children with speech, language and communication needs, Law et al. (2012) identified 23 interventions that specifically targeted language. These interventions are displayed in Table 6.2. Although most of these interventions treat more than one aspect of language, several interventions target specific language skills. These skills may involve morphosyntax (e.g. Morphosyntactic Intervention), vocabulary (e.g. Word Wizard) or semantics (e.g. Colourful Semantics). In several interventions, there is an emphasis on developing awareness of language and of one's comprehension

Table 6.2 *Language interventions in children*

Intervention	Description
The Becky Shanks Narrative Intervention (Shanks, 2001)	Focuses on understanding and using story grammar to support children to tell verbal narratives and stories
Broad Target Recasts	A specific intervention programme based on recast technique – a more experienced speaker responds to what a child says by expanding, deleting or changing their utterances while maintaining the meaning
Colourful Semantics	Uses coloured visual prompt cards to 'show' the structure of a sentence, thus linking the structure of a sentence (syntax) and its meaning (semantics)
Comprehension Monitoring	Develops the child's ability to recognize and react to not understanding what has been said (meta-awareness)
The Derbyshire Language Scheme (Knowles and Masidlover, 1982)	Published by Derbyshire County Council, this intervention uses individual and group activities to improve a child's use and understanding of language. Teaching activities are linked to approximately 200 language objectives.
Earobics	A comprehensive, computerized intervention programme for training phonological awareness and auditory-language processing
Every Child A Talker (ECAT)	ECAT targets practitioners and parents and is designed to help them establish environments that will optimally support a child's language and communication development.
Fast ForWord (Scientific Learning Corporation, 2016)	A computerized intervention programme that aims to improve children's reading and oral language skills
Focused Stimulation	A technique used to draw a child's attention to specific aspects of grammar or vocabulary; a particular word, phrase or grammatical form is targeted and used repeatedly while interacting with the child
Language For Thinking	Supports the development of higher-level language such as verbal reasoning and inferencing; students progress through levels of questioning, from concrete questions about the here and now ('What is this?') to abstract questions where they are

Table 6.2 (*cont.*)

Intervention	Description
	asked to predict or justify why something has happened ('What would happen if ...?')
Let's Learn Language	A parent language promotion training programme that aims to reduce early language delay and behaviour problems related to early language delay; promotes child-centred interactions, with children taking the lead and parents modelling language when responding to their children
Let's Talk Programme	Developed by specialist teachers and SLTs, this programme aims to raise awareness of speech, language and communication in primary schools and to develop the confidence and skills of teaching staff in identifying and responding to children with speech, language and communication needs. Training is delivered to key staff in a school via language groups for children.
Living Language	A theoretically derived and highly structured developmental programme which teaches spoken language and is intended to mirror the way that children normally learn language. Children are taught the words and constructions that they need to know to relate to people they come into contact with and to learn from their environment, especially in school.
Milieu Teaching/Therapy	Involves manipulating or arranging stimuli in a preschool child's natural environment to create a setting that encourages them to engage in a targeted behaviour (e.g. a desirable toy may be placed out of reach to encourage a child to request it). Four strategies are used to encourage a student to demonstrate a targeted behaviour: modelling; mand-modelling; incidental teaching; and time-delay.
Morphosyntactic Intervention	Targets morphosyntactic aspects of language through three main activities: auditory awareness activities; focused stimulation activities; and elicited production activities; clinicians provide children with

Table 6.2 (*cont.*)

Intervention	Description
	different levels of support, from the highest level where forced choice tasks are used (e.g. 'The man jumps or runs?') to the lowest level where the clinician indirectly demonstrates for the child how to use target language within an activity or conversation
The Oral Language Programme	Includes direct instruction to develop vocabulary, inferencing, expressive language and listening skills
Phonology with Reading Programme	This intervention is inspired by research on reading difficulty which indicates that combining phonological training with reading is successful in facilitating reading development in poor readers. This intervention consists of three components: letter-sound knowledge; phonological awareness; and reading books at the instructional level. Phonological awareness training is the key component.
Shape Coding	Uses a combination of shapes, colours and arrows to 'code' phrases, parts of speech, and words and word endings, respectively; designed to 'show' the structure of a sentence and link the structure of a sentence and its meaning
Strathclyde Language Intervention Programme (McCartney, 2007)	Promotes the language development of children with specific language impairments; includes comprehension monitoring, vocabulary development, grammar and narrative therapy
Talk Boost	Aimed at children with delayed language development between 4 and 7 years and provides support for them to close the gap/ catch up with their peers; focuses on listening, vocabulary, sentence building, storytelling and conversations; includes a training package for teaching and support staff
Talking Time (Dockrell et al., 2006, 2010)	An interactive oral language intervention package designed to support language and to foster communication with and between preschool children; the aim is to develop children's language before they reach

Table 6.2 (*cont.*)

Intervention	Description
	primary school. Three key skills are targeted: vocabulary development; the ability to make inferences; and the ability to recount a narrative.
Visualizing and Verbalizing (Bell, 1987)	Designed to help understanding of language in language-impaired students; aims to improve listening and reading comprehension by focusing on mental imagery skills
Word Wizard	Teaches targeted vocabulary from the National Curriculum to children with specific language impairment who are taught in mainstream schools; uses word meanings, speech sounds and repetition to help children learn new vocabulary
Enhancing Language and Communication in Secondary Schools (ELCISS)*	Aims to enhance language and communication in secondary school children with primary language and communication impairment through narrative/storytelling and vocabulary enrichment
Language 4 Learning*	Developed for use with preschool children with delayed language development to promote pre-literacy and oral language skills; carried out by SLT assistants under the direction of experienced SLTs; children treated at home with parents

* Enhancing Language and Communication in Secondary Schools (ELCISS) and Language 4 Learning were not included in the 23 language interventions identified by Law et al. (2012). They are described by the authors as 'up-and-coming' interventions because they are under development and there is insufficient evidence to judge their value.

of language. Interventions like Earobics and Phonology with Reading Programme emphasize phonological awareness, while Comprehension Monitoring develops children's awareness of their understanding of language. A number of interventions aim to establish environments that are supportive of children's language learning (e.g. Every Child a Talker). Others involve computerized interventions (e.g. *Fast ForWord*), interventions delivered through parents, teachers and SLT assistants (e.g. Let's Learn Language) and interventions that have a focus on educational settings (e.g. Enhancing Language and Communication in Secondary Schools). Some interventions have a visual component (e.g. Shape Coding), while others emphasize language-related cognitive skills like reasoning and **inferencing** (e.g. Language for Thinking). With such diversity of content and approach, it is not possible to examine each of these language interventions in detail. However, some general remarks are in order.

Of all language skills addressed by the interventions in Table 6.2, those that target vocabulary are most common. This reflects the fact that the use and understanding of vocabulary are not only essential to a child's communicative success but also central to a child's ability to access the curriculum. The first challenge of any vocabulary intervention is the choice of words to be targeted in intervention. It is argued that these words should be 'aligned with the curriculum' and have the most 'meaningful and functional impact on children' (Steele and Mills, 2011: 359). This can be seen in Word Wizard in Table 6.2, which teaches targeted vocabulary from the National Curriculum to children with specific language impairment. Dockrell et al. (2006) used data from parental questionnaires and age of acquisition norms to identify target vocabulary in their Talking Time intervention. Instructional strategies to teach targeted vocabulary can also vary between interventions. Core vocabulary in Talking Time is developed by play-acting around themes such as 'Going on Holiday'. This encourages incidental word learning in which children are learning vocabulary as a by-product of an activity that is not explicitly geared to vocabulary learning. Word Wizard uses word meanings, speech sounds and repetition to help children learn new vocabulary. The aim of these strategies is to establish phonological and semantic representations of target words. The features of an effective vocabulary intervention have been examined in several studies. In one such study, a meta-analysis of vocabulary intervention on word learning in young children, Marulis and Neuman (2010) reported greater effects of combined pedagogical strategies that included explicit and implicit instruction.

Vocabulary interventions address a specific aspect of language within a relatively circumscribed context, namely, a child in a therapeutic or instructional relationship to an SLT or teacher. A quite different approach to language intervention is one which involves a range of agencies and practitioners, and which emphasizes the need to establish environments that are conducive to children's language learning. These programmes are community- or population-based interventions. Several interventions in Table 6.2 exhibit features of this type. The aim of Every Child a Talker (ECAT) is to 'create a developmentally appropriate, supportive and stimulating environment in which children can enjoy experimenting with and learning language' (Department for Children, Schools and Families, 2008: 3). ECAT can be implemented in Early Years settings, with a childminder or at home with parents. Let's Learn Language is based on the Hanen programme 'You Make the Difference'. It is a parent language promotion programme that targets toddlers with few or no spoken words at 18 months of age. This community-based intervention aims to reduce early **language delay** and early behaviour problems that are linked to language delay. The Let's Talk Programme is a school-based language training programme for staff in schools. It was developed in a city in the Midlands in the UK through inter-agency collaboration between Children's Community Health Services, the Children's Speech and Language Therapy Service and the city's Special Needs Teaching Service as part of the Local Education Authority. Training is given to key school staff in how to facilitate and increase opportunities for children's language development and in how to increase their ability to identify children with delayed and impoverished language. Increasing awareness of effective teacher talk is also emphasized.

Interventions for adult-onset language disorders such as aphasia are also too numerous to address in detail. Many interventions for people with aphasia address impairment-level deficits such as word-finding difficulties or **anomia**. Most people with aphasia experience anomia, which can be treated using semantic and phonological therapies. Semantic treatments include circumlocution-induced naming, personalized cueing and semantic feature analysis (Maddy et al., 2014). In circumlocution-induced naming, instead of cues, the person with aphasia is required to describe and 'talk around' (**circumlocution**) a pictured object, etc. for as long as it takes until the name of it occurs to the client. Semantic feature analysis is a systematic cueing technique whereby people with aphasia are asked to produce words that are semantically related to the target word they cannot recall, e.g. for the target word *cup*, cues might involve questions about its use ('What do you do with it?'). Activation of the semantic network surrounding the target word is presumed to increase the likelihood that the word will be retrieved. Treatments for anomia often result in poor generalization, with gains restricted to those words that are directly targeted in an intervention. Best et al. (2013) used cueing therapy in the rehabilitation of noun retrieval/production in 16 participants with chronic aphasia. Intervention resulted in significant improvement on naming treated items for 15 of 16 participants. Generalization to untreated items occurred only in participants who were classified as having relatively less of a semantic difficulty and more of a phonological output deficit. The reader is referred to Whitworth et al. (2014) for further discussion of impairment-level interventions for people with aphasia.

Of course, the real significance of interventions for impairment-level deficits in people with aphasia lies in their impact on a client's communication and participation in a range of activities. Best et al. (2008) found that therapy which targeted **word retrieval** in people with aphasia not only improved participants' word finding in picture naming but also increased their ratings of their communicative activity and life participation. The activities and participation of people with aphasia, and the environmental and personal factors that help or hinder participation, are features of the ICF framework (WHO, 2001). This framework has had a profound influence on interventions for people with aphasia. Alongside therapies for impairment-level deficits, it is now equally important for intervention to increase the participation of people with aphasia. A **total communication** intervention, which emphasizes the use of whichever means of communication is available to the client, is one way in which participation can be increased. Rautakoski (2011) adopted a total communication approach, which involved use of residual speech, spontaneous non-verbal communication, and low- and high-tech devices, in an intervention for people with severe or moderate aphasia. A further way in which increased participation of the person with aphasia can be achieved is to modify the communicative behaviours of conversational partners. Conversational partner training is a component of several aphasia interventions (see Whitworth et al., 2014, for review). Eriksson et al. (2016) used one such intervention – Supporting Partners of People with Aphasia in Relationships and Conversation (Lock et al., 2001) – in a study of six dyads consisting of a person with aphasia and a significant other. Improvements in functional communication in the person with aphasia were reported as a result of the intervention.

> **KEY POINTS: Clinical Interventions: Language**
>
> - An extensive range of interventions is available to treat language disorders in children and adults. The selection of an appropriate intervention is guided by several considerations including a client's language disorder, medical diagnosis, psychiatric status and academic, social and occupational functioning.
> - Some language interventions address specific language levels (e.g. vocabulary intervention), while others attempt to stimulate a range of expressive and receptive language skills (e.g. syntax and semantics). The aim of intervention is to achieve generalization of language gains made in clinic to everyday communication in a range of contexts.
> - Many interventions involve direct therapy with child or adult clients. Parents and spouses have a vital role to play in providing additional stimulation between sessions and monitoring a client's language skills. Other interventions aim to establish environments that are conducive to language learning in children. These interventions often involve many agencies and practitioners and are community-based programmes.
> - The focus on the client's environment has resulted in the development of conversational partner training in interventions for clients with aphasia. Certain behaviours on the part of conversational partners can limit a client's participation in conversation. These behaviours can be modified in therapy. Also, partners can be trained in how to reveal the communicative competence of clients with aphasia.
> - Any language intervention must be able to demonstrate that it results in a positive impact on a client's activities and participation and, more generally, well-being and quality of life. The evidence base that language interventions can achieve these types of outcomes for clients is relatively strong, but there is still a need for more research in this area.

6.5 Clinical Interventions: Fluency

Interventions for the treatment of stuttering and cluttering may not be as numerous as those for speech and language, but they are no less varied. Key factors in the selection of an intervention are the age of the client and the duration of stuttering. For very young children, dysfluency may resolve spontaneously without the need for direct intervention. In this case, intervention may take the form of education and guidance about parental speaking patterns and environmental modifications that may improve a child's fluency. For an adult who has stuttered since childhood, the attainment of normal fluency may not be an attainable goal, but the client may benefit from an intervention that encourages less effortful stuttering. Aside from the age of the client and duration of stuttering, other factors to be considered in the selection of an intervention include the client's intellectual functioning. Interventions that address the cognitive and affective components of stuttering require a self-reflective capacity which may not be present in the child or adult with Down syndrome and intellectual disability. This has particular relevance given the increased prevalence of stuttering and other fluency disorders in individuals with genetic syndromes such as Down syndrome and fragile X syndrome (Van Borsel and Tetnowski, 2007). A further component of the planning of intervention concerns the use of individual versus group therapy. While individual therapy allows an SLT to deliver treatment that is tailored to the particular needs of a client, group therapy can serve an important role in providing psychosocial support to clients. These and other important considerations in fluency intervention will be addressed further below.

Indirect treatments are the intervention of choice for young children who stutter. The focus of SLTs in these treatments is on modifying environmental and parental factors that may be contributing to a child's dysfluency. The rationale for indirect intervention is twofold. First, approximately 70% of children who display a lack of fluency in the preschool years eventually acquire fluent speech production (Sidavi and Fabus, 2010). With such a high percentage of spontaneous recovery, many clinicians prefer to adopt a policy of 'wait and see' before instituting direct treatments. Second, there is also a concern that by making young children aware of their lack of fluency, this may serve to perpetuate dysfluency beyond the early years. During indirect intervention, SLTs instruct parents in how to manage demands in the child's environment that may exceed a child's limited capacities for fluent speech production. For example, a parental communicative style in which questions are used extensively places linguistic demands on children that may exceed their limited capacity for language production. Parental separation and family bereavement place significant emotional demands on children. A family routine in which structured activities dominate and there are limited opportunities for rest and leisure can fatigue young children and place excessive demands on their immature motor speech production systems. SLTs can instruct parents in how to manage each of these demands. For example, parental questions can be replaced by comments that place fewer linguistic demands on children. On occasion, SLTs may also train a child's capacities for fluency (e.g. improving word-finding capacity). One such indirect treatment is Parent–Child Interaction Therapy as practised by the Michael Palin Centre for Stammering Children in London.

The Lidcombe Program (Harrison and Onslow, 1999; Onslow et al., 2003) is a direct intervention that targets the stuttered speech of preschool children. It is a behavioural treatment which is based on the premise that stuttering is an operant behaviour that can be targeted by verbal contingencies. Verbal contingencies are comments produced by parents when a child stutters or does not stutter. Parents provide verbal contingencies to their child during structured conversations that are designed for this purpose and during everyday conversations. The Lidcombe Program uses five verbal contingencies. Three contingencies are used for stutter-free speech: praise (*that was lovely smooth talking*); request for self-evaluation (*was that smooth?*); and acknowledge (*that was smooth*). Two verbal contingencies are used for unambiguous stuttering: acknowledge (*that was a stuck word*) and request self-correction (*can you say that smoothly*). Verbal contingencies for unambiguous stuttering are used much less frequently than verbal contingencies for stutter-free speech. During weekly visits to clinic, for 45–60 minutes, SLTs train parents in how to conduct the treatment and also ensure that it is being implemented properly.

Several studies have examined the clinical effectiveness of direct and indirect treatments of preschool children who stutter. De Sonneville-Koedoot et al. (2015) compared the effectiveness of direct treatment (the Lidcombe Program) with indirect treatment (the RESTART Demands and Capacities Model based treatment) in 3- to 6-year-old preschool children who stutter. At 18 months follow-up, the percentage of non-stuttering children for direct treatment was 76.5% versus 71.4% for indirect treatment. Children who received direct treatment showed a greater decline in percentage of syllables stuttered at 3 months than children who received indirect treatment. At 18 months, stuttering frequency was 1.2% for direct treatment and 1.5% for indirect treatment. However, no differences between the treatment approaches were significant. According to the authors, these findings indicate that treatment effects are explained by factors which these interventions have in common (e.g. an increase in one-on-one time that parents spend with their child) rather than by the unique features of each intervention. These findings also suggest that factors other than the clinical effectiveness of an intervention (e.g. parental preference) may be decisive in the selection of an intervention in a particular case.

For school-age children and adolescents, a combination of fluency-shaping and stuttering-modification techniques may be used. Blomgren (2013) states that the premise of fluency-shaping approaches to treatment is that speakers who stutter habitually use speech production strategies that are outside of their motor speech control abilities. The goal of fluency-shaping treatment is to promote a new speech production pattern that is conducive to fluent speech. A key component of any fluency-shaping treatment is a reduction of speech rate through the use of **prolonged speech** (also known as 'stretched speech' or 'smooth speech'). The person who stutters is also instructed in how to make motor speech movements with less articulatory pressure and to initiate vocal fold vibration in a gradual, controlled manner. Stuttering-modification approaches have a different emphasis: the reduction of speech-related **avoidance behaviours**, fears and negative attitudes. The goal is to modify stuttering moments. By decreasing tension associated with stuttering, stuttering is less severe, and there is reduction of the fear of stuttering and avoidance behaviours. The person who stutters is encouraged to reduce **struggle behaviours**, tension and the rate of stuttering – in effect, to stutter more fluently. Laiho and Klippi (2007) used stuttering-modification treatment in a study of 21 children/adolescents who stutter. In two-thirds of participants, the percentage of syllables stuttered decreased as a result of the intervention, a finding that was also replicated with avoidance behaviour and struggle behaviour. The quality of stuttering became milder, with many children having shorter moments of stuttering and more **repetitions** and **prolongations** instead of **blocks** by the end of therapy.

There is now clear evidence that even preschool-age children who stutter are aware of their speech difficulties and have negative speech-associated attitudes (Clark et al., 2012). Also, significant affective problems, such as disabling levels of social anxiety, are often found in people who stutter, and particularly among adults who stutter (Iverach and Rapee, 2014). Interventions that address these cognitive and affective aspects of stuttering may be used alongside fluency-shaping and stuttering-modification treatments. One such intervention is cognitive behavioural therapy (CBT). Menzies et al. (2009) describe four core components of CBT for the treatment of anxiety in adults who stutter: (1) exposure; (2) behavioural experiments; (3) cognitive restructuring; and (4) attentional training. During exposure, the person who stutters enters a situation that they have included in a 'fear hierarchy' (e.g. use of the telephone). After entering the situation, the individual reflects on the validity of their expectations of harm in that situation. Behavioural experiments involve social situations in which the client is asked to produce stuttering voluntarily. The person who stutters is asked to predict the outcomes of stuttering before engaging in the experiment and later reviews the outcomes of the experiment. During cognitive restructuring, people who stutter are encouraged to challenge negative beliefs and judgements, predominantly about the evaluations of others. Having identified and systematically modified any negative thoughts related to stuttering, clients are then encouraged to use these 'reframes' in everyday situations. Attentional training reduces the frequency of threat-related intrusive thoughts by increasing the client's capacity to attend to alternative cognitive targets. By increasing a client's ability to control where attention is placed, clients can reduce their bias towards negative aspects of the social environment.

A range of devices is now available for the treatment of people who stutter. These devices use **delayed auditory feedback** (DAF) and **frequency altered feedback** (FAF) to emulate **choral speech**. One such device is called SpeechEasy™. This device works by delaying what the speaker says by a few milliseconds (range from 0ms to 220ms) and by altering the pitch perception of the user's voice (pitch can be raised or lowered in 500 Hz increments). The device has a similar appearance to a hearing aid. It is custom fit, powered by hearing aid batteries and is worn in one ear. As well as the personal use of devices by clients who stutter, other devices are available for SLTs to use as a training tool with clients in clinic. SpeechCoach™ is one such device that uses DAF and FAF to recreate the choral speech effect. There is growing evidence of the clinical effectiveness of devices that work by means of DAF and FAF. Van Borsel et al. (2003) reported that DAF was an effective means of reducing stuttering in nine adults who stutter when it was employed as the only treatment approach outside of a therapeutic environment. Devices that achieve DAF and FAF may also be used with children who stutter. The manufacturers of SpeechEasy™ recommend its use with children as young as 8 years of age, although an SLT must assess if a particular child is a suitable candidate for the use of this device.

Cluttering interventions have received much less investigation than stuttering interventions. Delayed auditory feedback can also be used to treat people who clutter (St Louis et al., 1996). Other treatment techniques include the use of pausing and overemphasis. Anomalies of speech rate – rapid and/or irregular speech rate – are a consistent feature of cluttering. Pausing involves inserting pauses at natural places in connected speech to slow down the rate of speech. Excessive over-coarticulation of sounds (i.e. collapsing syllables such as 'com-muny' for *community*) is also a feature of cluttering. Overemphasis involves exaggerating the articulation of speech to prevent over-coarticulation and increase speech clarity. Healey et al. (2015) compared the use of pausing and overemphasis to treat the occurrence of over-coarticulation in the conversational speech of a teenage male. Although a decrease in over-coarticulation resulted from the use of both strategies, pausing brought about a greater reduction in over-coarticulation in conversational speech than overemphasis. The subject was also more likely to implement pausing than overemphasis in **carryover**. People who clutter have been reported to have pragmatic language difficulties. For example, they have been described as being verbose, as using non-specific language, as not giving background information, and as taking less communicative responsibility by not posing 'mending' questions when something is not clear (see Scaler Scott, 2017, for further discussion of pragmatics in cluttering). For these clients, some components of a pragmatic language intervention would also appear to be warranted. Van Zaalen and Reichel (2015) recommend that special attention is given to improving pragmatic skills such as turn-taking, topic maintenance, and story-narrating abilities in the treatment of people who clutter.

KEY POINTS: Clinical Interventions: Fluency

- The selection of an appropriate fluency intervention is guided by a range of factors including the age of the client, the duration of stuttering, a client's intellectual functioning and communicative requirements (e.g. speaking on a telephone at work).
- For preschool children who stutter, an indirect intervention may be chosen over a direct intervention. An indirect intervention identifies the motor, cognitive, linguistic and affective demands on the child in his or her environment, and considers how these demands can be modified in order to encourage fluent speech production. SLTs work directly with the parents rather than the child.
- Preschool children who stutter may also be treated using a direct intervention such as the Lidcombe Program. In this program, parents are taught how to deliver verbal contingencies to children in response to stutter-free speech and unambiguous stuttering. There is evidence to support the clinical effectiveness of this program as well as of indirect treatment.
- For older children who stutter, a combination of fluency-shaping and stuttering-modification techniques may be used. Fluency-shaping techniques encourage a new speech production pattern that is conducive to fluent speech. Prolonged speech (also known as 'smooth speech' or 'stretched speech') is a fluency-shaping technique which emphasizes a reduction of speech rate. Stuttering-modification therapy promotes a less effortful form of stuttering.
- Cognitive and affective aspects of stuttering may be addressed by means of cognitive behavioural therapy. Devices that alter the speech signal through delayed auditory feedback and frequency-altered feedback (e.g. SpeechEasy™) emulate choral speech and may be used as fluency training tools or for a client's personal use.
- Cluttering treatments may also use delayed auditory feedback, and techniques such as pausing (to address rate anomalies) and overemphasis (to address over-coarticulation). Intervention may also need to consider aspects of pragmatics that may be impaired in people who clutter.

6.6 Clinical Interventions: Voice

The treatment of voice disorders involves the use of surgical procedures, chemotherapy and **radiotherapy**, hormonal and pharmacological treatments and **voice therapy**. More often than not, two or more of these interventions are combined in the treatment of clients with voice disorders. Adults with laryngeal cancer, for example, may require a partial or total laryngectomy depending on the location and extent of a laryngeal tumour. A tumour that is diagnosed early may be treated by radiotherapy alone, while chemotherapy is used to treat a tumour that has spread beyond the tissues of the larynx. Voice therapy must establish an alaryngeal method of communication for the client through the use of an electrolarynx, **oesophageal speech** or **voice prosthesis**. The client who undergoes gender reassignment surgery may also require surgical intervention (e.g. **cricothyroid approximation**) in order to achieve an acceptable speaking voice. The female-to-male transsexual may receive hormonal treatment in the form of androgen therapy that facilitates the lowering of vocal pitch. Voice therapy is undertaken alongside these surgical and hormonal treatments in order to ensure that any modifications of the client's voice do not result in vocal abuse and misuse. Children with dysphonia related to vocal nodules may require microlaryngeal surgery in order to remove vocal fold lesions. However, if the vocally abusive behaviours (e.g. screaming) that led to the development of nodules are not addressed in voice therapy, then these benign lesions are likely to re-emerge. These scenarios illustrate that there are multiple approaches to the treatment of voice disorders and that the results of surgical and other interventions can be maximized through voice therapy.

As with other interventions in communication disorders, interventions for voice disorders can be direct or indirect. In a review of interventions for preventing voice disorders in adults, Ruotsalainen et al. (2007: 2) characterized direct and indirect interventions in the following terms:

> Direct techniques focus on the underlying physiological changes needed to improve an individual's technique in using the vocal system and may aim to alter vocal fold closure (adduction), respiratory patterns or resonance, pitch or articulatory tension ... Indirect techniques concentrate on contributory and maintenance aspects of the voice disorder and may involve relaxation strategies, counselling, explanation of the normal anatomy and physiology of the vocal tract, explanation of the causal factors of voice disorders and voice care and conservation.

On one estimation, direct voice therapy accounts for more than 75% of treatment time in voice therapy sessions (Gartner-Schmidt et al., 2013). A direct voice intervention typically includes one or more of the following therapies: vocal function exercises; Lessac-Madsen Resonant Voice Therapy (LMRVT); general resonant voice therapies; confidential voice; stretch and flow phonation; flow phonation; accent method; laryngeal massage; manual circumlaryngeal therapy; facilitating techniques; and semi-occluded vocal tract. These techniques differ in the physiological adjustments they aim to achieve and the client groups who may benefit from their use. For example, LMRVT aims to minimize the impact stress of the vocal folds while maximizing vocal output. A resonant voice is produced by vocal fold movement that ranges between a barely adducted and a barely abducted position. The client is trained in how to configure the oral cavity in such a way that allows high-frequency energy in the sound source to be reinforced in the **vocal tract** (Myers and Finnegan, 2015). LMRVT is designed for individuals with hyper- or hypo-adducted voice problems associated with conditions such as nodules, polyps, non-specific phonotraumatic changes, paralysis, paresis, atrophy, **bowing** and **sulcus vocalis** (Verdolini, 2004). A quite different physiological adjustment is the focus of stretch and flow phonation which is used to treat clients with voice disorders related to hyperfunctional aetiologies. The aim of this technique is to initiate volitional control over vocal subsystems, while maintaining a perception of minimal muscular effort during phonation. The client is instructed in how to better control respiratory patterns to support voice production, coordinate respiratory and laryngeal function while focusing on oropharyngeal resonance, and reduce physiological effort while phonating (Watts et al., 2015).

A widely used direct treatment which targets vocal loudness is the Lee Silverman Voice Treatment (LSVT). Developed by Ramig et al. (1995), this intervention uses intensive, high phonatory effort exercises to increase vocal fold adduction. LSVT does not encourage shouting or yelling but through a systematic hierarchy of exercises encourages the client to achieve an improved, healthy vocal loudness with no strain. As well as stimulating the motor system to achieve improved phonatory, respiratory and articulatory activity, LSVT includes sensory awareness training to help clients with Parkinson's disease realize that their voice is too soft and that a louder voice is within normal limits. The treatment is administered in 16 sessions over a single month (four individual 60 minute sessions per week). There is evidence to suggest that LSVT is a clinically effective treatment of **hypophonia** in clients with Parkinson's disease. Mahler et al. (2015) reported data that supported the efficacy of LSVT to increase vocal loudness and functional communication in people with Parkinson's disease. Improved vocal sound pressure level was achieved post-treatment. Treatment effects in these clients were maintained for up to 2 years. Wight and Miller (2015) conducted an audit of outcomes for 33 people with Parkinson's disease who completed LSVT in a routine hospital outpatient setting. Significant intensity gains for reading and monologues were achieved post-therapy but were not maintained at 12 and 24 months. Significant intensity increases on prolonged vowel occurred post-therapy and were maintained at 12 and 24 months. LSVT has other clinical applications, including the treatment of speech in children with dysarthria due to cerebral palsy (Levy, 2014) and decreased facial expressivity (**hypomimia**) in clients with Parkinson's disease (Dumer, 2014).

Indirect intervention addresses a range of factors that contribute to and maintain voice disorders. Lifestyle factors such as alcohol consumption and smoking can damage the laryngeal epithelium and lead to the development of laryngeal carcinoma. Many clients do not understand the interaction of these factors in the pathogenesis of laryngeal cancer, namely, that alcohol consumption causes dehydration of the laryngeal mucosa, which is then more vulnerable to the carcinogenic effects of tobacco smoke; such clients can benefit from a clear explanation of their interaction by an SLT. Cigarette smoking is also known to increase acid reflux events, most probably by means of reducing lower oesophageal sphincter pressure (Kahrilas and Gupta, 1990). If the **upper oesophageal sphincter** (called the cricopharyngeus) is also not functioning normally, a bolus can spill into the larynx and pharynx, causing laryngopharyngeal reflux (LPR). The airway epithelium, including the epithelium of the larynx, is fragile and more easily damaged by gastric reflux than the oesophageal epithelium. The corrosive effect of reflux on this epithelium leads to the development of a number of laryngeal pathologies including laryngeal cancer. Certain diets are also associated with reflux disease. For example, the lower oesophageal sphincter is weakened by caffeine, alcohol, chocolates and peppermints, while carbonated beverages such as sodas can bring acidic contents into the throat. During indirect treatment of clients with dysphonia, the SLT can provide education and advice about these factors. For the management of reflux disease, this may include the recommendation to pursue pharmacological treatment or the need to use more than one pillow in bed at night.

Factors such as smoking and laryngopharyngeal reflux are included in a wider discussion of good vocal hygiene during indirect treatment of clients. Vocal hygiene also includes information about the need for adequate hydration and the effects of dehydration on the laryngeal mechanism. Inadequate hydration results in thickened mucous, which speakers then attempt to remove from the laryngeal mechanism by means of frequent throat clearing and other phonotraumatic behaviours. A well-humidified environment is vital for good vocal hygiene. Clients are often unaware, for example, of the effects on laryngeal tissues of a car heater running at high temperatures during a long journey. During vocal hygiene, SLTs also want to make clients aware of the effects of prescription medications on the voice. For example, aspirin can cause **vocal fold haemorrhages** (see Figure 6.2), while antihistamines for the treatment of allergies and hayfever can have a drying effect on the laryngeal mechanism. Inhalation of fumes in the workplace is detrimental to vocal health, as are dusty environments

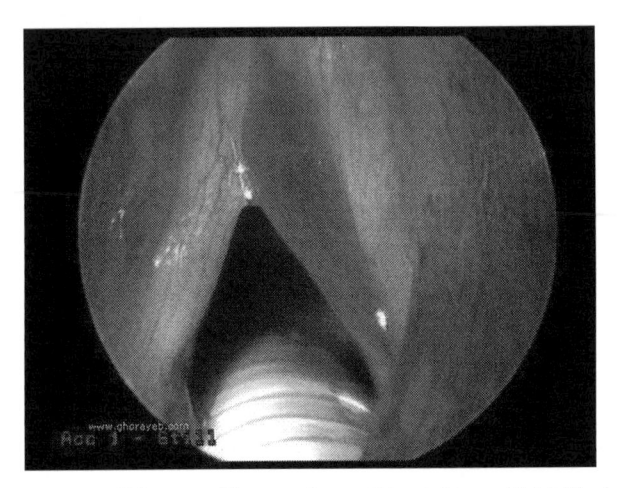

Figure 6.2 *Submucosal haemorrhage of the right vocal fold. The haemorrhage was caused by traumatic endotracheal intubation and not by ingestion of aspirin. (Reproduced with permission from Otolaryngology Houston, www.ghorayeb.com). (A colour version of this image is also available in the plate section.)*

and environments where pollutant levels are high (e.g. cyclists among heavy city traffic). SLTs must also make clients aware as part of vocal hygiene that increases in vocal intensity by shouting or speaking above high ambient noise levels can have damaging consequences for the voice. This is a particularly important consideration for fitness instructors, who must speak over background music and other noise in gyms, although it may apply with equal relevance to other professional voice users (e.g. teachers). Simple modifications such as the use of a microphone during an exercise class can minimize the occurrence of phonotraumatic behaviours. Clear explanations of laryngeal anatomy and physiology must accompany each of these aspects of vocal hygiene.

Other components of indirect treatment include relaxation techniques, psychosocial counsel and motivational issues. Relaxation techniques are used to reduce muscular tension and to energize muscle systems that are used in voice production. Of the many techniques used to facilitate relaxation, one that allows clients to contrast muscle tension with relaxation is Jacobson's Progressive Relaxation. The client may begin by curling his/her toes as hard as possible and keeping them contracted for 15 seconds. The client will then slowly relax them, feeling the sharp contrast between the tightness when they were contracted and the heaviness when they were relaxed. Carryover of the relaxed state to voice production is not easily achieved. This technique has been found to be useful with clients who have **muscle tension dysphonia** and for some hyperfunctional voice users (Heuer et al., 2006). Many clients with voice disorders present with significant psychosocial issues that must be addressed during therapy. Voice disorders are associated with low self-esteem and confidence, poor voice-related quality of life and increased levels of anxiety and depression (Cohen et al., 2006; Dietrich et al., 2008). Adults may believe that their professional advancement or job security is threatened by a voice disorder. Adolescents with voice disorders may experience poor self-esteem at an important period in their psychosocial development. SLTs must attend to these psychosocial issues alongside direct treatment of the voice disorder. Finally, motivational issues are also a component of indirect treatment. Voice therapy demands behaviour change as long-established vocal behaviours are replaced by new vocal behaviours. Clients must be highly motivated in order for these changes to occur. This extends to regular attendance at therapy sessions and completion of homework exercises.

Voice therapy with clients who have undergone laryngectomy involves establishing some form of alaryngeal communication. This can be achieved through the use of an electrolarynx, the development of oesophageal speech or the use of **surgical voice restoration** (voice prosthesis). An electrolarynx is an electromechanical device that transmits a tone. When held against the neck or cheek, this tone is transmitted into the oral cavity where it is shaped into speech sounds by movement of the articulators. Electrolaryngeal speech can be acquired relatively quickly and easily. However, there may be some discomfort for clients in using the electrolarynx when neck tissue is tender following surgery or radiotherapy. One further drawback is that voiceless consonants are perceived as voiced consonants owing to the continuous nature of the sound source. During oesophageal speech, air that is transported into the oesophagus is released through the upper oesophageal sphincter, which then vibrates. Oesophageal speech can be an effective method of communication for alaryngeal clients. However, the resulting voice quality is not acceptable to all clients and the technique is not easily acquired. Also, because the air supply that generates oesophageal speech is considerably reduced compared to a pulmonary airstream, this form of alaryngeal communication is characterized by short utterance lengths and increased pause times. The development of surgical voice restoration has largely overcome this issue. When the client's **neck stoma** is occluded, a pulmonary airstream is directed through a prosthesis that connects the trachea to the oesophagus. The upper oesophageal sphincter then vibrates as it does during oesophageal speech. Surgical voice restoration permits extended speech production. However, clients must be able to clean and maintain the prosthesis. All three methods of alaryngeal communication are illustrated in Figure 6.3.

KEY POINTS: Clinical Interventions: Voice

- Voice disorders may be treated using surgical procedures, hormonal and pharmacological treatments, radiotherapy and chemotherapy, and voice therapy. Voice therapy is used to maximize the outcomes of surgical procedures and other forms of treatment.
- Direct and indirect techniques are used in voice therapy. Typically, these techniques are used in combination in the treatment of clients with voice disorders.
- Direct techniques intervene on the physiological changes that need to take place for vocal improvements to occur. This may take the form of less effortful vocal fold adduction during phonation or improved respiratory patterns for voice production.
- Indirect techniques focus on factors that contribute to and maintain voice disorders. They include vocal hygiene and relaxation techniques. Vocal hygiene addresses lifestyle factors (e.g. smoking) and behaviours (e.g. phonotraumatic behaviours such as screaming) that are detrimental to good vocal health.
- Voice therapy for clients who have undergone laryngectomy must establish a form of alaryngeal communication. This can be achieved through the use of an electrolarynx, oesophageal voice or surgical voice reconstruction (voice prosthesis). Clients may use more than one of these methods of communication, e.g. electronic larynx and oesophageal voice.

6.7 Clinical Interventions: Swallowing

For many children and adults, swallowing is impaired as a result of illnesses, injuries and disorders arising in the developmental period (e.g. cerebral

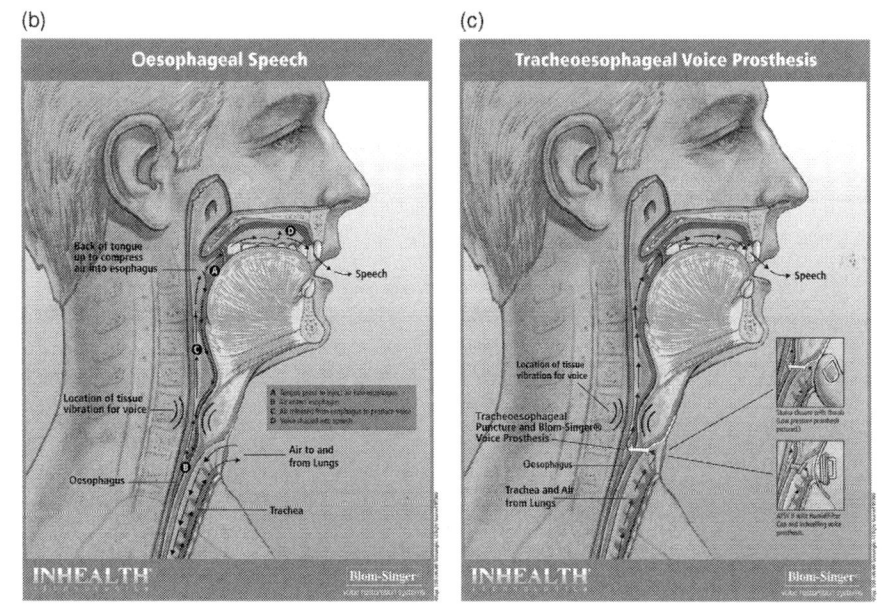

Figure 6.3 *Three methods of alaryngeal communication: (a) electronic/artificial larynx; (b) oesophageal speech; and (c) tracheoesophageal voice prosthesis (reproduced with permission of InHealth Technologies, www.inhealth.com)*

palsy, childhood brain tumour) or on account of events that have their onset in adulthood (e.g. stroke, motor neurone disease). Each of these conditions has the potential to compromise swallowing and along with it an individual's physical well-being and quality of life (Davis, 2007). Prompt and aggressive treatment of dysphagia is necessary in order to avoid serious and potentially fatal consequences such as choking, **aspiration pneumonia**, dehydration and malnutrition. In recent years, the treatment of dysphagia has become an increasingly important part of the work of SLTs. Dysphagia can be treated using compensatory strategies, direct therapy and indirect therapy (Logemann, 1991). Compensatory strategies are designed to limit the symptoms of swallowing problems without necessarily directly changing swallowing physiology. Such strategies include postural changes, modification of bolus volume and consistency as well as rate of food presentation. Direct therapy techniques are designed to change swallowing physiology. These techniques include swallow manoeuvres, oral sensory stimulation procedures and the use of maxillofacial prosthetics, medication and surgical procedures. Indirect therapy procedures aim to improve the neuromuscular processes that are necessary for swallowing (e.g. control and strength of lip and tongue muscles) without actually producing a swallow. Indirect therapy is used when a client cannot safely consume an oral food or liquid diet (Provencio-Arambula et al., 2007). Several of these interventions will be addressed further in this section.

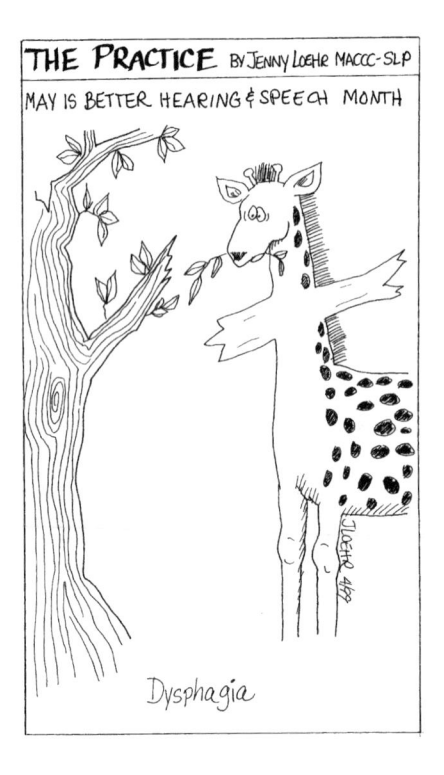

Swallowing disorders in children and adults can be effectively compensated. Logemann (2006) observes that while postural changes do not affect the motor disorder that causes dysphagia, they nevertheless can compensate for this disorder while spontaneous recovery occurs or while sensory stimulation and exercise programs are implemented. Logemann identifies five postural changes that are used in the treatment of dysphagia: head back; chin down; head rotated to damaged side; lying down on one side; and head tilt to stronger side. Each of these postures affects a specific aspect of swallowing. For example, the head-back posture uses gravity to clear the oral cavity in a client who displays inefficient oral transit of a bolus on videofluoroscopy. The chin-down posture pushes the tongue base backward towards the pharyngeal wall. This technique may be used with clients who display reduced post-propulsion motion of the tongue base, resulting in residue in the **valleculae** (the space between the pharyngeal surface of the tongue and the **epiglottis**). Compensatory head postures have been shown to be effective in the treatment of clients with dysphagia. Solazzo et al. (2012) reported that compensatory postures guaranteed safe oropharyngeal transit in 88% of patients with aspiration or no transit in their study. Some head postures were more effective than others. A chin-down posture, head-turned posture and a hyperextended head posture achieved a safe swallow in 56%, 25.3% and 6.7% of patients, respectively.

Characteristics of the bolus such as volume and consistency are known to affect events during swallowing. For example, an increase in bolus volume increases the opening duration of the upper oesophageal sphincter in healthy subjects, while an increase in bolus consistency from thick liquid to honey thick results in longer pharyngeal transit duration (Nascimento et al., 2015). Findings such as these inform the dietary modifications that are recommended by SLTs and others in the management of clients with dysphagia. One such recommendation is that in order to slow the oropharyngeal transit of the bolus, and in so doing reduce the risk of aspiration, liquids should be thickened. It is common practice, for example, in the treatment of feeding difficulties in infants to add thickening agents to formula or expressed breast milk (Dion et al., 2015). In its global guidelines, the World Gastroenterology Organisation (2014) recommends modifying the consistency of food to thicken liquids in the treatment of oropharyngeal dysphagia. It should be noted, however, that there is limited clinical evidence and a lack of clinical practice guidelines to support this widely adopted practice (see Logemann, 2006, and Dion et al., 2015, for discussion). Also, while reducing the risk of penetration aspiration, thickened liquids can increase the risk of dehydration (Logemann, 2006) and post-swallow residue in the pharynx (Steele et al., 2015). As well as the viscosity and consistency of food, dietary modifications for clients with dysphagia must also attend to sensory properties of food such as taste. There is evidence, for example, that a sour bolus can improve swallowing response in clients with neurogenic dysphagia (see Loret, 2015, for review). SLTs must work closely with dieticians to ensure not only that dietary modifications are safe but that they also meet a client's nutritional needs.

Direct interventions are designed to change swallowing physiology. They include swallow manoeuvres such as tongue holding, supraglottic swallow, effortful swallow and the Mendelsohn manoeuvre (Logemann, 2006). Each manoeuvre addresses a specific component of disordered swallowing. For example, the supraglottic swallow (and super-supraglottic swallow) is used with clients who demonstrate reduced airway protection. The effortful swallow is used with clients who present with clinically significant residue in the valleculae and/or **pyriform sinuses** as well as in clients with reduced airway closure (Vose et al., 2014). Clients receive guidance and instruction from SLTs in how to use each technique. To perform a supraglottic swallow, the client is instructed to hold his or her breath before and during the pharyngeal swallow. This is designed to close the true vocal cords before and during swallowing to prevent the entry of food into the airways (Bodén et al., 2006). Notwithstanding their widespread use, there is limited evidence to support the clinical effectiveness of these techniques. McCabe et al. (2009) reported limited evidence of the positive effects of behavioural swallowing interventions, including swallowing manoeuvres, in clients with dysphagia post-cancer treatments. Ashford et al. (2009) examined seven behavioural treatments for clients with dysphagia secondary to neurological disorders such as stroke, dementia, Parkinson's disease and brain injury. Four of the seven treatments examined were swallowing manoeuvres. The results of this systematic review indicated that research supporting behavioural interventions for neurogenic dysphagia involving postures and manoeuvres was 'young and sparse'.

Each of the techniques and modifications described above assumes that clients are oral feeders or that they will resume oral feeding following recovery from illness or injury. Where oral feeding is judged to be unsafe, is unlikely to improve or may get worse, nutrition and medication may be delivered directly into the stomach by means of a tube. A nasogastric tube (NG tube) may be passed into the stomach via the nasal cavities. Alternatively, a gastrostomy tube may be placed through the abdominal wall directly into the stomach (**percutaneous endoscopic gastrostomy**, or PEG tube) (see Figure 6.4). An internal retention balloon is inflated inside the stomach and holds the tube in place.

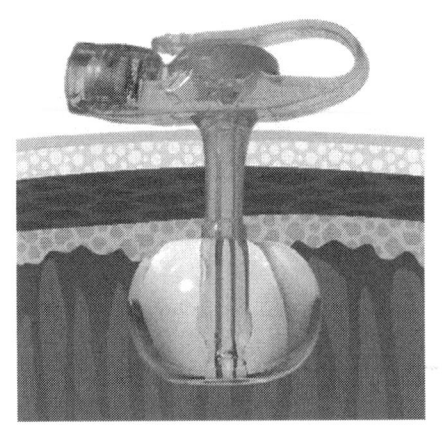

Figure 6.4 *A PEG tube – the MiniONE® Balloon Button (Image courtesy of Applied Medical Technology, Inc.)*

Nutrition is administered through an external feeding port that should be closed when the tube is not in use.

Both NG tubes and PEG tubes have advantages and disadvantages. NG tubes can be quickly and easily passed. They have low procedure-related mortality, although the tube may be inadvertently placed into the lungs. They also need to be replaced frequently because of displacement or blockage. PEG tubes are more cosmetically acceptable to clients and are less irritating. They do not require replacement for several months and have more nutritional benefit than NG tubes. They may be accompanied by minor complications (e.g. tube obstruction and leakage) and major complications (e.g. gastric haemorrhage). SLTs play a vital role in the management of clients with dysphagia who are tube fed. They can work on improving the neuromuscular control of swallowing in tube-fed clients. Children who are tube fed can develop a lack of interest in food and high levels of anxiety around feeding and mealtimes. SLTs can work with tube-fed children to give them pleasant oral sensory experiences around food. SLTs also have an important role in monitoring change of swallowing over time. By treating dysphagia and maximizing the safety of oral intake, speech and language therapy can result in PEG tube removal (Jarvis and Rogers, 2008).

CASE STUDY: Dysphagia Intervention

An 83-year-old male was referred to speech-language pathology by his primary care physician. He complained of having difficulty initiating a swallow approximately six–seven times per meal. He also had mild intermittent coughing after a swallow. He had a history of Parkinson's disease and dysphagia. A previous modified barium swallow conducted on 30 August 2010 revealed decreased laryngeal elevation, premature spillage, pharyngeal delay of 1–2 seconds, piecemeal deglutition, and residue in the valleculae and the pyriform sinuses. No aspiration or penetration was observed. Swallowing therapy was recommended.

On 20 October 2010, a speech-language pathology evaluation including a bedside swallow study was undertaken. The patient displayed an inability to trigger a swallow response intermittently with all consistencies of food and liquids. He also exhibited slowed oral transit time, stasis in both lateral sulci, stasis on the tongue, decreased laryngeal elevation and intermittent coughing with per oral intake. Oro-pharyngeal exercises were commenced on 20 October 2010. These exercises included chin tuck against resistance exercises, jaw opening against resistance exercises and oral motor exercises until muscles fatigued. There were two–three sets of exercises per session. Each session lasted 30 minutes and sessions were conducted three times a week.

After 4 weeks of therapy conducted three times per week, incidences of difficulty initiating swallowing had reduced from six–seven times per meal to only one–two times per meal. Coughing occurred only occasionally. Upon discharge from therapy 10 days later, there were no further incidents of difficulty initiating swallowing, and no further coughing during or after per oral intake. Oral transit time had decreased, and oral stasis was reduced to within normal limits (Alternative Speech and Swallowing Solutions, www.alternativespeech.com).

> **KEY POINTS: Clinical Interventions: Swallowing**
>
> - Dysphagia in children and adults can lead to choking, aspiration pneumonia, dehydration and malnutrition. It must be aggressively treated to avoid these adverse consequences.
> - The three main approaches to the treatment of dysphagia are the use of compensatory strategies, direct therapy and indirect therapy.
> - Compensatory strategies do not change swallowing physiology but limit the symptoms of dysphagia. They include postural changes (e.g. chin down) as well as dietary modifications involving bolus volume, consistency and taste.
> - Direct therapy is designed to alter swallowing physiology. Direct therapy techniques include the use of swallow manoeuvres (e.g. supraglottic swallow), medication, maxillofacial prosthetics and surgical procedures.
> - Indirect therapy is used with clients who cannot safely consume liquids and food orally. The aim is to strengthen muscles involved in swallowing.
> - For clients with severe neurological impairment (e.g. following a stroke) or structural damage (e.g. post-cancer treatment), non-oral feeding may be necessary. This can be achieved through use of a nasogastric tube or a percutaneous endoscopic gastrostomy (PEG tube). Each form of tube feeding has advantages and disadvantages, some of which can be life threatening.
> - There is limited evidence of the clinical effectiveness of some dysphagia treatment techniques (e.g. thickening of liquids), notwithstanding their widespread use in clinical practice.

6.8 Evidence-Based Practice

Throughout this chapter, mention has been made of studies that support (or fail to support) the use of a particular intervention in clients. This is because speech and language therapy, like other health disciplines, subscribes to evidence-based practice in medicine. A widely used definition of evidence-based medicine is taken from Sackett et al. (1996):

> Evidence based medicine is the conscientious, explicit, and judicious use of current best evidence in making decisions about the care of individual patients. The practice of evidence based medicine means integrating individual clinical expertise with the best available external clinical evidence from systematic research.

In order to practice evidence-based medicine, SLTs must be aware of what the best available evidence in the field states about the clinical effectiveness of an intervention, and must be capable of integrating this evidence with their own expertise to arrive at decisions about patient care. Clinical decisions that are not supported by the best available evidence are not only likely to put the well-being of patients at risk but also likely to represent a waste of limited resources such as clinician time and equipment costs. Clearly, there is an ethical imperative on all health and medical professionals to avoid harm to patients, while increasing pressures on healthcare budgets require resources to be directed at those interventions that are likely to produce the most cost-effective gains for clients.

In this section, evidence-based practice in the context of speech and language therapy is addressed. Three issues will be examined. First, the issue of what constitutes high-quality evidence in SLT is of paramount importance if therapists are to use this evidence to ground their decision-making. Some remarks about what constitutes high-quality evidence in SLT are therefore necessary. Second, in order for there to be evidence that a particular intervention in SLT is effective, it must be possible to measure treatment effects and outcomes that have been achieved as a result of the intervention. The notion of outcome in SLT is complex and requires examination. Third, it was described at various points in the chapter that some SLT interventions, and even some widely adopted SLT interventions, are not supported by evidence or at least not by high-quality evidence. This raises the issue of the status of these interventions and whether their continued use is justified given their lack of supporting clinical evidence. It also suggests that there needs to be greater effort on the part of SLTs to undertake the type of research that could be used to demonstrate the effectiveness of SLT interventions. Both of these issues will be addressed further in this section.

To the extent that evidence-based practice requires SLTs to base their clinical decision-making on evidence, it is vital that this conforms to the highest possible standards of accuracy and rigour. For evidence to satisfy such standards, it must be obtained by means of research that upholds scientific standards such as objectivity and reproducibility. In relation to demonstrating the effectiveness of a clinical intervention, the 'gold standard' of scientific research is a **randomized controlled trial**. Sibbald and Roland (1998) state that 'randomised controlled trials are the most rigorous way of determining whether a cause-effect relation exists between treatment and outcome and for assessing the cost effectiveness of a treatment'. They further state five important features of a randomized controlled trial: (1) there should be random allocation of subjects to intervention groups; (2) patients and trialists should remain unaware of which treatment was given until the study is completed (a double blind study); (3) all intervention groups should be treated identically except for the experimental treatment; (4) patients are analysed within the group to which they were allocated irrespective of whether they experienced the intended intervention; and (5) the focus of analysis is on estimating the size of the difference in predefined outcomes between intervention groups. Although many studies in SLT examine the effectiveness of interventions, few studies conform to the standards of a randomized controlled trial. In a randomized controlled trial of a language intervention (*Language for Learning*) in preschoolers with language delay, Wake et al. (2012) describe the weaknesses of studies included in two Cochrane systematic reviews and the 'limited evidence' of treatment effectiveness that emerges from these studies in consequence:

> Most studies are small (under 20 in each arm) with limited follow-up, many of the studies are not protocol driven and detail of the interventions was often lacking. Unsurprisingly there are few replications and heterogeneity is high. Most of the studies were 'efficacy' trials, carried out in controlled environments with therapies often administered by the person developing the intervention. Very few could be construed as 'effectiveness' trials with the potential to be rolled out across a service. The underlying populations were often not well-characterised, and little is ever reported about the children's developmental history. Finally, very few of these studies included any form of economic analysis, making it impossible to establish the costs and benefits of the interventions.

In the absence of high-quality evidence obtained through randomized controlled trials, SLTs resort to various practices. Some of these practices are not consistent with the principles of evidence-based medicine. For example, in their survey of practice patterns in the management of paediatric dysphagia among Canadian SLTs, Dion et al. (2015) reported that some areas of practice did not reflect recent published research or experts' opinion. Also, even when high-quality evidence is available, busy clinicians do not have time to synthesize the often conflicting findings of the many treatment studies that are published in an area. This is where systematic reviews can be most beneficial to SLTs. Roulstone et al. (2015: 83) remark that 'systematic reviews are a way of making sense of the extended body of literature and subsequently making objective judgements across the range of papers. From these they hope to provide a fuller answer about "what works" by providing a map of the areas of uncertainty, the quality and weight of evidence and areas where there is a lack of relevant research'. In this chapter, eight systematic reviews have been reported in SLT areas ranging from interventions for preventing voice disorders in adults to non-speech oro-motor treatments for children with developmental speech sound disorders.

GROUP EXERCISE: SLT and Critical Thinking

Critical thinking is the ability to evaluate the rational merits of arguments, claims and evidence. This area of study is typically associated with subjects like philosophy and psychology where the logical features of arguments and their supporting evidence are evaluated. Given the centrality of evidence-based practice to the work of SLTs, it is relevant to ask if SLTs might not also benefit from the type of instruction that is offered in a critical thinking course. After all, SLTs must display sound clinical decision-making, advance valid arguments in support of a particular course of action

> and be able to detect flawed reasoning that might lead to erroneous decisions about a client's care. These logical skills go beyond the type of training that typically occurs in a research methods course, for example. In a group, discuss the potential benefits to the work of SLTs of a more rigorous approach to teaching rational evaluative skills such as occurs in a critical thinking course.

Of course, no evidence of the effectiveness of an intervention is possible if investigators do not establish in advance of a study exactly what outcomes may be expected to be achieved by means of treatment. Outcomes must exhibit certain properties. They must be measurable in order for investigators to record them with any accuracy at all. Outcomes may be realized on completion of a course of therapy, e.g. a reduction of percentage of stuttered syllables following group therapy for children who stutter. Alternatively, outcomes may be realized some months or even years after an intervention has taken place. In this way, investigators may want to establish if an early language intervention in children can result in improved literacy scores at 16 years of age. Some outcomes may relate to aspects of speech and language, such as percentage of intelligibility to unfamiliar listeners or scores on a test of **receptive syntax**. Other outcomes may describe behaviours that are known to be influenced by language and communication skills. This includes psychological well-being (e.g. depression scores), **social functioning** (e.g. number of friendships), academic attainment (e.g. number of GCSE or high school qualifications) and occupational status (e.g. unskilled employment). These latter outcomes have assumed considerable prominence in recent years as speech and language therapy attempts to demonstrate the long-term benefits to society and the economy of the interventions that it provides. The measurement of long-term outcomes is particularly challenging for investigators. In longitudinal studies, participants are often lost to follow-up. Also, any particular outcome is likely to be influenced by factors other than the treatment that subjects received. An individual's employment status at 25 years of age may well reflect the effects of an early language intervention. However, it is equally likely to reflect academic attainment or social skills at 16 years.

Several systematic reviews in SLT have produced conclusions that may unsettle clinicians as they contemplate their clinical significance. Typically, these conclusions are worded in the following terms: there is no evidence that intervention *X* produces outcome *Y* (where *Y* represents some gain for a client, such as improved language test scores or better social integration). For example, in a Cochrane systematic review Lee and Gibbon (2015) concluded that there is no strong evidence that non-speech oro-motor treatments are an effective treatment or an effective adjunctive treatment for children with developmental speech sound disorders. It should be noted, however, that a lack of evidence that a treatment is effective is not the same as evidence that a treatment is not effective. In fact, many 'no evidence' conclusions of systematic reviews simply reflect a lack of randomized controlled trials in an area or at least a limited number of these trials – there were only three such trials in the systematic review conducted by Lee and Gibbon. There are two lessons to emerge from these reviews. The first is that interventions which are currently in use but which are not supported by clinical evidence should not necessarily be abandoned. These interventions may indeed be effective – and presumably many clinicians believe that they are – but the limited research that has been conducted to date has not been able to demonstrate their effectiveness. The second lesson is that SLTs need to undertake many more research studies which can produce the type of high-quality evidence that is needed to address questions about the clinical effectiveness of interventions. Lee and Gibbon make the same point in the conclusion of their review: 'Well-designed research is needed to carefully investigate non-speech oral motor treatment as a type of treatment for children with speech sound disorders.'

KEY POINTS: Evidence-Based Practice

- Like all health disciplines, SLT subscribes to the principles of evidence-based medicine. These principles require clinicians to base their decisions about patient care on high-quality clinical evidence as well as their own expertise.
- Evidence-based practice in SLT is justified by the need to provide clients with the best possible outcomes in the most cost-effective manner possible. Healthcare providers require adherence to evidence-based practice in the SLT services that they commission.
- SLTs must assess the quality of the evidence that they use in clinical decision-making. Many studies that examine the effectiveness of SLT interventions are not randomized controlled trials and their evidence is limited in consequence. Systematic reviews are valuable in helping clinicians assess the quality of evidence in a clinical area.
- Studies which examine the effectiveness of SLT interventions must be clear from the outset about the outcomes to be measured. Some outcomes can be achieved and measured upon completion of a course of therapy, while others relate to treatment effects that are experienced months or even years after intervention has taken place. Some outcomes relate to aspects of speech and language, while other outcomes describe behaviours or performance in areas (e.g. employment status) that are known to be influenced by communication skills.
- Many systematic reviews have revealed a lack of evidence to support the effectiveness of SLT interventions. However, a lack of evidence that an intervention is effective is not the same as evidence that an intervention is not effective. Accordingly, clinicians should not discontinue use of these interventions. The lesson to emerge from these reviews is that SLTs must undertake more high-quality research studies in order to demonstrate the effectiveness of the interventions they use.

WEBSITE: Intervention and Outcomes

After reading the chapter, visit the website and test your knowledge of intervention and outcomes by answering the short-answer questions for this topic.

Suggestions for Further Reading

Cummings, L. (ed.) 2014. *Cambridge handbook of communication disorders*, Cambridge: Cambridge University Press.

Part D in this edited volume examines the management of developmental and acquired communication disorders. In dedicated chapters, the most recent approaches to SLT intervention in the following areas are addressed: developmental and acquired motor speech disorders; developmental language disorders; acquired aphasia; disorders of voice; and disorders of fluency.

Speyer, R. 2012. 'Behavioural treatment of oropharyngeal dysphagia: Bolus modification and management, sensory and motor behavioural techniques, postural adjustments, and swallow manoeuvres', in O. Ekberg (ed.), *Dysphagia: diagnosis and treatment*, Heidelberg, New York, Dordrecht and London: Springer, 477–92.

This chapter provides an extended discussion of the behavioural treatments of dysphagia examined in this chapter, including postural adjustments, swallow techniques, dietary modifications and motor and sensory treatments.

Dodd, B. 2007. 'Evidence-based practice and speech-language pathology: Strengths, weaknesses, opportunities and threats', *Folia Phoniatrica et Logopaedica* **59**:3, 118–29.

This article reviews the literature on evidence-based practice in speech-language pathology. The discussion addresses challenges that evidence-based practice poses for clinicians. It also considers opportunities that evidence-based practice makes possible for the profession.

QUESTIONS: Intervention and Outcomes

(1) Each of the following statements describes a clinical scenario in which SLT intervention is warranted. For each statement, indicate whether a direct or an indirect intervention should be undertaken:
 (a) A 60-year-old man with aphasia reports reduced conversational participation since his stroke. He also describes poor adjustment to his disability and a desire to share his experiences with other people who have aphasia.
 (b) A child with cleft palate uses a glottal stop in place of oral plosives. Speech is also hypernasal. Therapy to address these speech defects is initiated.
 (c) The spouse of a man with motor neurone disease reports significant difficulty understanding him and poor compliance with augmentative and alternative

communication (AAC). The SLT recommends environmental modifications to improve the client's comprehensibility.
  (d) A woman commences therapy after a laryngectomy for treatment of laryngeal cancer. Intervention focuses on the use of an electrolarynx and oesophageal speech.
  (e) A child with SLI has significant problems with expressive language. A classroom assistant engages in structured language tasks with the child under guidance from an SLT.
(2) Each of the following statements describes a client with a speech disorder. For each client, a speech intervention is warranted. Indicate whether that intervention should have a phonological focus, a motor speech programming and planning focus, or a motor speech execution focus:
  (a) Jack is 6 years old. He produces distorted consonants and vowels and his speech errors are inconsistent. An SLT evaluation reveals no neuromuscular weakness of the tongue, lips, jaw or soft palate.
  (b) Mary is 60 years old and is in recovery from a stroke. Her speech is moderately hypernasal and her tongue and lip movements are weak.
  (c) Sally is 8 years old and has a repaired palatal cleft. Many of her articulations are backed and she uses a glottal stop in place of all oral plosive sounds.
  (d) Dan is 7 years old and has cerebral palsy. His speech is moderately unintelligible. Tongue movements have reduced range and strength. Some oral articulations are masked by nasal emission.
  (e) Mike sustained a head injury in a motorbike accident. Since the accident, he has produced speech sound errors such as omissions and substitutions and has exhibited prosodic difficulties. His errors are most evident during volitional speech production.
(3) Respond with *true* or *false* to each of the following statements about language interventions:
  (a) Generalization in anomia therapies is often limited to directly trained words.
  (b) Parental questionnaires may be used to identify vocabulary to be targeted in intervention.
  (c) A total communication intervention emphasizes the use of spoken language.
  (d) Circumlocution-induced naming is a phonological therapy for anomia.
  (e) Some language interventions aim to increase a client's metalinguistic awareness.
  (f) Language interventions typically address either expressive language or receptive language skills.
  (g) Community-based language interventions can involve multiple agencies and practitioners.
  (h) Conversational partner training is typically used with children who have language delay.
  (i) Some language interventions target the development of story grammar.
  (j) Focused Stimulation is a pragmatic language intervention.
(4) Group therapy is used extensively by SLTs to treat children and adults who stutter. Describe three advantages of group therapy over individual therapy with these clients.

(5) The following statements describe different types of voice therapy in clients. For each statement, indicate if the voice therapy is a *direct treatment* or an *indirect treatment*:
   (a) A 55-year-old woman with muscle tension dysphonia is instructed in how to use relaxation techniques by an SLT.
   (b) An SLT encourages the use of yawn-sigh phonation in a client who engages in hyperadduction of the vocal folds.
   (c) An SLT makes a client with persistent dysphonia aware of the role of hydration in maintaining good vocal health.
   (d) A client with Parkinson's disease is instructed in the use of techniques to increase subglottal air pressure for speech production.
   (e) A child who has had microlaryngeal surgery for the removal of vocal nodules receives education from an SLT about the damaging consequences of phonotraumatic behaviours such as screaming.

(6) Examine the case study on dysphagia intervention in section 6.7, and then answer the following questions:
   (a) This 83-year-old man complained that he had mild intermittent coughing after swallow. What is the clinical significance of coughing in this context?
   (b) The modified barium swallow performed on this client revealed piecemeal deglutition but no aspiration or penetration. Explain what is meant by the terms *piecemeal deglutition*, *aspiration* and *penetration*.
   (c) A bedside swallow study showed stasis in both lateral sulci and stasis on the tongue. What is stasis and why does it occur?
   (d) This client received treatment for his dysphagia. Did the intervention include the use of swallow manoeuvres?
   (e) Did this client's intervention make use of exercises to improve neuromuscular processes that control swallowing?

(7) Respond with *true* or *false* to each of the following statements about evidence-based practice in SLT:
   (a) Evidence-based practice applies only to the management of clients with acquired communication disorders.
   (b) Systematic reviews evaluate the quality of evidence in a clinical area.
   (c) Most studies that examine the effectiveness of SLT interventions take the form of randomized controlled trials.
   (d) Establishing the effectiveness of an intervention requires SLTs to study a range of outcomes.
   (e) Outcomes in SLT intervention research relate only to aspects of communication and swallowing.
   (f) When a systematic review concludes that there is no evidence to support the effectiveness of an intervention, the intervention may be taken to be not effective.
   (g) Evidence-based practice in SLT also relies on the expertise of individual clinicians.
   (h) Systematic reviews of interventions for voice disorders are less reliable than systematic reviews of interventions for language disorders.
   (i) Evidence-based practice operates exclusively in the allied health professions.
   (j) Outcomes in SLT intervention research must be measurable.

7 The Profession of Speech and Language Therapy

7.1 Introduction

Like any health discipline, speech and language therapy must address a range of professional issues and challenges. Many of these issues reflect the wider healthcare context in which SLT must operate. This context is characterized by the need to provide high-quality clinical services to a growing number of clients with complex needs when health spending[1] is decreasing in real terms. These competing demands create considerable challenges for SLTs who must respond by working flexibly across contexts ranging from acute hospital settings to community-based facilities. Other contexts require therapists to understand how SLT is integrated with the education system and the criminal justice system. The complex needs of many clients, particularly older people with several health conditions, require SLTs to work within **multidisciplinary teams** in the assessment, diagnosis and treatment of individuals with communication and swallowing disorders. Clients with head trauma, for example, encounter SLTs within a rehabilitation team that also includes neurologists, **neuropsychologists**, **physiotherapists**, **occupational therapists** and specialist nurses. As knowledge of communication and swallowing disorders has increased, SLTs have found themselves working alongside a growing number of medical and health professionals in multidisciplinary teams. For example, gastroenterologists are now as involved in the management of certain clients with voice disorders as SLTs and otolaryngologists. Decisions about patient care across large teams that involve many different professionals require excellent communication and strong **collaborative working** practices. These issues will be addressed in this chapter within a wider examination of the role of SLTs within multidisciplinary teams.

Throughout this book, extensive reference has been made to professional bodies and associations such as the Royal College of Speech and Language Therapists (RCSLT), the American Speech-Language-Hearing Association (ASHA) and Speech Pathology Australia. The role of these bodies in the work of SLTs cannot be overemphasized. In earlier chapters, it was described how pre-registration courses are required by RCSLT to fulfil specific requirements across a range of foundational disciplines in SLT. As well as overseeing the clinical education of SLT students, professional bodies have a further important role to play when students graduate and enter the profession. For it is then that

continuing professional development (CPD) begins and runs throughout a therapist's clinical career. By undertaking CPD, therapists are continually renewing and updating their clinical skills and knowledge to reflect new developments in the field. Professional bodies have a key role to play in providing CPD activities such as workshops and seminars, in monitoring the standard of these activities and in ensuring that their members participate in them. To this end, regular audits of the CPD activities of its members are undertaken by the RCSLT, for example. But the work of professional bodies does not end with the clinical education of SLT students and CPD. For these bodies also prepare clinical practice guidelines for the management of clients with communication and swallowing disorders, lobby governments and federal agencies for better services for these clients, and improve public understanding of, and respect for, people with communication and swallowing disorders. These functions and other responsibilities of professional bodies will be examined in this chapter.

Charitable organizations are playing an increasingly important role in SLT. This role is threefold. First, many charities fund SLT clinical posts which serve the needs of clients that the charities aim to support. A brief survey of *Bulletin*, the professional magazine of the RCSLT, shows that between January and July 2016, the following charitable organizations advertised SLT positions: Autism Wessex; Ambitious about Autism; Scope (a charity that supports disabled people); Young Epilepsy; and SeeAbility (a charity that supports people with sight loss). As state-funded SLT services in the UK and elsewhere come under increasing pressure, it appears likely that charitable organizations will play an increasingly important role in the provision of SLT services in years to come. Second, charitable organizations also provide much-needed support to parents, spouses and carers of children and adults with communication and swallowing disorders. It is support services to these individuals that are most likely to be affected by reduced health spending by central government, and that charitable organizations have considerable experience and expertise in providing. Third, charitable organizations also have an important role to play in **advocacy** for people with **communication disorders**. This includes lobbying government for improved employment opportunities and social equality for people with communication disorders and influencing government policy relating to the provision of SLT services. Charitable organizations can also help improve society's perceptions of people with communication disorders through effective awareness-raising campaigns and educational activities. Each of these roles of charitable organizations will be examined further in this chapter.

7.2 SLT in Multidisciplinary Teams

The multidisciplinary team is a feature of modern healthcare systems. As knowledge specialization has taken place, the emphasis in healthcare is less on the individual clinician and more on the combined expertise of a group of clinicians who work together to assess, diagnose and treat clients. In this section, the role of SLTs in multidisciplinary teams will be examined. Several features of these teams are noteworthy. First, multidisciplinary teams emerge to address the clinical needs of clients. Many of the medical conditions which give rise to communication and swallowing problems in children and adults are complex genetic, psychiatric and neurodegenerative disorders that cannot be addressed by a single medical specialism. The clinical management of these conditions necessarily requires the combined expertise of several clinicians. Second, the constitution of multidisciplinary teams varies considerably with clinical context. The clinicians in a child development team are not the same clinicians as in a head and neck cancer team or in a head injury rehabilitation team. Yet, SLTs are able to contribute their clinical skills to each of these different teams. It will be argued that it is a sign of the remarkable versatility of the profession that this is possible. Third, for multidisciplinary teams to work well, they must be more than the sum of the individual working practices of each clinician in the team. Clinicians must communicate and share information with other members of the team through weekly case reviews. Decision-making must be informed by the viewpoints of all relevant experts and not simply reflect the views of a single clinician. These collaborative working practices can only be developed in a context of mutual trust and respect among members of the team. These practices will also be examined in this section.

It will not have escaped the reader of earlier chapters in this book that SLTs never work in isolation from other medical and health professionals. Even SLTs in independent or private practice must receive referrals from health visitors and physicians, read reports written by other clinicians and seek advice from, and refer clients to, other professionals. Multidisciplinary teams are ever present, even in the case where their members do not all occupy the same clinical space. The reason for this combined labour is clear enough – no individual clinician has the requisite knowledge and clinical skills to assess, diagnose and treat clients with communication and swallowing disorders. To illustrate this, imagine a client who presents at a voice clinic with persistent hoarseness. This client undergoes a laryngological examination by an otolaryngologist to establish if the client's dysphonia has an organic basis. Referral to an SLT may follow to address poor vocal hygiene and the phonotraumatic behaviours that emerged during the taking of a case history. But the involvement of other clinicians does not end here. For the otolaryngologist may have observed inflammation of the laryngeal muscosa during laryngoscopy and may decide that referral of the client to a gastroenterologist is also necessary in order to investigate possible reflux disease. Imagine that gastroesophageal reflux disease (GERD) is diagnosed and treated but that it, along with good vocal hygiene, achieve little improvement in the client's dysphonia. At this stage, it might be decided that a psychologist should evaluate the client in order to establish if a diagnosis of psychogenic dysphonia is warranted. The multidisciplinary team in this case involves several clinicians whose task it is to jointly determine which factors are playing a causal role in this client's voice disorder.

The management of a client with dysphonia is not unique in requiring the involvement of several professionals. Imagine the case of a child with a neurodevelopmental disorder such as autism spectrum disorder (ASD). A **psychiatrist** or psychologist may make the primary diagnosis of ASD. But this child will also have to be assessed by an SLT to establish the extent of any delay in language development. In the case where spoken language does not emerge, an SLT will need to institute an alternative communication system such as the *Picture Exchange Communication System* (Frost and Bondy, 1994). However, a number of other professionals will also be involved in the management of this child. An **educational psychologist** must assess this child to establish if learning will be compromised by the presence of an intellectual disability. Specialist teachers and classroom assistants must be able to implement recommendations of the psychologist and make whatever adjustments are required to facilitate this child's learning. Assessment and intervention by an occupational therapist is needed to help children with ASD perform activities of daily living (e.g. feeding, dressing), and improve fine motor skills (e.g. handwriting), play and social participation. Many children with ASD experience feeding difficulties and gastrointestinal problems. Referral to a gastroenterologist may be necessary to address these problems. Also, intervention by a **dietician** may be needed in order to make dietary changes and to ensure that the child's nutritional requirements are met. A **social worker** also has a vital role to play in helping parents of children with ASD access respite care and other support services. Once again, a wide range of professionals, which includes SLTs, is involved in the management of children with ASD.

It emerges that the individual clinical expertise that comprises multidisciplinary teams is determined by the primary medical diagnosis of the clients who are assessed and treated by the team. No-one would be surprised to discover, for example, that **oncologists** are key medical professionals in a head and neck cancer team, neurologists are integral to a head injury rehabilitation team, and that **paediatricians** are members of a child development team. However, it may be somewhat more surprising to discover that SLTs can contribute to each of these different teams. The inclusion of SLTs in multiple teams is in part the result of an expansion of the professional remit of speech and language therapy to include 'new' roles in areas such as the management of clients with dysphagia. Recently, the remit of SLT has expanded again to include a public health role in the tackling of social inequality related to childhood language disorder. But the involvement of SLTs in many different multidisciplinary teams is also an indication of how important communication and swallowing are to the successful rehabilitation of clients after illness and injury. Even more than physical disabilities, communication impairments have been shown to limit the social participation and reintegration of adults following events like stroke and TBI (see chapter 5 in Cummings, 2014a, for discussion). Interventions which lessen the negative impact of communication disorders are thus considered to be integral to the care that multidisciplinary teams provide. The involvement of SLTs in many different multidisciplinary teams attests to the remarkable versatility of speech and language therapy in improving the lives of children and adults with communication and swallowing disorders. Central to this versatility is the capacity of the profession to reinvent itself in order to respond to new challenges.

In any multidisciplinary team, the number of professionals and diverse clinical backgrounds of members can create challenges for the team. One of the most significant challenges concerns communication. The need for effective communication is of paramount importance, especially when one considers that poor communication is often the basis of medical errors, many of which can cause severe injury or even death (O'Daniel and Rosenstein, 2008). An area of SLT practice where poor communication between team members could directly compromise patient safety is the management of clients with dysphagia. Imagine that a client is admitted to a hospital ward following a stroke. An SLT receives a referral from a neurologist to investigate the client for possible dysphagia. A bedside assessment of the client raises a suspicion of aspiration, which is subsequently confirmed by means of a videofluoroscopic swallow study. As a result of assessment, it is decided that oral feeding is unsafe for this patient and should be discontinued. The decision to discontinue oral feeding and to institute some other method of delivery of nutrition to the patient (e.g. nasogastric tube feeding) must be communicated to all members of the dysphagia team. In the absence of effective communication between the SLT and other members of the dysphagia team, particularly nurses and dieticians, the patient is placed at high risk of aspiration, dehydration and malnutrition. It is with a view to averting these serious consequences of a lack of communication between the members of the dysphagia team that the RCSLT makes the following recommendation in its Dysphagia Training & Competency Framework:

> Where the multidisciplinary team is fragmented or disparate, the SLT has a duty to seek out relevant professionals and engage in communication with them and families/carers for the benefit and good quality treatment of the patient/client. (2014: 12)

Aside from patient safety, effective communication between members of the multidisciplinary team is important for other reasons. It is often the case that decisions about which course of treatment to pursue in a particular case are based on a number of competing considerations. For example, although surgical procedures can achieve pitch elevation in the male-to-female transsexual client, unrealistic expectations on the part of the client about post-surgical voice production may be reason enough not to pursue surgical intervention in a particular case. Clinical decision-making of this type can be arrived at only through communication between clinicians, with all relevant views able to be expressed and afforded respect. Communication between members of the multidisciplinary team is also necessary to establish if one aspect of a client's care is likely to impact positively or negatively on another aspect. For example, changes to a client's medications may have implications for the intelligibility of speech or for a client's compliance with an SLT intervention. Communication between members of the team may be necessary to identify unforeseen consequences of different therapies and to make adjustments wherever possible. Finally, there may be cases where SLTs have to act as advocates for the client and communicate the client's views to other members of the multidisciplinary team when the client is unable to do so. This is especially relevant for clients with neurodegenerative diseases such as motor neurone disease or with advanced head and neck cancers where communication may eventually not be possible. In such cases, SLTs may have to communicate a client's wishes about the continuation of care and end-of-life care to the team.

Effective communication between members of the multidisciplinary team can take different forms. It includes oral communication at weekly team meetings and in telephone calls to other clinicians, and written communication in the form of updating patient records and writing reports. Regular meetings are an important part of the work of multidisciplinary teams. If these meetings do not have a clear purpose or goal, or if they are poorly organized and conducted, their contribution to patient care can be limited. Raine et al. (2014) identified 21 indications of good practice for improving the effectiveness of multidisciplinary team meetings. These authors state that the primary objective of team meetings should be to agree treatment plans for patients. Other functions, they argue, are important but should not take precedence. It is during multidisciplinary team meetings that some of the tensions and conflicts in the wider team can become apparent. For example, tension can arise between the professional practices of individual team members and the goals of the multidisciplinary team. It is not uncommon, for example, for team members to report low team identification but high professional identification (Onyett et al., 1997). Some 'unlearning' of professional practices may need to occur in order for collaborative working to emerge between members of the team. Collaborative working practices between SLTs and a range of professionals including ENT consultants and **respiratory therapists** have been described (Gardner, 2014; Swigert, 2016). An area where the SLT and respiratory therapist can collaborate is in the management of clients with pneumonia. By familiarizing the respiratory therapist with the clinical signs of dysphagia, the SLT can help ensure referral of patients to speech and language therapy for a swallowing evaluation.

CASE STUDY: Head Trauma Rehabilitation Team

M.G. is a 50-year-old married man who was assaulted and experienced head trauma. As well as right frontal and parietal fractures, a CT scan revealed a left epidural and subdural haematoma. He was in a coma for approximately 10 days. When he regained consciousness, his swallowing was assessed at bedside and using videofluoroscopy and was judged to be unsafe. Enteral feeding via a PEG tube was initiated. There was no intelligible speech production, and M.G. appeared to have very limited auditory verbal comprehension.

M.G. spent 2 years and 9 months at an inpatient rehabilitation facility specializing in head injury. When he entered the facility, he was judged to be inconsistently responsive to general stimuli. When he left the facility almost 3 years later, he was rated to be confused but was responding appropriately to simple directions. M.G. returned home to live with his wife. He received 24-hour care in all areas including basic hygiene and grooming skills. He could say a few words but had severe anomia. He had good muscle strength in his left arm and leg and moderate to severe spasticity and contractures throughout his right extremities with synergistic movement patterns. He used a wheelchair and was taking anti-seizure medications.

M.G. also exhibited significant cognitive deficits. He had short-term memory loss and was unable to solve problems. He displayed poor initiation and concrete thinking. Additionally, he had right visual neglect and decreased visual acuity with moderate perceptual impairments. M.G. was unable to initiate, plan or organize an activity, and was dependent on others to direct his schedule. There was no recognition of his cognitive impairments.

SPECIAL TOPIC: Interprofessional Education and Interprofessional Practice

In multidisciplinary teams, clinicians work in parallel or sequentially in the management of clients. For example, the otolaryngologist may first perform a laryngological examination of a client with dysphonia and then refer the client to SLT for work on vocal exercises and vocal hygiene. A quite different model of collaborative working is envisaged in interprofessional education (IPE) and interprofessional practice (IPP). The World Health Organization (2010: 7) states that 'interprofessional education occurs when students from two or more professions learn about, from and with each other to enable effective collaboration and improve health outcomes'. IPE is a necessary first step in preparing students to become collaborative practice-ready health workers.

IPE and IPP are now widely adopted in healthcare as effective strategies that can help mitigate the global health workforce crisis. To this end, they have been adopted by the American Speech-Language-Hearing Association (ASHA) as one of its objectives in its 10-year (2015–2025) Strategic Pathway to Excellence plan. The desired outcome of this objective is that by 2025, IPE approaches to the clinical education of SLT students are adopted by academic programmes and that all ASHA members are engaged in interprofessional collaborative practice. There is evidence that this is being achieved. DiGiovanni and McCarthy (2016) described how IPE was instituted in their own institution, Ohio University. Launching an IPE initiative required the integration of several programmes across two colleges. Edwards et al. (2015) described a course assignment that encouraged interprofessional collaborative practice between SLTs and social workers in the management of children in need of early intervention services. Interprofessional collaborative practice between nurses and SLTs is also embedded in the management of clients with dysphagia (Dondorf et al. 2016).

KEY POINTS: SLT in Multidisciplinary Teams

- In modern healthcare, the multidisciplinary team is a cost-effective way of delivering high-quality clinical services to clients who have complex needs that span several specialisms.
- SLTs are members of many different multidisciplinary teams, including the dysphagia team, the head trauma rehabilitation team and the mental health team. The other members of these teams include dieticians and gastroenterologists (dysphagia), neurologists and neuropsychologists (head trauma), and psychiatrists and social workers (mental health).
- SLTs can contribute in various ways to multidisciplinary teams. They can contribute their expertise in communication and swallowing to team decisions about the treatment of clients, work with team members in the assessment and diagnosis of clients, and provide guidance to team members about the remit of SLT to increase referral to its clinical services.
- Large teams with members from a number of medical and health professions can create challenges that must be overcome if patient care is not to be compromised. For example, poor communication within teams can place patient safety at risk. The subordination of team goals to the professional practices and interests of individual members can compromise clinical decision-making.
- Collaborative working between members of the multidisciplinary team is of paramount importance and can be achieved through open discussion about the roles and responsibilities of members, sharing of information between members and joint attendance of members at training events.

7.3 SLT across Contexts and Countries

The contexts in which SLTs assess and treat clients are as varied as the multidisciplinary teams to which they belong. For most child clients, SLT is delivered in mainstream and special schools, although community clinics, health centres and clients' homes are also significant contexts for the delivery of paediatric SLT services. For many adult clients, SLT is accessed as a hospital inpatient or outpatient, at home or in residential facilities in the community. Less often, SLT services are available in youth offending institutions and in prisons. The contexts in which SLT is delivered are significant for a number of reasons. They can determine how the service is funded. In the UK, for example, most school-based SLT services are funded by education authorities while SLT in hospitals in the National Health Service are funded by the mainstream health budget. They can also determine the equipment and other resources that are available to clinicians. In acute hospital settings, investigative techniques such as videofluoroscopy are available to assess clients with suspected dysphagia. These same techniques are not available in residential care facilities where clients with dysphagia may have to be referred to more specialist facilities or assessed using

Table 7.1 *Data from ASHA's 2015 SLP Health Care Survey showing SLT services in a range of facilities*

Facility	Percentage
General medical, Veterans Affairs, or long-term acute care hospital	15.8
Rehabilitation hospital	10.2
Paediatric hospital	8.5
Skilled nursing facility	21.2
Home health agency or client's home	18.1
Outpatient clinic or office	23.6
Other	2.4

other techniques. The practice of SLT also varies across countries. The profession is known by quite different names in different parts of the world including speech and language therapy (UK and New Zealand), speech-language pathology (USA), speech pathology (Australia), and logopedics and phoniatrics (Sweden). Differences extend beyond the nomenclature of the profession. For example, in Brazil speech-language pathology and audiology are one profession (Fonoaudiologia) and are taught conjointly. The profession of SLT in different countries will be addressed further in this section.

Although it is widely acknowledged that SLT is practised in many different contexts, little objective data exists on the distribution of SLT services across settings. One exception is to be found in surveys conducted by ASHA. In its 2015 Health Care Survey, ASHA asked respondents to select the one type of facility that best describes where they worked most of the time (ASHA, 2015a). The percentages in Table 7.1 were obtained across seven categories of facility included in the survey. Beyond paediatric hospital, the data in Table 7.1 provides little information about the contexts in which SLT services are delivered to children. Another ASHA survey – the 2016 Schools Survey – shows that the majority of SLT services to children are delivered in elementary school (ASHA, 2016b) (see Table 7.2).

These figures are noteworthy in several respects. First, they reflect the chronic nature of many adult acquired communication and swallowing disorders. The adult who experiences a stroke and develops aphasia, dysarthria and dysphagia (or some combination of these disorders) is admitted initially to an acute care hospital. The priority in this setting is to achieve medical stabilization of the client and to perform an assessment of the client's communication, swallowing and other needs. In the event that SLT intervention is required, it is initiated in the acute care setting but continued for the most part in facilities that specialize in longer-term rehabilitation. One such facility is the skilled nursing facility that provides skilled nursing care to clients who no longer require the high level of medical support available in the acute hospital setting but who must undergo further treatment and recuperation before returning home. SLT is one of the services available to clients in skilled

Table 7.2 *Data from ASHA's 2016 Schools Survey showing SLT services in a range of facilities*

Facility	Percentage
Special day/residential school	3.8
Pre-elementary (preschool)	12.5
Elementary school	56.8
Secondary school (middle school, junior high, senior high)	14.2
Student's home	1.7
Administrative office	2.0
Combination from the above list	8.3
Other	0.8

nursing facilities.[2] For clients with conditions such as aphasia, SLT intervention can also be provided at home and in outpatient clinics, depending on the client's level of mobility. The high percentages of SLT provision in skilled nursing facilities, clients' homes and outpatient clinics reflect the duration of care that is required by clients with chronic conditions such as aphasia.

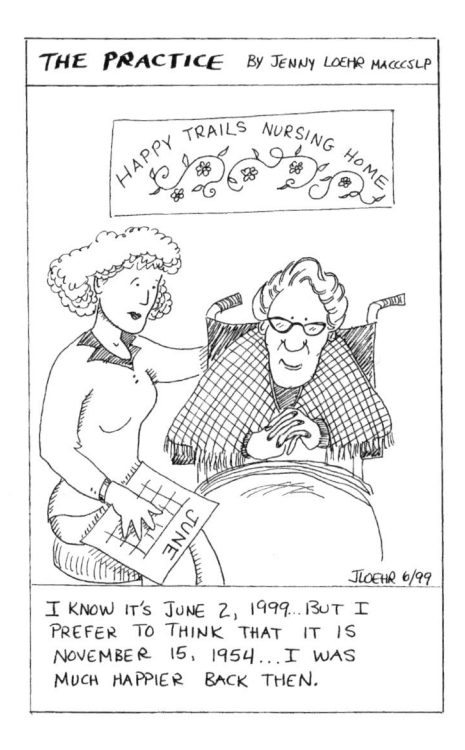

THE PRACTICE BY JENNY LOEHR MACCCSLP

HAPPY TRAILS NURSING HOME

I KNOW IT'S JUNE 2, 1999... BUT I PREFER TO THINK THAT IT IS NOVEMBER 15, 1954... I WAS MUCH HAPPIER BACK THEN.

A second noteworthy feature of these figures is the high concentration of paediatric SLT services in elementary school (56.8%) and the much lower concentration in preschool settings (12.5%). This distribution of provision suggests that many children with speech and language problems receive SLT interventions, possibly for the first time, when they have already started school. Clearly, if children enter school with such impoverished speech and language skills that they are unable to form peer relationships and access the curriculum, the priority for clinicians and educators must be to deliver intensive speech and language services in elementary school settings. However, recent clinical evidence suggests that intervention is most effective when it is delivered in the preschool years (Ullrich et al., 2014). This is the basis of the many early years language interventions that now exist (see Table 6.2 in Chapter 6). To improve outcomes in children with early language delay, the UK government has made SLT intervention in the preschool years a policy priority (Roulstone et al., 2015). In the USA, speech-language intervention in the preschool years is a provision under Part C of the 2004 Individuals with Disabilities Education Act (IDEA). Part C is a $436 million programme which serves infants and toddlers through age 2 with developmental delays or who have diagnosed physical or mental conditions with high probabilities of resulting in developmental delays. Children are eligible to receive services, including speech-language services, at a state's discretion. As further SLT interventions are developed, government legislation and policies that mandate their use in the preschool years may achieve a much-needed redistribution of SLT services in schools in years to come.

A third noteworthy feature of these figures concerns the percentage of respondents (14.2%) who identified secondary school as the setting where they undertook most or all of their work. This figure is only slightly higher than the percentage of respondents (12.5%) who identified preschool as their primary work setting in the 2016 Schools Survey. The high concentration of SLT services in elementary school drops back significantly in secondary school. A possible explanation of this decrease is that there is a widespread assumption that significant speech and language gains are possible only in the early school years and that improvements in speech and language skills as a result of intervention are less likely to occur during adolescence. This assumption is not supported by the results of clinical studies, which have shown that adolescent clients are able to make significant gains as a result of SLT intervention. Ebbels et al. (2014) reported significant gains in the comprehension of **coordinating conjunctions** following an intervention in 14 adolescents with severe receptive language impairments. These gains were maintained after 4 months. Bacsfalvi and Bernhardt (2011) found that 5 of 7 adolescents with **hearing impairment** continued to generalize their speech production or maintained their level of performance 2–4 years after speech intervention with **ultrasound** and electropalatography. If the reduced concentration of SLT services in secondary schools is related to the belief that minimal gains can be made by adolescents in therapy, then the findings of these studies and others like them suggest that this belief is mistaken.

There is a further reason why intensive SLT services should be available to adolescent clients. It is during adolescence that there is significant development of **social communication skills** of the type that are needed to forge strong bonds with peers and to establish group affiliations (Cummings, 2015). If these skills are compromised, there can be adverse, long-term consequences for an individual's **self-esteem** and psychological well-being (see chapter 5 in Cummings, 2014a, for discussion). Intensive SLT intervention in the adolescent years can help teenagers at risk of these consequences develop strong language skills that can be used, among other things, to negotiate conflict and resolve interpersonal difficulties. In the UK, a report by the children's communication charity I CAN highlights the importance of communication skills during adolescence and the limited opportunities that exist in secondary schools for the development of these skills:

> For most young people, language continues to develop throughout the school years and into adulthood. They develop the skills they need to problem solve, build effective relationships, negotiate and tell jokes. However, a significant group of young people find this difficult: those with speech, language and communication needs (SLCN). Despite the importance of communication, and the number of young people with SLCN, there is often limited opportunity in secondary schools for pupils to develop spoken communication skills. There is also limited understanding of, and support for, those with SLCN. Without support, poor communication can impact on a young person's academic success as well as their social and emotional development. (Hartshorne, 2011: 3)

With greater recognition of the role of language skills in the ability of adolescents to negotiate the increasingly complex relationships of their social world, a further redistribution of SLT services to include enhanced provision for adolescents in secondary schools may be possible.

Aside from the contexts in which SLT is practised, it is also important to consider the practice of SLT in other countries around the world. Like other health professionals, SLTs can and do pursue employment outside of the countries where they trained. Some indication of the extent of international movement of SLTs is provided by the figure that approximately 2,000 certified ASHA members live outside the United States (Lubinski and Hudson, 2013). That SLT has considerable global reach is indicated by the following facts and figures from Bleile et al. (2006). These authors reported that

- At least 55 countries have national associations
- Turkey is the country with the newest national association
- There are at least 24 international professional associations and groups
- The Asia Pacific Society for the Study of Speech, Language and Hearing is the newest international association
- At least 51 countries have student education programmes
- There are approximately 672 student education programmes worldwide

- Bangladesh has the newest student programme
- Sub-Saharan Africa is the region with fewest student education programmes
- Iceland and Singapore are countries which are developing student education programmes

Several important issues are raised by the fact that SLT has an increasingly global presence. The first issue concerns the extent to which the practice of SLT in different countries is shaped by linguistic and cultural influences in these countries. For example, countries with large bilingual populations may require different clinical competencies of SLTs than countries where SLTs work for the most part with monolingual populations. Also, negative perceptions of people with disabilities in some cultures can have damaging consequences for the referral of clients to SLT services and for the funding of services. The second issue concerns the extent to which there is international cooperation between SLTs who work in different countries. International cooperation can lead to sharing of knowledge and best practice which can enhance the professional development of therapists and the quality of clinical services that clients receive. The third issue is that, notwithstanding the growth of SLT worldwide, there are still many countries and populations in the world where SLT services do not exist at all or are under-developed. For children and adults with communication disorders in these countries, the lack of SLT services can limit educational achievement and employment opportunities and serves to perpetuate the impoverished conditions in which many of these individuals live. When viewed as an important part of international efforts to tackle global poverty, the provision of SLT services is an issue that assumes political and even ethical significance. Each of these points will be addressed further below.

As one might expect, SLT is shaped by the linguistic and cultural influences of the countries in which it is practised. An important linguistic influence on the delivery of SLT services is bilingualism. Bilingualism is the norm in many countries around the world.[3] However, most SLT services and education programmes have an English monolingual focus. In its practice portal on bilingual service delivery, the American Speech-Language-Hearing Association (2016c) states that 'some graduate schools offer bilingual specialty training programs, but it should be noted that the depth and breadth of training in this area is variable from program to program'. One of the most pressing challenges for those who provide clinical language services to bilingual clients is the availability of clinicians who are able to work in the languages spoken by clients. Some indication of the scale of this challenge is provided in a study by Mennen and Stansfield (2006), who reported that in one Scottish city, 53 languages other than English were spoken by the bilingual school-age population. Even when clinicians are available, there are other challenges for a bilingual SLT service to overcome. Most standardized language assessments are designed for monolingual English-speaking clients and use monolingual norms. In a report commissioned by RCSLT, Stow and Pert (2015: 10) state that

> When assessing a bilingual child, the very premise of [standardised] assessments is called into question. Although a few assessments have been adapted and re-standardised on languages other than English, or even developed especially for speakers of other languages, there is still a severe dearth of standardised assessments for speakers of major languages. The situation is even worse for minority language speakers.

Notwithstanding these difficulties, there is evidence that some SLT services are able to address the specific needs of bilingual clients. Of the three cities in Great Britain studied by Mennen and Stansfield (2006), two appeared to be offering a proportionate SLT service to both monolingual and bilingual children in terms of the relative numbers of children on SLT caseloads. However, only one service was confident that it was fully satisfying the RCSLT (1998) good practice guidelines on bilingualism.

Cultural influences can shape every aspect of SLT practice. For example, in today's Western societies, paternalism in healthcare is generally discouraged. Clinicians no longer take the view that clients should defer to them as experts in decisions about their healthcare. Instead, clients and their families are actively encouraged by SLTs and other health professionals to participate in decision-making about intervention. However, in some cultures, inclusivity in clinical decision-making around, for example, the setting of treatment objectives may be perceived to be a sign that a clinician lacks competence. Also, verbal and non-verbal communicative behaviours vary across cultures. These behaviours include facial expressions, eye gaze, body postures, turn-taking in conversation and rules of social interaction. Sensitivity to these cultural differences in communication is necessary, both for SLTs who are practicing in countries where they did not undertake their clinical training and for SLTs who have a culturally diverse caseload. Where cultural knowledge is lacking, there is a risk that a cultural difference in behaviour (e.g. the use of silence in conversation) may be misinterpreted as a disorder. Awareness of cultural preferences is particularly important in the management of clients with dysphagia, for example, where suggested dietary modifications must be sensitive to the food preferences of a particular culture. As forms of disability, communication and swallowing disorders may be negatively perceived and evaluated in certain cultures. SLTs must be aware of how these perceptions and judgements can affect referral to, and compliance with, SLT interventions. In short, SLTs must be aware of the cultural contexts in which SLT is practised in order to navigate successfully around these issues and to provide clients with culturally appropriate services.

International cooperation between SLTs does exist and is actively encouraged by professional associations (e.g. ASHA) and bodies such as the Standing Liaison Committee of Speech and Language Therapists/Logopedists in the EU (CPLOL). Cooperation permits the exchange of knowledge and best practice between clinicians and can facilitate the development of clinical services, particularly in countries of the world where SLT is still relatively under-developed. ASHA has an International Issues Board which consists of ten members who collectively represent the global diversity, knowledge and experience of SLT in different regions of the world. The Board is charged with facilitating ASHA's engagement with speech, language and hearing organizations worldwide with a view to promoting scientific and resource exchange and improving the science and practice of the professions concerned. CPLOL is composed of 35 professional organizations of speech and language therapists/logopedists in 32 countries and represents more than 80,000 professionals. One of its objectives is to promote within member countries of the EU the exchange of scientific knowledge and research in the fields of speech and language therapy-logopedics. While CPLOL facilitates scientific exchange between member countries of the EU, other organizations promote cooperation between countries with well-developed SLT services and countries where services are still in a formative stage. For example, Communication Therapy International (CTI) was established in 1990 by a small committee of SLTs who are mostly based in the UK but are interested in international work. The aim of CTI is to link people worldwide who have an interest in communication disability so that they can share ideas, experience, knowledge and resources.

Worldwide, there are many people with communication and swallowing disorders who do not have access to clinical services. Bleile et al. (2006) states that SLT is largely absent in three-quarters of countries and territories around the world, and that communication services are often provided by members of another discipline such as nursing, psychology or education. Unsurprisingly, these countries are also some of the most impoverished in the world. Bowen (2016) reports that there are only two internationally certified speech-language pathologists in Tanzania, while Makerere University in Kampala, Uganda, has the only bachelor's degree in SLT in East and Central Africa. In the absence of effective communication skills, children and adults in these countries are at a considerable social, academic and economic disadvantage. Poor communication skills compound the already difficult circumstances in which many of these individuals live and are a significant barrier to tackling poverty in these countries. However, international charitable organizations and national governments are undertaking considerable efforts to address this lack of SLT provision. Examples include the international children's charity Chance for Childhood, which funds SLT posts in Rwanda, and Yellow House, a non-profit organization that supports SLT for children with communication disabilities in Western Kenya. In 2016, the United States Agency for International Development (USAID), supported by the Vietnam Monitoring and Survey Services Project, conducted an assessment of speech therapy/pathology services in Vietnam. The assessment findings and recommendations have been used by USAID/Vietnam to design future assistance programmes for people with disabilities in the country.

CASE STUDY: Volunteering with Yellow House Children's Services

The following extracts are taken from the stories and experiences of volunteers who have worked for Yellow House Children's Services in Kenya. Examine these extracts and then answer the questions at the end of the chapter. Full-length volunteer accounts can be accessed at: www.yellowhousechildrens.org/past-volunteer-experiences.html

Jessie is an SLT who worked in Kisumu in Kenya in 2015:

> I have seen first-hand how important it is to have a speech therapy service available not only for the families accessing the clinics but also crucial for all the other professions who are working with children with communication difficulties. Professionals such as physiotherapists, occupational therapists, doctors, nurses and teaching staff are all being asked to support children with communication difficulties and not knowing how. With health and education professionals not knowing how to effectively support these children how do we expect families to cope?

Rachel is an SLT who worked in Western Kenya in April 2014:

> Disability is often viewed as inability, failure and shame in Kenya. Rarely do they celebrate the life of someone with a disability. This narrow minded belief means there is room for change and reform, which I played my small part in achieving. Being the person who plays with children, encourages them, laughs with them and values the person in them shows the public that there is life after disability. I tried to get them to see the person first and disability second. I did not succeed in doing this with every family or person I met. I like to believe I succeeded in one, maybe two families. At least that's two families who now have a child with a disability, rather than a 'disabled child'.

Sally is an SLT who worked in Kilifi in Kenya in July 2011:

> Kilifi Primary School is a mainstream school with a special education program for children with a diagnosis of either cerebral palsy or mental handicap ... As with the regular classes, the special education classes have a very repetitive, rote-learning approach to teaching which unfortunately does not cater well for those kids with communication and/or learning difficulties. I found myself quite overwhelmed by how 'behind' the teaching style was, and had to resist the temptation to try and change everything. I was lucky to develop a positive rapport with some of the special education teachers, who were willing to try new approaches, and not afraid to tell me when they thought such approaches would not work.

KEY POINTS: SLT across Contexts and Countries

- SLT is practised in clients' homes, schools and a range of medical and health facilities including hospitals and community clinics. SLT services vary markedly across countries, from well-resourced clinics in which highly qualified clinicians work to services that are non-existent or poorly equipped.

- There is little objective data on the contexts in which SLT is practised. The data that does exist shows that there is a concentration of SLT services in facilities that address long-term rehabilitation of clients and in elementary school.
- For the purpose of SLT service planning, it is important to ask if services are directed at areas of greatest need. It is argued that some redistribution of SLT services away from elementary school towards preschool and secondary school may better serve the needs of clients.
- SLT is a well-developed health profession in many countries of the world. However, in other countries there are little or no clinical services available to children and adults with communication and swallowing disorders. This lack of services reduces the life chances of people with these disorders and compounds the poverty in which many of them live.
- SLT is shaped by linguistic and cultural influences of the countries in which it is practised. International cooperation between SLTs around the world permits sharing of expertise and resources. The combined work of national governments and charitable organizations is vital for the planning and delivery of SLT services to the many under-served populations with communication disability around the world.

7.4 SLT Professional Bodies and Associations

Most SLTs become acquainted with the associations that represent their profession for the first time as students on SLT education programmes. This marks the start of an important professional membership for SLTs. The nature of that membership can vary, from practising status for those therapists who hold SLT positions to non-practising status for individuals who do not practise but nevertheless wish to retain an association with a professional body. Other categories of membership include newly qualified members, retired members and student members (see Table 7.3). Speech Pathology Australia has a separate membership category for those who are re-entering the profession. Professional bodies are integral to every aspect of SLT. They accredit undergraduate and

Table 7.3 *ASHA membership categories for year-end 2015*

MEMBER CATEGORY	NUMBER
Certified members (SLPs only)	156,254
Certified non-members (SLPs only)	2,287
NSSLHA (student) members	12,110
International affiliates	468
Members without certification	375
Associates	207

postgraduate courses at university, ensuring that these courses adhere to certain standards and that students receive the full range of clinical skills and knowledge to practise competently. Professional bodies oversee continuing professional development (CPD) of their members by providing CPD activities and monitoring compliance with these activities. They devise clinical guidelines for the profession, which are designed to ensure consistent standards of care for clients with communication and swallowing disorders. Professional bodies can influence national health policy, play a role in workforce planning and advocate for improved clinical services for clients and their families. They have an important role to play in raising public and professional awareness of communication disorders and in changing public perceptions of people with these disorders. They facilitate research through the publication of journals, and discuss professional issues with their members at conferences and in magazines. Each of these functions of professional bodies will be addressed further in this section.

Accreditation One of the key functions of professional associations in SLT is to accredit the undergraduate and postgraduate university courses that lead to the award of an SLT degree. This task is a sizeable one that continues to grow as new courses are developed. ASHA first accredited graduate education programmes in audiology and speech-language pathology in 1965. Today, it manages the **accreditation** of 266 master's programmes in speech-language pathology throughout the USA. In the UK, the RCSLT oversees the accreditation of 15 undergraduate SLT courses and 9 postgraduate courses. Accreditation is a rigorous process and necessarily so. It is designed to ensure that SLTs are trained to the highest possible standards and that clinical education is consistent across different institutions. The Council on Academic Accreditation in Audiology and Speech-Language Pathology is a semi-autonomous body within ASHA. The 18-member strong council consists of academics, a number of which must be research-qualified (PhD or EdD), clinical practitioners who are employed full-time in non-academic settings and a public member who is not involved with the professions of audiology and/or speech-language pathology. Members serve for a term of 4 years and undertake an average of 4–6 hours of work per week during certain periods of the year. As well as establishing accreditation standards, council members conduct evaluations of accreditation and reaccreditation applications to determine compliance with established standards, accredit qualified graduate programmes and monitor compliance over the period of accreditation through review of annual reports.

Continuing Professional Development (CPD) After qualification, SLTs must ensure that they continually update their clinical knowledge and skills in order to maintain membership of a professional association. CPD is the process by means of which this is achieved. CPD requirements vary across different professional bodies. To maintain the Certificate of Clinical Competence (CCC) with ASHA, individuals must accumulate 30 certification maintenance hours during each 3-year interval. For dual certificate holders, these hours are earned in either audiology or speech-language pathology. Members of the RCSLT must complete a minimum of 30 hours of CPD per year, while therapists with membership of Speech Pathology Australia must accrue 60 CPD points over 3 years (no less than 20 hours per year). As well as requiring a certain amount of continuing professional development, professional bodies also specify the types of activities which qualify as CPD. Activities accepted by ASHA for certification maintenance hours include formal training sessions sponsored by manufacturers on equipment used in the evaluation and treatment of clients; college or university coursework; and attendance at state association workshops, university scientific symposia and seminars offered through other professional associations. CPD activities are assigned different credits. For example, to maintain certification of Speech-Language & Audiology Canada, members must accumulate a minimum of 45 continuing education equivalents (CEEs) every 3 years. Each hour of attendance at a workshop is worth 1 CEE, while a conference presentation earns 4 CEEs.

Clinical Guidelines Another important role of professional bodies is to establish guidelines for the clinical management of clients with communication and swallowing disorders. These guidelines are intended to ensure that all clients in SLT receive a consistent standard of care, which is based on the best available clinical evidence. The second edition of the RCSLT's *Clinical Guidelines* was published in 2005. It contains 12 clinical guidelines, which are underpinned by a core guideline. The 12 guidelines are a combination of population-based and disorder-based guidelines:

Children

- Preschool children with communication, language and speech needs
- School-aged children with speech, language and communication difficulties

Children and adults

- Autistic spectrum disorders
- Cleft palate and velopharyngeal abnormalities
- Clinical voice disorders
- Deafness/hearing loss
- Disorders of fluency
- Disorders of feeding, eating, drinking and swallowing (dysphagia)
- Disorders of mental health and dementia
- Dysarthria

Adults

- Aphasia
- Head and neck cancer

In the management of any individual client, SLTs may need to consult more than one of these guidelines. For example, management of children with cerebral palsy may require SLTs to consult each of the following guidelines: preschool or

Table 7.4 *Clinical guidelines of Speech Pathology Australia*

CLINICAL GUIDELINES
Augmentative and alternative communication
Autism spectrum disorders
Dysphagia: General
Evidence-based practice for the management of stuttering
Evidence-based speech pathology practice for individuals with autism spectrum disorder
Fibreoptic endoscopic evaluation of swallowing (FEES): An advanced practice for speech pathologists
Laryngectomy
Speech pathology in mental health services
Speech pathology services in schools
Tracheostomy management
Videofluoroscopic swallow study (VFSS)
Working in a culturally and linguistically diverse society

school-aged children with speech, language and communication difficulties; clinical voice disorders; deafness/hearing loss; dysphagia; and dysarthria. As well as the 12 guidelines shown above, the RCSLT has published separate guidelines for adults with **learning disability**.

Speech Pathology Australia has also produced clinical guidelines for its members. Currently, there are 12 guidelines with a further two guidelines on **laryngology** and literacy in development. As can be seen in Table 7.4, some guidelines are based on disorders such as dysphagia and autism spectrum disorder, while others relate to investigative techniques like videofluoroscopy and fibreoptic endoscopic evaluation of swallowing. Still other guidelines address the contexts in which SLT is practised (e.g. schools and mental health services), or issues which affect the work of SLTs such as cultural and linguistic diversity. Speech Pathology Australia recommends that each of these guidelines is read in conjunction with its other core documents, including its code of ethics, scope of practice and parameters of practice.

Advocacy Professional associations also have an important role to play in influencing policy at all levels of government with a view to improving the lives of people with communication and swallowing disorders. The advocacy efforts of ASHA and its members are set out in its 'Blueprint for Action' document (ASHA, 2016d). This document is produced annually and includes the most pressing policy issues that face ASHA members at the federal and state levels. In the 2016 'Blueprint for Action', SLTs ranked funding and practice issues for school-based and early intervention services, Medicaid reimbursement, scope of practice, demonstrating value and quality services, and federal education as the most important advocacy efforts for the profession. The RCSLT has a Policy and

Public Affairs Team which influences policy and legislation in the interests of people with communication and swallowing disorders across the UK. In 2015, to support the communication skills of children in socially disadvantaged areas, the RCSLT influenced the draft statutory guidance to the Children and Young People (Scotland) Act. In the same year, the RCSLT also influenced the guidance accompanying the Health and Social Care (Safety & Quality) Act to ensure that health and adult social care bodies share information about an individual's speech, language and communication needs where this might facilitate the provision of care. Speech-Language & Audiology Canada (SAC) publishes a quarterly newsletter – *SAC in Action* – which updates members on its advocacy activities. Among the issues addressed in the summer 2016 issue were two new SAC position statements, which are designed to influence decision-makers and become advocacy tools for SAC members and associates, and lobbying by SAC for communication health services to be included in federal investments in health care.

Education and Awareness Like many individuals with disabilities, children and adults with communication and swallowing disorders can face bullying and discrimination at school, in the workplace and in their local communities. A significant function of professional bodies is to challenge these behaviours and negative perceptions of individuals with communication disorders through public education activities. These activities take many different forms. Professional bodies can make fact sheets and other literature on communication disorders available to the public through their websites. For example, ASHA has an extensive set of information resources on speech, language, hearing and swallowing disorders that can be accessed online by the public. Many of these resources are available in both English and Spanish. Professional bodies may use education campaigns to increase public understanding of communication disorders and to raise awareness of the services that SLT is able to offer individuals with these disorders. In 2010, the RCSLT launched its Giving Voice campaign, which aims to 'give voice' to people with speech, language and communication needs and ensure that their needs and those of their families and carers are met. Through locally organized 'Giving Voice' activities, members of RCSLT have succeeded in raising awareness of communication disorders and the SLT profession among the general public. Professional bodies also play an important role in the education of other professionals about the work that is performed by SLTs. For example, Speech Pathology Australia has developed a GP Education Kit to help promote SLT with **general practitioners** and other professionals.

Research SLTs do not merely assess and treat clients with communication and swallowing disorders. It is part of their professional remit to contribute to the knowledge base of their discipline by conducting research. Professional bodies support the research activities of their members in several ways. One form of support is the publication of scholarly journals in the field. ASHA, for example, publishes four international journals in speech-language pathology and audiology: *American Journal of Audiology*; *American Journal of Speech-Language*

Pathology; *Journal of Speech, Language, and Hearing Research*; and *Language, Speech, and Hearing Services in Schools*. The RCSLT publishes the *International Journal of Language & Communication Disorders*. All these journals are available to members of professional bodies as part of their annual subscription. Aside from scholarly journals, professional bodies also support the research of their members through the provision of research grants. Speech Pathology Australia offers clinician and student research grants of up to $5,000 and $10,000. Since 2007, Speech-Language & Audiology Canada has offered its members clinical research grants worth $2,500 with the aim of increasing the clinical evidence base in the fields of speech-language pathology and audiology in Canada. Other ways in which professional bodies give prominence to research is through their magazines. For example, in its professional magazine *Bulletin*, the RCSLT addresses a wide range of research issues in its Research and Development Forum. Special interest groups are another important vehicle for the promotion of research by professional bodies. ASHA has 19 such groups in areas ranging from craniofacial and velopharyngeal disorders to augmentative and alternative communication.

KEY POINTS: Professional Bodies and Associations

- SLTs around the world are represented by professional associations. These associations perform a number of important functions beyond being the professional voice of their members. These functions include the following: accreditation; continuing professional development; clinical guidelines; advocacy; education and awareness; and research.
- Accreditation of undergraduate and postgraduate courses in SLT is necessary to ensure that students receive the skills and clinical knowledge that are needed to practise competently. Upon graduation, SLTs must also continually update their knowledge and skills in order to keep pace with developments in the field. Professional associations oversee accreditation and continuing professional development.
- To avoid inconsistencies in clinical care across regions and centres and ensure that clients receive a high standard of care, professional associations also devise clinical guidelines for the management of clients with communication and swallowing disorders. These guidelines base recommendations for treatment on the best available clinical evidence.
- Like other individuals with disabilities, children and adults with communication and swallowing disorders need other people and organizations to represent their views, and to influence health and social policy that has an impact on their lives. This key advocacy role is also performed by professional associations.
- People with communication disorders can experience bullying, discrimination and harassment. These intimidating behaviours often have their roots in a lack of understanding of communication disorders among

- the general public. Professional associations attempt to counter misconceptions and ignorance about people with communication disorders through educational activities and awareness-raising campaigns.
- SLTs also contribute to the knowledge base of their discipline by conducting research. Professional bodies support the research activities of their members by publishing scholarly journals, sponsoring academic conferences, providing research grants to members, and discussing research issues in their professional magazines.

7.5 SLT and Charitable Organizations

People with communication and swallowing disorders are able to seek advice and support from a growing number of charitable organizations. Many of these organizations have arisen to meet the needs of clients when these needs are not adequately addressed by pre-existing health and social services. Often, it is clients themselves or their family members who provide the impetus for the development of these organizations. Some charitable organizations are sponsored by individuals who have experienced communication disorders, either personally or in their immediate family. SLTs who work with clients who have speech, language and communication needs are often most acutely aware when established services are unable to offer clients the support they need. Several charitable organizations are the result of efforts by SLTs to improve the lives of children and adults with communication disorders. Aside from their origins, charitable organizations also have several roles or functions in supporting people with communication disorders. Considerable anxiety can attend the diagnosis of a communication or swallowing disorder. A key function of charitable organizations is to alleviate this anxiety by providing easily understood information about communication and swallowing disorders to clients and their families. Charitable organizations also provide information for professionals like teachers, health visitors and general practitioners. They act as advocates for clients with communication disorders, fund research into these disorders and raise public awareness of communication disorders. Each of these aspects of the work of charitable organizations will be examined further in this section.

Several charitable organizations that provide support for people with communication and swallowing disorders are displayed in Table 7.5. These organizations can be broadly classified into two types. There are charities that have a specific communication disorder as their focus. These organizations often carry the name of the communication disorder in question. The Tavistock Trust for Aphasia and the Childhood Apraxia of Speech Association of North America represent people with aphasia and children with apraxia of speech, respectively.

Table 7.5 *Charities that support people with communication and swallowing disorders*

Charitable organization	Description
Action for Stammering Children	The charity behind the Michael Palin Centre for Stammering Children in London. ASC commissions the delivery of specialist services from this centre for children and young people who stammer.
Afasic	A parent-led organization founded in 1968 to help children and young people with speech and language impairments and their families. There are local groups throughout the UK. Afasic is a founding member of The Communication Trust, a coalition of 50 not-for-profit organizations.
British Voice Association	An association of multidisciplinary professionals who work to promote voice in the broadest sense. Assists people with voice problems, ranging from severe pathology and cancer to subtle difficulties of artistic performance.
Cancer Laryngectomee Trust	Established in 1985 by Sydney Norgate, a laryngectomee, this charity aims to provide support and understanding for all people in the UK who are about to have, or have had, a laryngectomy.
Childhood Apraxia of Speech Association of North America (CASANA)	Founded in 2000, CASANA's mission is to strengthen the support systems in the lives of children with apraxia so that each child is afforded their best opportunity to develop speech and communication.
Cleft Lip and Palate Association (CLAPA)	Established in 1979 as a partnership between parents and health professionals, CLAPA supports people and families affected by cleft lip and/or palate in the UK. The charity provides non-medical services to complement the medical care provided by specialist cleft teams.
Headway	Established in 1979, Headway provides support services and information to brain injury survivors, their families and carers, as well as to professionals in the

Table 7.5 (*cont.*)

Charitable organization	Description
	health and legal fields. Headway has more than 125 groups and branches across the UK.
I CAN	A children's communication charity that supports children with severe and complex speech, language and communication difficulties in the UK. The core of I CAN's work is delivered through two specialist schools, Dawn House and Meath Schools.
Mencap	Founded in 1946 by Judy Fryd, the mother of a child with learning disability. The charity changed its name to Mencap in 1969. Today, Mencap champions the needs of people with learning disability through its network of over 400 local groups across the UK.
Multiple Sclerosis Trust	Established in 1993 by Jill Holt and Chris Jones, both of whom have personal experience of MS, the Multiple Sclerosis Trust provides information and support to people with MS and supports professionals who work with clients and their families.
National Autistic Society (NAS)	The UK's leading charity for people with autism and their families. For over 50 years, NAS has provided information and advice to people affected by autism, and supported professionals, politicians and the public to understand autism better.
Parkinson's UK	Founded in 1969 under the name the Parkinson's Disease Society by Mali Jenkins, the sister of a PD sufferer. Parkinson's UK provides expert information on Parkinson's disease and funds research to ensure new and better treatments are delivered.
Scope	Established in 1952 under the name The Spastics Society by three parents of children with cerebral palsy. Changed its name to Scope in 1994. Today, the charity provides support, information and advice to more than a quarter of a

Table 7.5 (*cont.*)

Charitable organization	Description
	million disabled people and their families every year.
Smile Train	Smile Train is an international children's charity. It provides training, funding and resources so that local doctors in 85+ developing countries can provide free cleft repair surgery and comprehensive cleft care to children in their own communities.
Stroke Association	The leading charity for the 152,000 people who have a stroke each year in the UK. The Stroke Association funds research, provides support services and conducts campaigns to help these people and their families. In April 2015, Speakability – a national charity that supports people with aphasia and their carers – merged with the Stroke Association.
Tavistock Trust for Aphasia	A charity founded in 1992 by Robin Tavistock, the late 14th Duke of Bedford, who developed aphasia following a brain haemorrhage in 1988. The trust aims to improve the quality of life of people with aphasia by funding research and raising awareness of aphasia.

Many more charitable organizations represent a medical condition or disorder in which communication and swallowing are often compromised. Smile Train and Headway represent people with cleft lip and palate and traumatic brain injury, respectively. These latter organizations often have well-developed resources relating to communication and swallowing disorders, even though these disorders are not their primary focus. For example, the Multiple Sclerosis Trust is a charitable organization that represents people with multiple sclerosis. This organization has extensive online resources relating to dysphagia, dysarthria and language and cognitive problems in multiple sclerosis. Also among the organizations in Table 7.5 are charities that serve the needs of a large range of clients, and others that address a specific client group. For example, I CAN and Afasic represent all children with speech, language and communication needs. Meanwhile, Action for Stammering Children only works with children and young people who stammer. Finally, some charities in Table 7.5 are national organizations (e.g. British Voice Association), while others have international reach (e.g. Smile Train).

The charities in Table 7.5 fulfil several functions in their work with clients and their families. One of their most important functions is to provide free, accessible information about communication and swallowing disorders to people from different backgrounds. Some individuals may access this information because they have been recently diagnosed with a communication disorder or know someone with a communication disorder. For the most part, these readers lack knowledge of conditions such as aphasia, dysarthria and dysphagia and the medical problems (e.g. stroke) that can cause these conditions. Terminology like *anomia, aspiration* and *cerebrovascular accident* has to be clearly explained or, for certain readers, avoided altogether. For example, the Stroke Association in the UK provides information leaflets that have been written for children aged 9 years and older who may have a parent or a grandparent with aphasia. Clear, accessible information is even more important if people with language disorders such as aphasia are to read and understand it. In the UK, the charity Connect produces information booklets that have been written specifically for people with aphasia. Of course, it cannot be assumed that it is only clients and their families who need information about communication and swallowing disorders. Knowledge of these disorders is often limited among medical, health and educational professionals. Charities have also responded to the need for information among professionals, with many providing online resources for these readers. For example, the brain injury charity Headway provides resources for general practitioners, while the National Autistic Society has online information for teachers, health workers and social care workers.

Advocacy is a vital function of all charitable organizations. However, it is an even more important function of those charities that represent people with communication disability who may not be able to express their own views and articulate their particular needs. Through lobbying politicians and policy-makers, charitable organizations are able to influence legislation and policy that affects the health and social services that clients and their families receive. Charities often undertake this important role alongside professional bodies (see section 7.4). In 2008, the children's communication charity I CAN, along with the Royal College of Speech and Language Therapists, conducted an independent review of *The Bercow Report*.[4] This review led to a detailed report that made recommendations for future action so that children and young people with speech, language and communication needs would remain a high priority for government. Often, the advocacy role of charities is stated in their mission and goals. For example, one of the goals of the Childhood Apraxia of Speech Association of North America is 'to facilitate better public policy and services for children affected by apraxia of speech'. One of the key strategic aims of the Cleft Lip and Palate Association is to be 'represented at the right places to influence decision making about cleft care in the UK'. Charities have had notable successes in advocacy. In 2017, a proposal to overturn the five mandated universal health visitor reviews for children aged 0–5 years in the UK was rejected. In an open letter in August 2016 to Viv Bennett (Chief Nurse at Public Health England), Bob Reitemeier (I CAN Chief Executive) emphasized the vital role that health visitor reviews play in detecting children with communication disability and the likely adverse consequences of any reduction of these reviews.

As public funding of research in many countries continues to decline, charitable organizations are playing an increasingly important role in funding research into communication and swallowing disorders. In the UK, charity funding of stroke research doubled from £6 million in 2007/8 to £13 million in 2011/12 (Stroke Association, 2014a). Today, the Stroke Association funds 11% of the total UK spend on stroke research (Stroke Association, 2014b). At least some of this research funding is directed towards studies that benefit people with communication and swallowing disorders (see Table 7.6).

Table 7.6 *Titles of research studies funded by the Stroke Association in the UK*

TITLE OF RESEARCH STUDY
Jargon busting: The cognitive and neurobiological mechanisms underpinning jargon aphasia and perseveration
Adapting a psychosocial intervention for people with post-stroke aphasia: A feasibility study
Predicting language outcome and recovery after stroke
Evaluating the implementation fidelity of self-managed computer therapy for aphasia post-stroke and exploring the factors associated with adherence
Evaluating the impact of therapeutic alliance between the rehabilitation clinician and stroke survivor: Focus on the speech and language therapist and the person with aphasia
Using transcranial direct current stimulation to alleviate anomia in chronic stroke aphasia
Direct current stimulation and remediation of comprehension deficits on stroke aphasia
Factors that influence the effectiveness of conversation training for people with aphasia: Who benefits most and which tasks really help people to learn new strategies?
Profiling chronic and recovered language comprehension networks post-stroke: Psychoacoustic, neuropsychological and fMRI investigations
IDEA Project – Inclusion in the Digital Economy for People with Aphasia
Evaluating the effects of a virtual communication environment for people with aphasia
Reading comprehension in aphasia: The development of a novel assessment of reading comprehension
Semantic assessment in aphasia
Improving the conversations of speakers with non-fluent aphasia

Aside from the direct funding of research studies, charities support research in other ways. For example, they can sponsor research symposia and conferences. The Childhood Apraxia of Speech Association of North America supports a Research Registry. This is a list of as many individuals with childhood apraxia of speech as possible. It contains information about each child's health and developmental history. The Registry is still in development. Once data is collected and enough children are registered, the list will enable authorized researchers to find suitable subjects for research projects and will offer families an opportunity to participate in research. Of course, each of these forms of research funding is possible only because of the financial support that charities receive from members of the public. In fact, the support of research funding is one of the main reasons why members of the public make donations to charities and engage in fundraising activities. In the case of large charities, combined donations can be very substantial indeed. For example, in the fiscal year 2015, the Smile Train raised more than $91 million in fundraising contributions (Smile Train, 2015).

Finally, charitable organizations also play a key role in raising public awareness of communication and swallowing disorders. Ignorance of these disorders is responsible for the victimization and discrimination that many people with communication disorders encounter in their daily lives. For example, there is widespread misunderstanding that adults with aphasia have reduced intellectual functioning. This might lead an employer not to recruit or promote these individuals. By raising public understanding of communication disorders, charities can challenge the many misconceptions that exist among the general public about people with communication disorders. The awareness-raising campaigns of charities take many different forms. Often, a particular day forms the backdrop to these campaigns. For example, on 14 May 2016, the Childhood Apraxia of Speech Association of North America (CASANA) held its fourth Apraxia Awareness Day. On this day, CASANA invited communities around the world to become aware of and educated about the needs, challenges and abilities of children affected by apraxia of speech. To help mark the day and raise the profile of apraxia of speech, CASANA urged individuals to engage in community and social media activities. Charities have also harnessed the publicity that surrounds commercially successful movies to increase public awareness of communication disorders. The *Hello* 2011 campaign by The Communication Trust to raise awareness of speech, language and communication needs in children drew on the heightened public interest in the topic that had been generated by the movie *The King's Speech*. Anita Kerwin-Nye, the Director of The Communication Trust, remarked in a press release on 7 January 2011: 'The *Hello* campaign will raise the profile of speech, language and communication development to unprecedented heights. We could not ask for a better way to capture the public's interest in this subject than with the release of the King's Speech.'

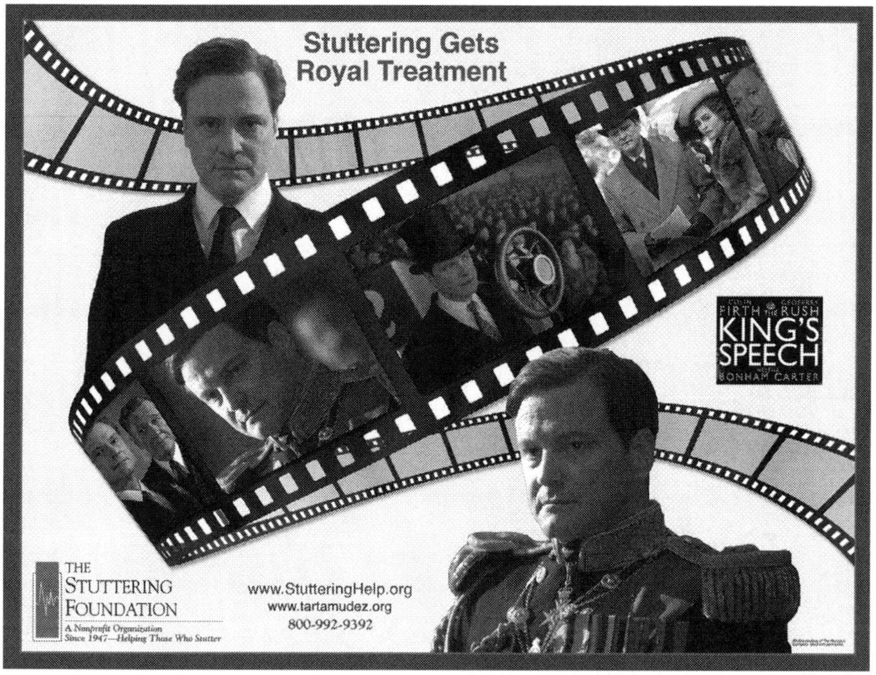

Figure 7.1 The King's Speech *has been used in awareness-raising campaigns by a range of charitable and non-profit organizations. (Reproduced with permission of The Stuttering Foundation of America)*

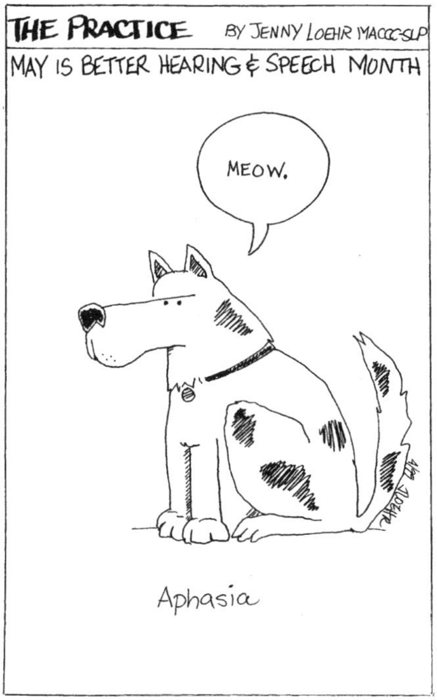

GROUP EXERCISE: Aphasia Awareness

A key function of charitable organizations and non-profit organizations with an SLT focus is to raise public awareness of communication disorders. In the extract below, Karen Tucker, executive director of the Adler Aphasia Center, is describing some of the ways in which supporters of the center can become involved in aphasia awareness month. Her comments appeared in 2011 in *Aphasia Advocate*, the newsletter of the center. Imagine that you and the other members of your group have been put in charge of an aphasia awareness-raising campaign. Use these comments as a starting point in a discussion of how you might proceed to organize such a campaign:

> June is Aphasia Awareness Month. I have an idea – grassroots. Let's start an aphasia chain – let's create a 'buzz' about aphasia. If each of you educate three people about aphasia, and those three tell someone, and so on and so forth, put it on your facebook pages, tweet it, who knows ... maybe it will show up on YouTube as a group line dance – you just never know today. But seriously, please help us to get the word out using your modes of communication. It can really make a difference in the lives of the 1,000,000 plus Americans of all ages that live with this condition.

KEY POINTS: SLT and Charitable Organizations

- There are many charities that support the needs of clients with communication and swallowing disorders and their families. Often, these charities exist to address needs that are not met by pre-existing health and social services.
- There are two main types of charities that support people with communication disorders. There are organizations that address a particular communication disorder such as stammering or aphasia. There are other organizations that address medical conditions such as stroke in which communication and swallowing may be compromised.
- Charities have four main purposes or functions, which are often stated in their mission or goals. These are to provide free, accessible information about communication and swallowing disorders, to act as advocates for clients and their families, to fund research into communication and swallowing disorders, and to raise public awareness of these disorders.
- The diagnosis of a communication or swallowing disorder is often accompanied by a demand on the part of clients and their families for information. Professionals such as health visitors and general practitioners also need access to information. Charities provide excellent online information fact sheets and booklets that are written for different types of reader.
- Advocacy is an important aspect of the work of charities. Clients with communication disorders are often unable to express their views and represent their interests to others. Charities can be a powerful voice for

> these individuals. They can influence policy and secure improved services for clients and their families.
> - Charities are playing an increasingly important role in the funding of research into communication and swallowing disorders. They award grants to academic and clinical researchers, sponsor research symposia and conferences, and develop research tools such as registries of subjects that can facilitate future research.
> - Charities also engage in awareness-raising campaigns with the general public. These campaigns are undertaken to overturn misconceptions about people with communication disorders that can lead to victimization and discrimination.

WEBSITE: The Profession of Speech and Language Therapy

After reading the chapter, visit the website and test your knowledge of the profession of speech and language therapy by answering the short-answer questions for this topic.

Suggestions for Further Reading

Kersner, M. and Wright, J. A. (eds.) 2012. *Speech and language therapy: the decision-making process when working with children*, Abingdon and New York: Routledge.

Two chapters in this edited volume address issues about SLTs working in multidisciplinary teams and across different contexts. Chapter 5 addresses the roles of SLTs working in community clinics, child development centres and hospitals. Chapter 9 discusses SLTs working with other practitioners.

Portland State University 2016. *Speech-language pathology in other countries*. Available online: www.pdx.edu/multicultural-topics-communication-sciences-disorders/speech-language-pathology-in-other-countries. Accessed 22 August 2016.

This website from Portland State University provides comprehensive information on the practice of SLT around the world. It describes the word for SLT, the required training and the scope of practice of SLT in 36 countries worldwide. Therapists in each of these countries are compared with speech-language pathologists in the USA. There is also information on how speech-language pathologists in the USA may be perceived by people from these countries.

Joffe, V. 2015. 'An international perspective: Supporting adolescents with speech, language, and communication needs in the United Kingdom', *Seminars in Speech and Language* **36**:1, 74–85.

This article examines the provision of SLT services to older children and young people with speech, language and communication needs in secondary schools in the UK. It develops the points raised in section 7.3 that SLT services are largely concentrated in the early years and that the provision of services to this age group of children does not reflect the extent of clinical need among this group.

QUESTIONS: The Profession of Speech and Language Therapy

(1) Use the information provided in the case study entitled 'Head Trauma Rehabilitation Team' to answer the following questions:
    (a) Name ten members of the multidisciplinary team that is providing care to M.G.
    (b) Which five members of the team that you identified in your response to (a) are involved in the management of M.G.'s dysphagia? Describe the specific role of each of these members.
    (c) The neurologist and radiologist each have at least two roles to play in the provision of M.G.'s care. For each of these medical specialists, state what these roles are.
    (d) Which of the team members that you identified in your response to (a) will assist M.G. in achieving independence in basic hygiene and grooming skills?
    (e) (i) Which of the team members that you identified in your response to (a) assesses M.G.'s cognitive skills?
        (ii) Are M.G.'s executive function skills impaired? Provide evidence for your answer.
        (iii) Which of M.G.'s cognitive deficits are related to parietal lobe damage?
        (iv) Which aspect of M.G.'s language is most likely to be affected by his concrete thinking?
        (v) Which aspect of M.G.'s cognitive performance is most likely to compromise self-monitoring?

(2) Examine the experiences of the SLTs who worked as volunteers for Yellow House Children's Services in Kenya (case study in section 7.3). Then answer the following questions:
    (a) All three SLTs are describing challenges of working with children with communication disorders in Kenya. Identify each of these challenges.
    (b) Which of the challenges identified in your response to (a) is most related to economic factors?
    (c) Which of the challenges identified in your response to (a) is most related to cultural factors?
    (d) Sally is describing some of the difficulties and tensions that can arise when knowledge and ideas are exchanged between professionals who work in different countries. What interpersonal factor was particularly important in Sally being able to encourage the Kenyan special education teachers to consider new approaches to classroom instruction?
    (e) The experiences reported by these SLTs show that they played key roles in the education of professionals and the public in Kenya. Describe what these roles were.

(3) Each of the following statements describes a function of a professional association in SLT. Which of the functions in italics applies to each statement? You should note that there may be more than one function in your response: *accreditation*; *advocacy*; *clinical guidelines*; *continuing professional development*; *education and awareness*; *research*
   (a) An SLT delivers a paper on motor speech disorders in adults at an international conference.
   (b) Paediatric SLTs attend a meeting with a health minister to lobby for improved early years SLT services for children at risk of language disorders.
   (c) An SLT is part of a working group that is reviewing clinical evidence with a view to updating standards of care for clients with dysphagia.
   (d) SLT students spend a day in a town centre handing out leaflets and talking to members of the public about people with communication disorders.
   (e) The SLT department in a university meets to discuss its preparedness for the upcoming validation of a new master's degree programme.
   (f) The SLT department in a local hospital receives a grant from the RCSLT to investigate the effect of the use of early videofluoroscopy on rates of aspiration pneumonia in clients with dysphagia.
   (g) During an interview on local radio, an SLT describes the varied caseload of therapists and what a career in speech and language therapy involves.
   (h) To update clinical knowledge, an SLT attends a workshop on augmentative and alternative communication (AAC) and reads a journal article on the topic.
   (i) An SLT conducts interviews with partners of people with aphasia as part of a study that examines the long-term social impact of aphasia.
   (j) SLTs sign a petition that calls for enhanced AAC provision for adults in long-term care facilities.
(4) Adults with Parkinson's disease can experience communication and swallowing disorders such as dysarthria and dysphagia. Parkinson's UK is the largest charity in the UK to provide support to people with Parkinson's disease and their families. Parkinson's UK expresses its mission in 'Our Vision and Values'. The following statements are taken from its mission. Relate each of these statements to one or more of the following functions of charities: *information*; *raising awareness*; *research*; *advocacy*.
   (a) We meet with Ministers, politicians and civil servants to raise key issues and influence policy appropriately.
   (b) We improve understanding of Parkinson's by changing attitudes and challenging myths.
   (c) We provide expert information on every aspect of Parkinson's so that people affected by the condition can stay in control of their lives.
   (d) We lead, influence and fund research to ensure new and better treatments in years rather than decades.
   (e) We organize events in the UK Parliaments and Assemblies and during the party conference season to raise awareness and build support.

Notes

Chapter 1

1 Crystal and Varley (1998) define elocution as 'the art of clear speaking in public, as judged by the cultural standards of the time; it aims to develop the speaking voice to its aesthetic and rhetorical peak, well beyond that which is necessary for the continuance of everyday communication' (13).
2 GCSE stands for General Certificate of Secondary Education. This is the school qualification that is taken by 16-year-olds in the UK.

Chapter 3

1 This increased prominence has occurred as a result of the inclusion of a growing number of communication disorders in DSM. For example, social (pragmatic) communication disorder was included for the first time in the fifth edition, DSM-5.

Chapter 5

1 An otolaryngologist is the only professional who is qualified and licensed to perform a laryngoscopy or strobovideolaryngoscopy for medical diagnostic purposes. This procedure can be undertaken by an SLT when the purpose is to assess vocal production and vocal function (ASHA, 1998).

Chapter 6

1 ASHA's 2013 *SLP Health Care Survey* confirms that individual intervention accounts for the larger part of the SLT workload. When respondents were asked what percentage of time they spent in individual treatment and group treatment, mean percentages of 72.0% and 1.4% were obtained, respectively.

Chapter 7

1 As an example, a survey of SLT provision conducted by the Scottish Parliament Health Committee in 2013 showed that although referrals to children's SLT services had grown, there had been an overall 8.8% decrease in funding for SLT in Scotland since 2011, with cuts coming from both health boards (up to 21.1%) and local authorities (up to 20.6%).
2 In the USA, speech-language pathology services in a skilled nursing facility are covered by Medicare Part A (Hospital Insurance) when they are needed to meet the client's health goal.
3 The Special Eurobarometer in 2012 showed that the majority of Europeans (54%) are able to conduct a conversation in at least one additional language. Furthermore, almost

all respondents in Luxembourg (98%), Latvia (95%), the Netherlands (94%), Malta (93%), Slovenia and Lithuania (92% each) and Sweden (91%) are able to speak at least one language in addition to their mother tongue. Outside Europe, it is estimated that close to 20% of the population in the USA is bilingual, a figure that has increased from 11% in 1980 and 14% in 1990. English-Spanish bilinguals represent about half of all bilinguals in the USA (Grosjean, 2012).

4 *The Bercow Report* (2008) involved 10 months of extensive evidence gathering and analysis, as well as consultation with a wide range of stakeholders. The report made recommendations to Government about the steps that it should take to transform provision for, and the experiences of, children and young people with speech, language, and communication needs and their families.

Answers

Chapter 1

Case study

(1) Michael's wife was able to describe his pre-morbid communication skills for the SLT. She was also able to describe how Michael was communicating at home following his accident.

(2) Following his accident, Michael does not appear to be motivated to communicate with members of his family. This suggests the presence of depression. Also, his wife reports that he has experienced growing social isolation as a result of his communication difficulties. Michael has evidently displayed poor psychosocial adjustment to his communication disorder. This is an area that family members can positively influence by providing him with support.

(3) An intervention of this type is adopted in Michael's case when the SLT decides to institute conversational partner training.

(4) Michael's family members have an important role to play in ensuring his successful use of an alternative communication system when he was mute and severely dysarthric.

(5) Michael's wife can be encouraged to make greater use of back-channel behaviour (e.g. 'hm', 'yes') as a means of explicitly signalling to Michael that she is listening to, and understanding, what he is saying. This will help reduce Michael's tendency to use repetition in conversation as a means of ensuring his message is communicated.

End-of-chapter questions

(1) (a) research;
 (b) education;
 (c) assessment;
 (d) mentoring;
 (e) diagnosis;
 (f) treatment;
 (g) advocacy
(2) (a) social impact;
 (b) psychological impact;

(c) occupational or vocational impact;
(d) academic impact;
(e) behavioural impact;
(f) forensic impact
(3) (a) semantics;
(b) otorhinolaryngology;
(c) developmental psychology;
(d) phonetics;
(e) neurology;
(f) psychiatry;
(g) pragmatics;
(h) educational psychology;
(i) physiology;
(j) epidemiology
(4) Part (A):
(a) developmental speech disorder;
(b) developmental language disorder;
(c) acquired language disorder;
(d) acquired speech disorder;
(e) developmental language disorder
Part (B):
(a) receptive-primary language disorder;
(b) expressive-secondary language disorder;
(c) receptive-secondary language disorder;
(d) expressive-primary language disorder;
(e) expressive-secondary language disorder
(5) (a) implement intervention;
(b) focus of intervention;
(c) provide support;
(d) provide information;
(e) receive training
(6) Three aspects of *Stoke Speaks Out* which qualify it as a speech and language intervention which fulfils a public health role:
(a) The intervention targets a population, namely, all 7-year-old children and their families in Stoke-on-Trent, rather than individuals.
(b) The intervention has a prevention element at its heart as it aims to avert the social disadvantage and other harmful consequences (e.g. poor mental health) of communication disorders.
(c) The intervention embodies health promotion in that it encourages people to be proactive and undertake positive behaviour change in relation to communication development and disorders.

Chapter 2

Case study

(1) poor turn-taking and poor topic maintenance
(2) 'Put the cup beside the spoon'; 'Put the pencil on top of the box'
(3) noun morphology – mouses; verb morphology – eated
(4) 'man car' (man's car)
(5) eated – over-regularization error

End-of-chapter questions

(1) Part (A):
   (a) alveolar plosive [d] → glottal plosive [ʔ]; alveolar nasal [n] → uvular nasal [ɴ]
   (b) consonant cluster reduction [st] → [s]
   (c) velar plosive [k] → velar fricative [x]
   (d) voicing [p] → [b]
   (e) devoicing [v] → [f]

   Part (B):
   (a) Child with Down syndrome
   (b) Girl with a repaired central cleft of hard and soft palates
   (c) Boy with developmental dysarthria
   (d) Adult with apraxia of speech and child with Down syndrome
   (e) Girl with a repaired central cleft of hard and soft palates

(2) (a) velar assimilation
   (b) velar fronting
   (c) stopping
   (d) velar fronting; prevocalic voicing
   (e) gliding of liquid
   (f) prevocalic voicing; devoicing
   (g) consonant cluster reduction; voicing; labial assimilation
   (h) consonant cluster reduction
   (i) final consonant deletion
   (j) consonant cluster reduction; nasal assimilation
   (k) labial assimilation
   (l) consonant cluster reduction; velar assimilation
   (m) palatal fronting
   (n) weak syllable deletion
   (o) cluster simplification
   (p) deaffrication
   (q) affrication
   (r) backing
   (s) initial consonant deletion
   (t) gliding of fricative; consonant cluster reduction

Answers   307

(3) (a) The child has incorrectly applied the inflectional suffix -s for plural nouns to the non-count noun *furniture*.
   (b) The child has incorrectly applied the inflectional suffix -ed for past tense to the infinitive form of the verb when *eat* has an irregular past tense form (*ate*).
   (c) The child has used the inflectional suffix for the superlative form of an adjective (-est) when the suffix for the comparative form (-er) is required.
   (d) The child has incorrectly applied the inflectional suffix -ed for past tense to the infinitive form of the verb when 'drink' has an irregular past tense form (*drank*).
   (e) The child has applied the inflectional suffix for the comparative form of regular adjectives (-er) to an adjective which has an irregular comparative form (*worse*).

(4) (a) locative preposition;
   (b) relative clause in subject;
   (c) reversible passive;
   (d) postmodified subject;
   (e) comparative

(5) (a) *sweeps*: two-argument verb (Joey$_{AGENT}$ sweeps the floor$_{PATIENT}$)
   (b) *swims*: one-argument verb (A boy$_{AGENT}$ swims in the pool$_{LOCATION}$)
   (c) *gives*: three-argument verb (Mary$_{AGENT}$ gives a cookie$_{THEME}$ to her friend$_{GOAL}$)
   (d) *jumps*: one-argument verb (A girl$_{AGENT}$ jumps from the diving board$_{SOURCE}$)
   (e) *runs*: one-argument verb (A boy$_{AGENT}$ runs in the grass$_{LOCATION}$)

(6) (a) presupposition;
   (b) presupposition;
   (c) implicature;
   (d) presupposition;
   (e) implicature;
   (f) implicature;
   (g) presupposition;
   (h) implicature;
   (i) presupposition;
   (j) implicature

(7) The boy studied by McTear (1985) fails to use ellipsis. In exchange 1, the part of the boy's response in brackets should have been omitted: 'they are [friends of mine]'. Even the interjection of the adult on the boy's turn in exchange 2 fails to bring about the use of ellipsis. The adult's use of 'umhmm' is immediately followed by the boy's completion of the utterance 'play with him'.

(8) (a) h-dropping;
   (b) loss of historical /r/;
   (c) monophthongal realisation;

(d) h-dropping;
(e) loss of historical /r/;
(f) loss of historical /r/;
(g) monophthongal realisation;
(h) loss of historical /r/;
(i) h-dropping;
(j) monophthongal realisation
(9) (a) false;
(b) true;
(c) false;
(d) true;
(e) true
(10) (a) true;
(b) true;
(c) false;
(d) false;
(e) true
(11) (a) agent + action;
(b) action + affected;
(c) possessor + possession;
(d) entity + attribute;
(e) action + location;
(f) entity + attribute;
(g) recurrence;
(h) negation;
(i) nomination;
(j) entity + location

Chapter 3

Case study

(1) otolaryngology; psychiatry; neurology; gastroenterology
(2) epidemiology
(3) aetiology
(4) inflammation of the laryngeal mucosa
(5) otolaryngology; neurology

End-of-chapter questions

(1) Part A:
(a) prevalence;
(b) incidence;
(c) prevalence;
(d) incidence;
(e) prevalence

Answers 309

Part B:
(a) infectious;
(b) genetic;
(c) neurological;
(d) genetic;
(e) infectious
(2) (a) anatomy;
  (b) physiology;
  (c) anatomy;
  (d) physiology;
  (e) anatomy;
  (f) anatomy;
  (g) anatomy;
  (h) anatomy;
  (i) physiology;
  (j) physiology. In (e), vocal nodules can compromise vocal fold physiology but the primary deficit is still a structural (anatomical) defect of the folds.
(3) (a) spastic quadriplegia cerebral palsy: developmental; non-progressive
  (b) multiple sclerosis: acquired; progressive
  (c) traumatic brain injury: acquired; non-progressive
  (d) cerebellar agenesis: developmental; non-progressive
  (e) cerebrovascular accident: acquired; non-progressive
  (f) Möbius syndrome: developmental; non-progressive
  (g) meningitis: acquired; non-progressive
  (h) nerve damage during laryngectomy: acquired; non-progressive
  (i) penetrating head injury: acquired; non-progressive
  (j) Duchenne muscular dystrophy: developmental; progressive
(4) (a) true;
  (b) false;
  (c) false;
  (d) true;
  (e) true;
  (f) true;
  (g) false;
  (h) false;
  (i) false;
  (j) true
(5) Part A:
  (a) Ménière's disease;
  (b) noise-induced hearing loss;
  (c) sensory presbycusis;
  (d) conductive hearing loss
  Part B:
  (a) tympanometry;

(b) pure tone audiometry bone conduction testing;
(c) acoustic reflex test;
(d) speech audiometry
(6) parts (c), (f) and (i)
(7) (a) infectious diseases;
(b) palliative care;
(c) paediatrics;
(d) endocrinology;
(e) gastroenterology;
(f) oncology;
(g) gerontology;
(h) geriatrics;
(i) maxillofacial surgery;
(j) orthodontics

Chapter 4

(1) (a) clinical psychologist;
(b) clinical neuropsychologist;
(c) developmental psychologist;
(d) cognitive neuropsychologist;
(e) educational psychologist
(2) Part A: (b), (c), (e) and (f)
Part B: wanted (cognitive ToM); discovered (cognitive ToM); angry (affective ToM); heard (cognitive ToM); decided (cognitive ToM); happy (affective ToM); frightened (affective ToM); see (cognitive ToM)
(3) (a) false;
(b) true;
(c) true;
(d) true;
(e) false
(4) (a) phonological output lexicon;
(b) orthographic input lexicon;
(c) abstract letter identification;
(d) letter-to-sound rules;
(e) auditory phonological analysis
(5) parts (a), (c) and (e)
(6) (a) Yes, Ms S presented with low mood and feelings of anxiety.
(b) The absence of an organic abnormality is not sufficient for a diagnosis of psychogenic dysphonia. There must also be the presence of psychological factors.
(c) This finding indicates that, notwithstanding her dysphonia, Ms S retains the capacity for normal phonation.

(d) On initial presentation at hospital, Ms S reported low mood. This was subsequently confirmed by a score of 15 on the Beck's Depression Inventory, indicating the presence of mild depression.
(e) No, the speech pathologist also used a psychological intervention with Ms S. In voice therapy, Ms S received counselling during which the abuse of her voice in the context of her family problems was subjected to psychotherapeutic examination.

Chapter 5

Case study

(1) A diagnosis of dysarthria is not warranted as Bob is able to produce intelligible speech sounds. A diagnosis of apraxia of speech is not warranted as Bob is able to sequence speech sounds.
(2) The picture description task allows the SLT to examine Bob's monological discourse skills. By engaging Bob in conversation, the SLT is able to assess his dialogical discourse skills.
(3) Bob's performance on formal assessment tasks is so compromised because he is unable to use contextual information to facilitate him on these tasks.
(4) When an SLT says /kə/ to elicit the production of the word *car*, a phonemic cue is used. A semantic cue (e.g. 'You can drive to work in this') may also be used to elicit the production of *car*.
(5) Videofluoroscopy is an imaging technique which is considered to be the 'gold standard' in the assessment of dysphagia. It is the most reliable and accurate assessment of the presence of aspiration in a client.

End-of-chapter questions

(1) (a) formal;
   (b) informal;
   (c) informal;
   (d) formal;
   (e) informal
(2) Part A:
   (a) pep for 'pet': Feature (2) Exhibits phonemic perseverative errors
   (b) moan for 'man': Feature (5) Exhibits phonemic vowel errors
   (c) lelo for 'yellow': Feature (1) Exhibits phonemic anticipatory errors
   (d) Arifca for 'Africa': Feature (3) Exhibits phonemic transposition errors
   (e) ben for 'pen': Feature (4) Exhibits phonemic voicing errors
   Part B:
   (a) consonant cluster reduction
   (b) consonant cluster reduction; final consonant deletion

(c) consonant cluster reduction; fronting
(d) stopping; final consonant deletion
(e) consonant cluster reduction; stopping; final consonant deletion
(f) liquid gliding
(g) fronting
(h) fronting
(i) deaffrication; stopping
(j) final consonant deletion
(k) weak syllable deletion
(l) final consonant deletion
(m) consonant cluster reduction
(n) consonant cluster reduction
(o) deaffrication

(3) (a) sentence comprehension;
    (b) word structure;
    (c) word classes;
    (d) pragmatics profile and/or pragmatics activities checklist;
    (e) reading comprehension;
    (f) semantic relationships;
    (g) word definitions;
    (h) sentence assembly;
    (i) pragmatics profile and/or pragmatics activities checklist;
    (j) sentence comprehension

(4) (a) false;
    (b) false;
    (c) true;
    (d) true;
    (e) true;
    (f) false;
    (g) true;
    (h) false;
    (i) false;
    (j) true

(5) (a)-(iii);
    (b)-(vi);
    (c)-(v);
    (d)-(i);
    (e)-(iv);
    (f)-(ii)

(6) parts (a), (c) and (e)

(7) (a) body structures and functions
    (b) environmental and personal factors
    (c) activities and participation
    (d) body structures and functions
    (e) environmental and personal factors

(f) activities and participation
(g) body structures and functions
(h) environmental and personal factors
(i) body structures and functions
(j) activities and participation

Chapter 6

(1) (a) direct intervention;
    (b) direct intervention;
    (c) indirect intervention;
    (d) direct intervention;
    (e) indirect intervention
(2) (a) motor speech programming and planning focus
    (b) motor speech execution focus
    (c) phonological focus
    (d) motor speech execution focus
    (e) motor speech programming and planning focus
(3) (a) true;
    (b) true;
    (c) false;
    (d) false;
    (e) true;
    (f) false;
    (g) true;
    (h) false;
    (i) true;
    (j) false
(4) Advantages of group therapy over individual therapy for children and adults who stutter:
    (a) Clients can practise strategies such as prolonged speech in the safety of the group before implementing them in everyday communicative contexts. Feedback can be offered by group members on the success or otherwise of strategies, and suggestions advanced for how to improve the use of techniques.
    (b) Group therapy more closely resembles everyday communication through the presence of multiple participants. Techniques and strategies are thus being developed in a context that is a better preparation for communication in the real world.
    (c) Stuttering can cause disabling levels of anxiety as well as significant practical difficulties in daily life (e.g. inability to make telephone calls). Clients in group therapy can derive significant support from learning about the experiences of others who stutter and hearing how they overcome challenges related to stuttering.

(5) (a) indirect treatment;
(b) direct treatment;
(c) indirect treatment;
(d) direct treatment;
(e) indirect treatment
(6) (a) Coughing is an important potential indicator of aspiration due to oropharyngeal dysphagia. However, the absence of coughing is not a sign that aspiration is not occurring. A client may silently aspirate, i.e. aspirate food and liquids in the absence of coughing.
(b) During piecemeal deglutition, a bolus of a large volume is divided into two or more parts, which are swallowed successively. Aspiration is when food and liquid enter the airway below the true vocal folds. Penetration is when food and liquid enter the laryngeal vestibule but, unlike in aspiration, they do not descend below the level of the true vocal folds.
(c) Oral stasis is when food gathers in the buccal or lateral sulci (space between the cheeks and adjacent teeth), the floor of the mouth, or in the mid-tongue depression. Stasis in both lateral sulci can occur when the muscles of the cheek have insufficient tone and food gathers as residue. Stasis may also be a sign of a poorly formed bolus which fragments easily in the oral cavity.
(d) Swallow manoeuvres were not part of this client's dysphagia intervention.
(e) This client's intervention did make use of exercises to improve the neuromuscular processes that control swallowing.
(7) (a) false;
(b) true;
(c) false;
(d) true;
(e) false;
(f) false;
(g) true;
(h) false;
(i) false;
(j) true

Chapter 7

(1)
(a) (i) speech and language therapist;
(ii) neurologist;
(iii) dietician;
(iv) radiologist;
(v) physiotherapist;

(vi) neuropsychologist;
(vii) occupational therapist;
(viii) critical care nurse;
(ix) gastroenterologist;
(x) pharmacist

(b) (i) speech and language therapist: assesses the safety of oral feeding and recommends alternative forms of feeding if oral feeding is unsafe
(ii) dietician: assesses patient's nutritional requirements and whether these are met through oral feeding, NG tube feeding or PEG tube feeding
(iii) critical care nurse: provides vital monitoring and aftercare for patients with PEG tubes to avoid serious complications such as peritonitis
(iv) gastroenterologist: assesses suitability of patients for PEG tube feeding and inserts tube using endoscopy
(v) radiologist: conducts a videofluoroscopic swallow study along with SLT

(c) Neurologist: assesses nature and extent of M.G.'s open head injury and manages post-traumatic seizures
Radiologist: interprets CT scan of M.G.'s head injury and conducts videofluoroscopic swallow study

(d) occupational therapist

(e) (i) neuropsychologist
(ii) M.G.'s executive function skills are impaired. He displays poor planning, organization, and initiation.
(iii) Neglect and perceptual impairments are related to parietal lobe damage.
(iv) Understanding of pragmatic aspects of language such as idioms and metaphors are most likely to be affected by M.G.'s concrete thinking.
(v) M.G.'s inability to recognize his cognitive impairments is most likely to compromise self-monitoring.

(2) (a) Jessie is describing a challenge that arises when SLT services are poorly developed or non-existent in a country. Other medical and health professionals are called upon to address communication difficulties in children when they lack the requisite expertise to do so. Rachel is describing a challenge that is related to negative societal perceptions in Kenya of individuals with communication disorders and other disabilities. Sally is describing a challenge that is related to differences in pedagogical practice.

(b) The challenge that is most related to economic factors is the one described by Jessie. In the absence of a well-funded healthcare system, which includes SLT services, clinicians in other disciplines are compelled to support children with communication disorders.

(c) The challenge that is most related to cultural factors is the one described by Rachel. Disability is perceived as a weakness or deficiency within Kenyan culture, leading to social exclusion and other forms of disadvantage for individuals with disabilities.

(d) positive rapport

(e) Education of professionals: The SLTs encouraged special education teachers to consider new approaches to teaching that would be beneficial for children with communication disability. By working with other professionals such as doctors and physiotherapists, the SLTs had the opportunity to raise awareness of communication disorders in children.

Education of the public: By challenging cultural stereotypes around disability, the SLTs were able to have a positive influence on poor public perceptions of people with disabilities.

(3) (a) continuing professional development and research;
(b) advocacy;
(c) clinical guidelines;
(d) education and awareness;
(e) accreditation;
(f) research;
(g) education and awareness;
(h) continuing professional development;
(i) research;
(j) advocacy

(4) (a) advocacy;
(b) raising awareness;
(c) information;
(d) research;
(e) raising awareness and advocacy

Appendix

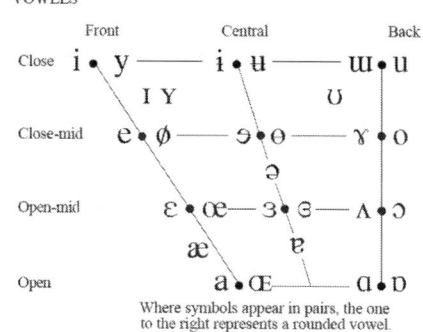

IPA Chart, www.internationalphoneticassociation.org/content/ipa-chart, available under a Creative Commons Attribution-Sharealike 3.0 Unported License. Copyright © 2005 International Phonetic Association.

Glossary

abduction: The opening of the vocal folds during the phonatory cycle. The folds are fully abducted during breathing.

academic impact: A communication disorder can adversely affect the academic performance of a child or an adult. Academic impact may be measured in the number of qualifications achieved by an individual at different stages of formal education.

acalculia: see *dyscalculia*

accent: The pronunciation of a linguistic variety. All speakers have accents which can reveal information about the regional and social identity of speakers.

accreditation: A process in which an individual or organization is evaluated and then awarded certification to demonstrate that high standards of quality, competence and integrity are met.

achalasia: A motility disorder of the oesophagus that is characterized by abnormal peristalsis – the wave-like muscle contractions that move food along the oesophagus – and complete or partial failure of the lower oesophageal sphincter to relax during deglutition. It is a cause of oesophageal dysphagia in children and adults.

acid laryngitis: see *reflux laryngitis*

acoustic neuroma: Also known as vestibular schwannoma, an acoustic neuroma is a benign tumour. It is the most commonly occurring tumour in the head and neck. When of sufficient size, it can appear on a CAT or MRI scan but is often detectable before then using an auditory brainstem response test. Symptoms include hearing loss, tinnitus and imbalance.

acoustic reflex test: A test that is based on the signal threshold level at which the stapedial muscle contracts. The lowest signal intensity that is capable of eliciting this acoustic reflex is known as the acoustic reflex threshold. The acoustic reflex test is a sensitive indicator of cochlear pathology.

acquired communication disorder: A communication disorder that has its onset after the period in which speech and language skills are normally acquired. Such a disorder can be found in adolescents and in adults.

active articulator: This is an articulator that performs most of the movement required to articulate speech sounds. The lower lip and tongue are both active articulators. Active articulators are attached to the jaw, which can move during articulation. See also *passive articulator*.

adduction: The approximation or closing of the vocal folds during the phonatory cycle and swallowing.

advocacy: Vulnerable children and adults may be unable to represent themselves or express their views effectively to others. This is particularly true if an individual has a communication disorder. An advocate acts on behalf of these clients by representing their interests to others on medical, legal and other matters.

aetiology: The medical or other causes of a disorder. Causes may range from organic problems (e.g. a laryngeal tumour in a voice disorder) through to psychological and behavioural factors (e.g. psychological trauma in psychogenic dysphonia). Many communication disorders have a mixed aetiology, with organic, psychological and behavioural factors all contributing to the development of these disorders.

affix: Affixes are bound morphemes, i.e. they can only occur when attached to some other morpheme such as a root or stem or base. Affixes include prefixes (*disagree*), suffixes (*walking*) and infixes where an affix is inserted into the root itself.

agrammatic aphasia: A type of non-fluent aphasia in which the speaker retains content words but omits function words and inflectional morphemes from his or her speech. The verbal output of speakers with agrammatic aphasia has the appearance of a telegram, e.g. 'Man ... walk ... dog' for *The man is walking the dog*.

agrammatism: Reduced or limited grammatical structure which is most often found in the presence of aphasia. See *agrammatic aphasia*.

AIDS dementia complex: Also referred to as AIDS-related dementia, AIDS encephalopathy and HIV encephalopathy. The condition is characterized by a progressive deterioration in cognitive function, including language, which is accompanied by motor abnormalities and behavioural changes. The association of cognitive changes with motor and behavioural signs is denoted by the word *complex*.

allophone: An allophone is a phonetic variant of a phoneme in a particular language.

alogia: see *poverty of speech*

Alport syndrome: This is a genetic condition that occurs in approximately 1 in 50,000 newborns. It is characterized by kidney disease, hearing loss and eye abnormalities. The hearing loss is high frequency in nature and is usually progressive during childhood.

Alzheimer's dementia: The most common form of dementia, accounting for 50% to 75% of all dementia cases. Alzheimer's dementia is characterized by prominent episodic memory impairment, with secondary deficits in word-finding skills, spatial cognition and executive functions. See *Alzheimer's disease*; *dementia*.

Alzheimer's disease: A neurodegenerative disease that is the most frequent cause of dementia. Amyloid plaques and neurofibrillary tangles develop in the brains of individuals with Alzheimer's disease.

amplification: The use of hearing aids, cochlear implants and other devices to give children and adults with hearing loss as much access to the auditory environment, and speech in particular, as possible.

amyotrophic lateral sclerosis: see *motor neurone disease*

anaphoric reference: A form of cohesion in which there is reference to a preceding textual unit (known as the antedecent). In the following example, the pronoun 'it' in the second sentence refers to the noun phrase 'a red dress' in the first sentence: *Mary bought a red dress. It was very expensive.*

anatomy: The study of the structure of the body. This includes macroscopic structure (gross anatomy) and microscopic structure (histology and cell biology). Applied to speech-language pathology, anatomy includes the study of the oral articulators (e.g. tongue), larynx, lungs and structures of the brain.

androgen therapy: A testosterone preparation used in the treatment of the female-to-male transsexual to induce virilization, including a deepening of the voice, cessation of menses and production of male-pattern body hair growth and physical contours.

anomia: A word-finding difficulty in which a client is unable to evoke, retrieve or recall a particular word. In anomic aphasia, there are relatively severe word-finding problems in the context of fluent, grammatically well-formed speech production and relatively intact auditory comprehension.

anxiety: An emotion characterized by feelings of tension, worried thoughts and physical symptoms such as increased blood pressure. Anxiety has a close relationship to communication disorders. Anxiety may be a consequence of conditions such as stuttering and aphasia. Communication impairment is a feature of anxiety disorders like selective mutism.

Apert syndrome: A genetic disorder caused by mutations in the FGFR2 gene. Features include premature fusion of certain skull bones (craniosynostosis), fusion of fingers and toes (syndactyly), conductive hearing loss, and cognitive abilities which can range from normal to mild or moderate intellectual disability.

aphasia (dysphasia): An acquired language disorder in which the expression and/or reception of language (spoken, written and signed) is compromised. Aphasia can be broadly classified as fluent and non-fluent types. Fluent aphasia is further subdivided into Wernicke's, anomic, conduction and transcortical sensory aphasia. Non-fluent aphasia is further subdivided into Broca's and transcortical motor aphasia. A further non-fluent aphasia – global aphasia – is characterized by severe impairment of all language functions.

aphonia: Literally, the complete absence of voice. Clients with conversion aphonia are able to whisper but are unable to achieve phonation.

apraxia of speech: A motor programming disorder which has its onset in adulthood typically following a stroke. Speech intelligibility is reduced in the absence of neuromuscular weakness. As well as speech errors involving consonants and vowels, AOS speakers display inconsistent errors, have more difficulty with volitional speech production than automatic speech production, and can display articulatory groping. Apraxia of speech may occur in isolation or alongside oral apraxia.

apraxic agraphia: A peripheral writing disorder which is considered to result from a lesion in the parietal and/or prefrontal lobe of the language-dominant hemisphere.

argument structure: The lexical representation of argument-taking lexical items such as verbs and prepositions. The argument structure indicates the number of arguments a lexical item takes (e.g. three arguments in the preposition 'x is between y and z'), the syntactic expression of the arguments and their semantic relation to the lexical item.

Arnold-Chiari malformation: The name given to a Type II Chiari malformation. This occurs when part of the cerebellum (the cerebellar tonsils) protrudes through the foramen magnum, the opening found in the occipital bone at the base of the skull. It is usually accompanied by a myelomeningocele, a form of spina bifida.

articulation disorder: A disorder that affects the phonetic level of speech production. Errors may be classified as substitutions (e.g. [w] for /r/), omissions, distortions or additions. Articulation disorders may have an organic aetiology (e.g. brain injury) or they may be of unknown origin.

Asperger's syndrome: A neurodevelopmental disorder in which there are impairments of social communication and restricted, repetitive patterns of behaviour, interests and activities. Asperger's syndrome was included as a disorder separate from autism for the first time in 1994 in the fourth edition of the *Diagnostic and Statistical Manual of Mental Disorders* (DSM-4). Since the publication of the fifth edition (DSM-5) in 2013, the diagnostic label 'Asperger's disorder' has been superseded by the label 'autism spectrum disorder'.

aspiration: The entry of food and liquid into the trachea and lungs. Aspiration occurs in clients with dysphagia and can cause pneumonia. If aspiration occurs without any outward signs of swallowing difficulty, it is called 'silent aspiration'.

aspiration pneumonia: see *aspiration*

atherosclerosis: The formation of fatty plaques on the inside wall of arteries. This can lead to a constriction in the flow of oxygenated blood to tissues. Atherosclerosis is a cause of cerebrovascular accidents.

atresia: The failure of the external auditory canal to form either fully or partially during embryological development. Atresia may occur in isolation or as part of a syndrome. It may be accompanied by microtia of varying grades and an abnormal middle ear cavity.

atrophy: The wasting or loss of muscle tissue through either lack of use (disuse atrophy) or damage of a nerve that innervates a muscle (neurogenic atrophy). Vocal fold atrophy can occur in clients with vocal fold paralysis.

attention: A state of focused awareness on a subset of the perceptual information available in the environment. Attention is an executive function that is mediated by the frontostriatal circuit in the brain. There are different types of attention. For example, selective attention is the differential processing of multiple sources of information that are available simultaneously.

attention deficit hyperactivity disorder (ADHD): A disorder that is diagnosed on the basis of symptoms of inattention and hyperactivity-impulsivity. DSM-5 recognizes four types of ADHD depending on the pattern and duration of inattentive and hyperactive/impulsive symptoms: combined presentation; predominantly inattentive presentation; predominantly hyperactive/impulsive presentation; and inattentive presentation.

audiogram: A graph that displays the results of pure-tone hearing tests. The frequency (pitch) of sound is measured in Hertz (Hz) and is represented on the horizontal axis. The intensity (loudness) of sound is measured in decibels (dB) and is represented on the vertical axis. An audiogram illustrates the type, degree and configuration of hearing loss.

audiology: The study of hearing. Also, audiology is the name of the profession concerned with the prevention, diagnosis and rehabilitation of auditory problems.

audiometry: The use of a range of tests to measure the function of the hearing mechanism. This includes tests of mechanical sound transmission (middle ear function), neural sound transmission (cochlear function) and speech discrimination ability (central integration). See *auditory brainstem response audiometry*; *immittance audiometry*; *speech audiometry*.

auditory brainstem response audiometry: This technique measures evoked potentials of the auditory nervous system. Signals are delivered to each ear independently through electrodes that are taped to the skull. These electrodes are used to detect microvolt sensory responses from the auditory nerve and brainstem. Slight modifications of the auditory brainstem response technique permit measurement of the middle latency response, an evoked response that occurs between the brainstem and auditory cortex.

augmentative and alternative communication (AAC): When spoken communication skills are severely impaired and are unlikely to improve, a type of AAC may be considered for use with a client. AAC may take high- and low-tech forms such as a communication board attached to a client's wheelchair or the use of synthesized speech output.

aural rehabilitation: On a holistic definition, aural rehabilitation is the reduction of hearing-loss-induced deficits of function, activity, participation and quality of life through a combination of sensory management, instruction, perceptual training and counselling (Boothroyd, 2007).

autism spectrum disorder: A neurodevelopmental disorder in which there are persistent deficits in social communication and social interaction and restricted, repetitive patterns of behaviour, interests or activities. These symptoms must be present in the early developmental period and cause clinically significant impairment in social, occupational or other important areas of functioning.

auxiliary verb: A verb that occurs with a main or lexical verb (e.g. *The girl is singing*). Modal auxiliary verbs express obligation (*You must attend the lecture*), permission (*You may travel with us*), ability (*Sally can swim two miles*) and prediction (*Jack will become a surgeon*).

avoidance behaviour: People who stutter engage in a range of behaviours to avoid a moment of stuttering and the loss of control and listener penalty that is associated with it. They may substitute words that they can say for the ones they fear stuttering on. They may talk around a word (circumlocution) and not say it at all. They may pause and pretend to think, and they may avoid talking and situations where talking is necessary altogether.

Babinski reflex: The Babinski reflex occurs in children up to 2 years old. When the sole of the foot is firmly stroked, the big toe moves upwards or towards the top surface of the foot and the other toes fan out. As children mature, the reflex disappears. Its presence in an adult is a sign of neurological disorder.

basilar membrane: The membrane that forms the floor of the cochlear duct, the chamber separating the scala vestibuli (upper) from the scala tympani (lower). The cochlear hair cells are located on the basilar membrane.

Beckwith-Wiedemann syndrome: A paediatric overgrowth syndrome caused by mutation or deletion of imprinted genes within the chromosome 11p15.5 region. Clinical features are highly variable and include rapid growth prenatally and in the early years, although adult height is usually in the normal range. This growth may be manifested as hemihypertrophy (overgrowth of one side of the body) and/or macroglossia (large tongue). Other features include hypoglycaemia (low blood glucose), abdominal wall defects, visceromegaly (enlargement of abdominal organs) and renal anomalies. There is a predisposition to tumour development. The incidence is estimated to be 1 in 13,700.

bedside assessment: A short, usually informal assessment of a client's communication skills and swallowing that is conducted at bedside. A bedside assessment is undertaken when a client is too frail or unwell to undergo more extensive assessment and to give the SLT preliminary information about a client's difficulties on which to base a more extensive assessment at a later time. Some standardized, norm-referenced assessments have versions that can be used at bedside, e.g. *Western Aphasia Battery – Revised* (Kertesz, 2006).

behavioural impact: A communication disorder may have adverse consequences for the behaviour of children and adults. In children, communication impairments may lead to disruptive behaviour in the classroom or challenging behaviour at home. In adults, communication impairments may lead to aggressive behaviour with family members and carers in the case of clients with conditions like dementia and traumatic brain injury.

bifid uvula: A bifid uvula is one of the cardinal signs of a submucous cleft palate (other signs are a translucent line in the midline of the soft palate and a short palate, and a V-shaped notch at the back of the hard palate). A bifid uvula may also occur in isolation in about 0.1–3% of the population (Wales et al., 2009).

bilingual aphasia: Aphasia in an individual who speaks two languages. Because bilingualism is the norm rather than the exception in many parts of the world, the prevalence of bilingual aphasia is on the increase. Bilingual aphasia raises unique management issues for SLTs (e.g. cross-linguistic effects of therapy).

bilingualism: The use of two languages by an individual. Bilingualism is very prevalent and is increasing. It is estimated that two-thirds of children globally are brought up in a bilingual environment (Crystal, 2003).

bipolar disorder: Formerly known as manic depression, this is a psychiatric disorder in which the patient's mood alters between manic episodes (characterized by euphoria, restlessness, poor judgement and risk-taking behaviour), depressive episodes (characterized by depression, anxiety and hopelessness) and episodes of normal mood (known as euthymia).

blending: A non-morphemic word-formation process in which two lexemes are merged into one, e.g. in_formation_ + _entertain_ment → in_fotain_ment.

block: A feature of stuttering in which a speaker becomes 'stuck' on a sound in a word and cannot move to the next sound. Attempts at producing the sound may or may not be audible.

bolus: A bolus is orally processed food particles which are in a ready-to-swallow state. During the oral stage of swallowing, food particles are incorporated with saliva and formed into a bolus through the action of the teeth and tongue.

bowing: The vocal folds close at the front and back but fail to adduct in the middle. Bowing is most commonly caused by presbylarynx ('old larynx') but may also result from lack of innervation to the vocal folds. See also _presbylarynx._

brain tumour: A benign or malignant neoplasm of the brain. Brain tumours may be primary in nature, if they originate in the brain, or secondary in nature, if they are a metastasis from a tumour elsewhere in the body. Most primary brain tumours in adults originate in the cerebrum, while in children they mostly arise in the cerebellum or brainstem. Secondary brain tumours may be related to cancers of the lung, breast, kidney, stomach, colon and melanoma skin cancer. Brain tumours are treated with a combination of surgery, radiotherapy and chemotherapy.

brainstem: The brainstem is the most caudal part of the brain. It is structurally continuous with the spinal cord and consists of the midbrain, pons and medulla oblongata. The brainstem contains cranial nerve nuclei and other nuclei and can be damaged by neurodegenerative diseases (e.g. Parkinson's disease) and cerebrovascular accidents.

breathiness: A vocal quality in which the voice is perceived to be weak. Breathy voice arises when the folds are not fully approximated so that complete closure does not occur during the vibratory cycle. There is considerable glottal leakage with some audible aspiration noise.

Broca's area: Broca's region is constituted mainly of Brodmann area 44. It is located in the posterior inferior frontal gyrus and is anterior to the primary motor cortex on the precentral gyrus. Broca's area is known to mediate the production of language but also contributes to comprehension.

candida albicans: A fungus that resides as a lifelong, harmless commensal in most individuals. *C. albicans* can cause infections that range from superficial infections of the skin to life-threatening systemic infections. Immunocompromised individuals such as patients with HIV can experience *C. albicans* infections that affect the oropharynx and/or oesophagus.

canonical babbling: A stage in speech-language acquisition that typically occurs between 5 and 10 months. A canonical syllable consists of at least one full vowel and one full consonant and exhibits rapid formant transitions and adult-like timing. Canonical syllables can occur in isolation (e.g. /da/) or in reduplicated sequences (e.g. /dada/). Canonical babbling is delayed in children with a range of developmental disorders (e.g. autism spectrum disorder).

carryover: see *generalization*

case history: Recording of all information relevant to a client's disorder through the use of informants such as patients, parents, spouses and carers. A case history can include information about pregnancy and labour, the attainment of milestones during the developmental period, previous illnesses and injuries, and current state of health.

cell biology: The study of cell structure and function.

central auditory processing: The processing of auditory signals from the ear by the auditory centres in the brain. Central auditory processing includes sound localization, auditory discrimination and recognition of temporal aspects of audition.

central nervous system: The part of the nervous system that consists of the brain and spinal cord.

cerebral palsy: A neurodevelopmental disorder that results in impairment of gross and fine motor skills. Speech production is often compromised. Cerebral palsy is caused by a range of factors in the pre-, peri- and post-natal periods that cause damage to the brain's motor centres.

cerebrovascular accident (CVA): The medical term for a stroke. CVAs may be caused by a blood clot (embolus) in one of the blood vessels in the brain or leading to the brain (embolic stroke) or by a haemorrhage (haemorrhagic stroke) in one of these vessels.

CHARGE syndrome: CHARGE stands for coloboma (a hole in one of the structures of the eye), heart defect, choanal atresia (blockage of one or both nasal passages), retarded growth and development, genital abnormality and ear abnormality. It occurs in approximately 1 in 8,500 to 10,000 individuals.

More than half of all cases of CHARGE syndrome are caused by mutations in the CHD7 gene.

chemotherapy: The use of cytotoxic drugs to destroy cancer cells.

child language acquisition: Also known as first language acquisition. This is the study of the stages that young children pass through on their way to acquiring the phonology, morphology, syntax, semantics and pragmatics of their native language. Different theoretical approaches to language acquisition (e.g. nativism, social interactionism) are also studied in child language acquisition.

childhood apraxia of speech: A motor speech disorder that has its onset in the developmental period. There is disruption of the programming of motor movements for speech production in the absence of neuromuscular deficits. Both consonant and vowel sounds are affected. There is often no clear aetiology of the disorder.

cholesteatoma: A middle ear disorder in which a benign accumulation of epithelium grows above and behind the upper part of the eardrum in the region known as the attic. As it grows, cholesteatoma may erode away the ossicles.

choral speech: Choral speech is speaking in unison. It is a phenomenon that immediately induces fluent and natural-sounding speech in almost all people who stutter, regardless of audience size, linguistic content and situation. Devices such as SpeechEasy™ use the choral speech effect on stuttering to help people who stutter achieve fluency.

circumlocution: A linguistic behaviour in which a client talks around a target word, e.g. the client who says 'the thing you tell the time with' for *watch*. Circumlocution is most evident in clients with aphasia where it is related to lexical retrieval deficits. However, it may also be used by people who stutter as a means of avoiding stuttered words, e.g. saying 'officer of the law' for *policeman*.

cleft lip and palate (CLP): A disorder of embryological development that results in a cleft of the upper lip, alveolus, hard and soft palates. Clefts may be unilateral or bilateral and can affect the primary palate only, the secondary palate only or both primary and secondary palates. Some clefts of the palate are described as submucous in nature, because the mucous membrane covering the palate may be intact and conceal an absence of muscle and bone beneath it.

clinical neuropsychology: A branch of neuropsychology that examines brain-injured individuals, most often with a view to undertaking rehabilitation. Clinical neuropsychologists are key members of the multidisciplinary team that assesses and treats individuals who sustain a traumatic brain injury.

clinical pragmatics: The branch of linguistic pragmatics that studies developmental and acquired pragmatic disorders in children and adults. The assessment and treatment of these disorders are also examined by clinical pragmatists.

clinical psychology: The branch of psychology that focuses on the understanding, assessment and treatment of psychological and behavioural problems and disorders. Among the clients treated by clinical psychologists are individuals with substance and other addictions, suicidal impulses, head injuries and compulsive eating.

clipping: A non-morphemic word-formation process in which there is deletion of parts of a lexeme at the end (e.g. *exam* from *examination*), the front (e.g. *phone* from *telephone*) or on both sides (e.g. *fridge* from *refrigerator*).

cluttering: A fluency disorder characterized by increased rate of speech, disorganized language and (somewhat disputed) a lack of awareness of communication difficulties on the part of the speaker. Cluttering is most often found alongside stuttering but sometimes occurs in a pure form.

cochlea: An inner ear structure that contains the organ of Corti. The action of the stapes footplate against the oval window displaces fluid in the cochlea. This displaced fluid triggers a neurophysiological response that leads to nervous impulses travelling to the brain via the vestibulocochlear nerve.

cochlear aplasia: A congenital malformation of the inner ear in which there is no cochlea and normal or malformed vestibule and semicircular canals.

cochlear hypoplasia: A congenital malformation resulting from an aberration in the development of the cochlear duct during the sixth week of gestation. A small cochlear bud of variable length (usually 1–3 mm) is seen to protrude from the vestibule on CT and MR imaging.

cochlear implantation: The use of a surgically implanted electronic device that is coupled to external components to provide useful hearing to children and adults with severe-to-profound sensorineural hearing loss.

cochleostomy: During cochlear implantation, a small hole called a cochleostomy is created in or near the round window of the cochlea through which the electrode array of the implant is inserted into the scala tympani.

cognitive behavioural therapy (CBT): A type of psychotherapy based on the view that the development and maintenance of psychological symptoms occurs as a result of the interaction between an individual's thoughts, emotions and behavioural responses. The therapist and client work collaboratively in CBT to identify and change thoughts and behaviours that may be maintaining symptoms.

cognitive development: The development in childhood and beyond of a range of intellectual skills related to thinking, reasoning, problem-solving and understanding.

cognitive module: A component of mental architecture in cognitive psychology. Modules may be innate, are specialized to process specific types of information or data (e.g. visual perceptual data) and are informationally encapsulated, among other features. The information processed by modules enters the mind's central system. Jerry Fodor first proposed the notion of domain-specific cognitive modules.

cognitive neuropsychology: A branch of cognitive psychology that investigates cognitive functions in individuals with brain damage with a view to understanding normal human cognition. Cognitive neuropsychology has had a profound influence on the SLT assessment of disorders such as aphasia.

cognitive psychology: The scientific study of higher mental processes such as perception, memory, language use, reasoning and problem-solving. An assumption of cognitive psychology is that the digital computer is a model of the mind and that mental processes involve rules operating upon mental representations.

cognitive-communication disorder: The term applied to any communication disorder that is related to cognitive deficits. The language and communication impairments of clients with traumatic brain injury and right-hemisphere damage are described as cognitive-communication disorders.

coherence: Although we can all recognize the difference between coherent and incoherent discourse, there is no widely accepted definition of coherence. Coherence may be defined as the extent to which spoken and written discourse holds together or makes sense as a unity. There is no specific set of linguistic features that confers coherence on a text. Proposed features include the use of adjacency pairs in conversation and discourse markers at the beginning and end of topic digressions.

cohesion: Certain grammatical and lexical features of sentences can link them to other sentences of a text. Forms of cohesion include anaphoric reference (e.g. *Paul likes marathons. He completes one every year*), substitution (e.g. *Jane bought an expensive sofa. It was the one in the shop window*), lexical reiteration (e.g. *The man and woman left the party early. The man was tired*) and ellipsis (e.g. *Would anyone like a drink? I would*).

collaborative working: Joint or integrated working by two or more individuals or organizations in pursuit of certain goals while maintaining their separate identities. In healthcare, collaborative working is a cost-effective way of managing patients with complex needs.

communication disorder: Any impairment of verbal and non-verbal communication. Communication disorders include speech, language, hearing, fluency and voice disorders. They are assessed and treated by speech-language pathologists.

communicative intention: A mental state that has particular significance in utterance interpretation. A hearer cannot be said to have understood a speaker's utterance unless he is able to establish the communicative intention that motivated the speaker to produce it.

complementary distribution: A mutually exclusive relationship between the allophones of a single phoneme in which one allophone occurs in an environment to the exclusion of all other allophones.

componential analysis: An approach to the study of word meaning in semantics. Componential analysts analyse word meaning in terms of semantic components or primitives, e.g. *mother* [FEMALE] [PARENT].

compounding: A morphemic word-formation process in which two free lexical morphemes are combined (e.g. *blackbird*).

comprehensibility: Comprehensibility refers to the ability of the listener to understand the acoustic signal given all the different clues (grammar, physical context, topic of conversation, etc.) there may be to intelligibility.

computerized axial tomography: A technique in which an X-ray source produces a narrow, fan-shaped beam of X-rays to irradiate a section of the body. On a single rotation of the X-ray source around the body, many different 'snapshots' are taken. These are then reconstructed by a computer into a cross-sectional image of internal organs and tissues for each complete rotation. This technique is commonly known as a CAT scan.

conductive hearing loss: Hearing loss which is related to damage and disease of the outer and middle ear, leading to compromised conduction of sound waves. Causes of this type of hearing loss include the failure of the ear canal to develop during embryological development (resulting in complete atresia of the canal), the development of middle ear disease such as otitis media ('glue ear') and ossification of the ossicular chain in otosclerosis.

confrontation naming: The presentation of an object or picture of an object which a subject is required to name. Confrontation naming is used to assess lexical retrieval.

consonant cluster reduction: A syllable simplification process which is found in the speech of normally developing children and children with speech sound disorders. Combinations of two and three consonants are reduced to a consonant singleton either syllable-initially (e.g. *string* [rɪŋ]) or syllable-finally.

constancy under negation: A feature of presuppositions that distinguishes them from entailment. While an entailment is cancelled by negation, a presupposition survives negation. For example, *John groomed the poodle* entails *John groomed the dog*. However, *John did not groom the poodle* does not entail that *John groomed the dog*. However, *The doctors managed to save the baby's life* presupposes that *The doctors tried to save the baby's life*. Also, the negated sentence *The doctors did not manage to save the baby's life* still presupposes that *The doctors tried to save the baby's life*.

continuing professional development (CPD): In order to maintain professional competence, an individual must continually update and extend their knowledge and skills in an area. Continuing professional development or CPD is the process through which this is achieved.

contrastive function: A property of phonemes. Phonemes such as /p/ and /b/ can be said to have a contrastive function or be in contrastive distribution. These phonemes contrast in English to generate different meanings. This can be seen in minimal pairs such as *lap* [lap] and *lab* [lab] and *pin* [pIn] and *bin* [bIn].

conversation analysis: The origins of conversation analysis are in an American sociological movement of the 1970s called ethnomethodology, defined as the study of 'ethnic', that is, participants' own methods of production and interpretation of social interaction. For the conversation analyst, analysis proceeds in an essentially inductive fashion. Many extracts of naturally occurring conversation are examined with a view to establishing recurring structural patterns. Conversation analysis has been applied in various ways to the study, assessment and treatment of communication disorders.

conversational repair: Trouble sources can arise during conversation and need to be repaired by participants. Repair strategies can take the form of a request for clarification followed by reformulation of a speaker's utterance. Repair work is often achieved collaboratively, especially in clients with communication disorders.

cooperative principle: A principle proposed by H. P. Grice to capture certain rational expectations between participants in verbal and non-verbal exchanges. This principle is the basis upon which speakers and hearers can derive implied meanings (so-called implicatures) from utterances in conversation.

coordinating conjunction: A closed grammatical class consisting of the words *and*, *but* and *or*. Coordinating conjunctions can be used to link nouns (*Mary likes wine and cheese*), adjectives (*The dog is wet and dirty*) and clauses (*Sally wanted the blue dress, but it was out of stock*).

correct information unit: A discourse measure proposed by Nicholas and Brookshire (1992). A correct information unit is a word that is intelligible in context, accurate in relation to the eliciting stimulus and relevant to and informative about the eliciting stimulus.

cranial nerve: Twelve paired sets of nerves that arise from the brain or brainstem and leave the central nervous system through cranial foraminae. These nerves control motor and sensory functions of the head and neck. Several cranial nerves are important for speech, hearing and swallowing.

cranial radiotherapy: Radiotherapy of the brain and its surrounding tissues. The use of radiotherapy to prevent or delay the spread of cancer to the brain is known as prophylactic cranial radiothcrapy.

cricothyroid approximation: A surgical procedure which is used to raise the pitch of the voice in male-to-female transsexuals. Titanium sutures are used to draw the cricoid and thyroid cartilages of the larynx together. This stretches the vocal folds, which elevates the pitch of the voice.

cricothyroid joint: A synovial joint formed from the articulation of the inferior cornua of the thyroid cartilage with facets on the cricoid lamina.

cueing: The delivery of a verbal or non-verbal prompt to elicit a response (usually a target word) from a client. In order to elicit the target word *watch* from an adult with aphasia, for example, an SLT may produce the initial sound of the word (phonemic cue), may say 'This is the thing you use to tell the time' (semantic cue) or may gesture looking at a watch on her wrist (gestural cue).

cytomegalovirus: The most common cause of congenital infection in the USA. Congenital cytomegalovirus (CMV) infection is the leading cause of sensorineural hearing loss in young children and can also cause significant intellectual disability. CMV is also a common opportunistic infection in individuals with HIV infection.

deixis: Linguistic expressions can be used to 'point' to aspects of spatiotemporal, social and discoursal context. There are five types of deixis: personal (*I want to leave early*), social (*Wie heißen Sie?*), temporal (*Sally departed last week*), spatial (*Joe lives here*) and discourse deixis (*The next section will present a different view*).

delayed auditory feedback: A process that involves recording a person's speech and replaying it to the speaker via headphones after a short delay (≤ 500 ms). Delayed auditory feedback has strong effects on fluency. It can induce fluency in people with developmental stuttering, and dysfluency in normally fluent speakers.

delusion: A false and bizarre belief. Delusions are a positive symptom of schizophrenia.

dementia: A deterioration in higher cortical functions (e.g. language, memory) that can be caused by a range of diseases (e.g. vascular disease, Alzheimer's disease), infections (e.g. HIV infection) and lifestyle (e.g. alcohol-related dementia).

depression: A common mental disorder that is characterized by sadness, loss of interest or pleasure, feelings of guilt or low self-worth, disturbed sleep or appetite, feelings of tiredness and poor concentration. Depression has a close relationship to communication disorders. It may be a consequence of conditions such as aphasia. Communication impairment may also be a feature of the depressed speaker.

derailment: A feature of language in schizophrenia in which speakers suddenly move off topic into irrelevant or tangential discourse.

derivational morphology: A branch of morphology that examines word-formation types that use prefixes (e.g. *disapprove*) and suffixes (e.g. *kindness*).

developmental apraxia of speech: see *childhood apraxia of speech*

developmental communication disorder: A communication disorder that has its onset in the developmental period, a time when children are undergoing speech and language acquisition.

developmental period: A period of time during which cognitive, linguistic and other abilities are acquired by infants, children and young people. The developmental period can extend for many years according to certain definitions. In the USA, the Centers for Disease Control and Prevention (2012) state that a developmental disability can have its onset at any time during development up to 22 years of age. One developmental disability – intellectual developmental disorder – can have its onset at any point up to the age of 18 years (American Psychiatric Association, 2013).

developmental phonological disorder: A condition in which children misarticulate many more speech sounds than is expected for their age. The disorder occurs in the absence of factors such as neuromuscular impairment and intellectual disability that might otherwise explain speech sound errors. Errors are typically characterized in terms of phonological processes such as stopping, fronting and weak syllable deletion. The disorder is more commonly found in boys than in girls.

developmental psychology: The branch of psychology that studies human growth and development across the lifespan. Developmental psychologists study cognitive, emotional, social, personality and motor development from the emergence of skills in infancy through to ageing in older adults.

developmental verbal dyspraxia: see *childhood apraxia of speech*

diadochokinetic (DDK) rate: Rapid syllable repetitions, e.g. /pə, tə, kə/, can be used to examine alternating articulatory movements and are a test of oral diadochokinesis. DDK rates are a routine part of the assessment of many speech disorders, e.g. apraxia of speech.

Diagnostic and Statistical Manual of Mental Disorders (DSM): Published by the American Psychiatric Association in 2013, the fifth edition (DSM-5) is an internationally recognized, authoritative guide to all mental disorders. It contains descriptions, symptoms and diagnostic criteria for these disorders. It is the handbook used by all healthcare professionals who are involved in the diagnosis of conditions ranging from autism spectrum disorder to schizophrenia.

dialect: The pronunciation, lexemes, grammatical structures and discourse features of a particular variety of a language.

diaphragm: A large, dome-shaped muscle that draws air into the lungs during inhalation when it contracts and flattens. During exhalation, the diaphragm returns to its domelike shape, forcing air out of the lungs.

dietician: The health professional who assesses, diagnoses and treats diet and nutrition problems. Dieticians work closely with SLTs in the management of clients with dysphagia.

diffusion tensor imaging (DTI): An *in vivo* imaging technique that allows three-dimensional visualization of the white matter anatomy in the brain. Because DTI is highly sensitive to changes at the cellular and microstructural levels, the technique can be used to investigate developmental, ageing and pathological processes of the central nervous system that influence microstructural composition and architecture of the affected tissues.

diphthong: Vowels whose quality noticeably alters as the tongue moves in the course of their production, e.g. *boy* [bɔɪ]. The start of the diphthongal movement is indicated by the first vowel symbol. The end or general direction of movement is indicated by the second vowel symbol.

diplegia: A term used in relation to cerebral palsy, although it may also be applied to other types of brain injury. A child with cerebral palsy and spastic diplegia has muscle stiffness that is predominantly in the legs and less severely affects the arms and face.

discourse: In terms of linguistic analysis, discourse is the level of language above individual sentences. The focus of study is on extended extracts of language in spoken and written texts.

discourse analysis: The study of extended spoken and written text to reveal how it is systematically structured and socially organized. Discourse analysts study monologic discourse (e.g. narrative) and dialogic discourse (e.g. conversation).

disorganized speech: see *thought disorder*

distal aetiology: This describes factors that are further back in the causal chain which lead to a disease or disorder. These factors act via a number of intermediary causes. For example, children can have language impairment on account of intellectual disability that is related to genetic and chromosomal abnormalities (e.g. trisomy 21 in Down syndrome). In this case, genetic factors are distal factors that act via intellectual disability to cause these children's language impairment.

distinctive feature: A phonological unit below the level of the phoneme. A phoneme can be described in terms of a matrix of distinctive features. For example, the nasal phoneme /m/ might be represented as a feature matrix [+sonorant, −continuant, +voice, +nasal, +labial].

Down syndrome: A chromosomal disorder that results from an extra chromosome 21. The additional chromosome may be found in all cells (trisomy 21), in some cells (mosaic) or attached to another chromosome (translocation). Individuals with the syndrome exhibit physical problems (e.g. heart defects) and cognitive difficulties (intellectual disability). See *trisomy 21*.

Duchenne muscular dystrophy: An X-linked neuromuscular disease characterized by progressive muscle degeneration. It has an incidence of approximately 1 in 3,800–6,300 live male births. Dysarthria and dysphagia are features of this disease.

dysarthria: A speech disorder that is caused by damage to the central and peripheral nervous systems. Dysarthria can be developmental or acquired in nature and affects articulation, resonation, respiration, phonation and prosody.

dyscalculia: A specific learning difficulty that affects the ability to acquire arithmetical skills. Individuals with dyscalculia have difficulty understanding number concepts, number relationships and outcomes of numerical operations.

dysfluency: Any disruption in the flow of speech. The term is used most commonly of the iterations and perseverations of stuttered speech. However, dysfluency is also a feature of other communication disorders (e.g. aphasia).

dyskinesia: Abnormal, uncontrolled movement that is a feature of many movement disorders (e.g. cerebral palsy). Dyskinesia may be caused by long-term use of levodopa in the treatment of Parkinson's disease and neuroleptic drugs in the treatment of psychiatric disorders (tardive dyskinesia).

dyslexia: A reading impairment that has its onset in childhood (developmental dyslexia) or in adulthood (acquired dyslexia). There are different types of dyslexia. For example, the individual with deep dyslexia can read words with concrete meanings more easily than words with abstract meanings. In surface dyslexia, which is often found in semantic dementia, the reading of non-words is preserved while the reading of irregular words is impaired.

dysphagia: The term given to a swallowing disorder in children and adults. Dysphagia can arise following a stroke or other neurological injury (neurogenic dysphagia), as a result of structural causes (e.g. a tumour), as a complication of surgery (iatrogenic dysphagia) or on account of psychological factors (psychogenic dysphagia). The oral and pharyngeal stages of swallowing may be compromised (oropharyngeal dysphagia) or the impairment may occur in the oesophageal stage of swallowing (oesophageal dysphagia). In most cases, the disorder can be managed by dietary and other modifications. When dysphagia is severe, non-oral feeding is instituted as the only safe method of feeding.

dysphonia: Another term for a voice disorder. Dysphonias may be organic (i.e. have a structural or neurological aetiology) or functional in nature (i.e. have a psychogenic or hyperfunctional aetiology). Regardless of the origin of a dysphonia, its effect on the perceptual attributes of the voice may be captured by terms such as *hoarse*, *breathy* and *strain-strangled*.

dyspraxia: A developmental coordination disorder that affects physical coordination. Individuals with dyspraxia have poor fine and/or gross motor skills relative to their general level of intelligence. When the disorder affects speech production, it is called developmental verbal dyspraxia.

ear canal: Also known as the external auditory meatus, the ear canal is part of the external ear. Measured from the tragus base to the tympanic membrane, the ear canal is 2.35 cm in length. It amplifies sound an average of 10–15 dB in the 2500–4000 Hz frequency range (Ackley, 2014).

ecological validity: Applied to SLT assessment, ecological validity describes the extent to which assessment tasks resemble everyday communication. In general, formal assessments have poorer ecological validity than informal assessments.

educational psychologist: The professional who specializes in educational psychology. See *educational psychology*.

educational psychology: The application of psychology and psychological methods to the study of learning, instruction and assessment and other issues (e.g. motivation) that influence the interaction between teaching and learning.

electroencephalography (EEG): A non-invasive technique in which the brain's electrical activity is recorded by means of electrodes placed on the scalp. Given that this electrical activity is small – it is measured in microvolts – the signal must be amplified before a resultant trace can be made. Although EEG has good temporal resolution (brain activity can be recorded almost as soon as it happens), the technique cannot locate the source of a signal. Functional MRI (fMRI) has better spatial resolution than EEG.

electroglottography: A non-invasive technique that indexes the contact area between the vocal folds. Two electrodes are secured around the neck at the level of the larynx. The opening and closing of the folds causes variation in the electrical resistance of a small, high-frequency current that is passed between the electrodes. These changes in resistance are displayed onscreen. Electroglottography can be used to assess and treat voice disorders, the latter through the provision of visual feedback.

electrolarynx: The electrolarynx or artificial larynx is a battery powered electromechanical device that generates a tone. When the head of the device is held against the tissues of the neck or cheek, the tone is transmitted into the oropharynx. The tone is then shaped into speech sounds by movements of the articulators. The tone can also be transmitted via an intraoral adapter. The electrolarynx is most often used by patients who have had a laryngectomy for the treatment of laryngeal cancer. Less commonly, it may be used by clients who have laryngeal apraxia.

electropalatography: An instrumental technique that provides a visual display of tongue-palate contacts. Electropalatography is used in the assessment and treatment of a range of clients including children with cleft palate. Not all subjects can tolerate the artificial palate that must be worn in this technique.

ellipsis: A form of grammatical cohesion in which there is omission of elements that are required by grammatical rules. For example, the question *Who would like beans on toast?* may receive the elliptical response *I would*.

embryology: The study of the formation and development of the embryo (or foetus) from the point of conception up to the time when it is born as an infant.

endocrinology: The medical discipline that studies the endocrine system and its disorders.

endotracheal intubation: A medical procedure in which a tube is placed into the trachea through the mouth or nose. Endotracheal intubation can lead to the formation of contact granulomas (also known as contact ulcers and intubation granulomas).

ENT medicine: Also known as otorhinolaryngology, ENT (Ears, Nose and Throat) medicine is the medical discipline that assesses and treats developmental abnormalities and acquired pathologies of the ear, larynx, pharynx, nose and oral cavity.

entailment: A semantic relation between sentences. An expression *A* entails *B* if the truth of *A* guarantees the truth of *B*, and the falsity of *B* guarantees the falsity of *A*. The sentence *Jack bought five guppies* entails that *Jack bought five fish*.

epidemiology: The study of the distribution of diseases and disorders in populations. Epidemiologists investigate the prevalence (total number of cases in a population) and incidence (number of newly diagnosed cases, typically within a year) of disorders in populations. They also investigate the distribution of diseases according to factors such as gender, age, socioeconomic class and ethnicity.

epiglottis: A cartilaginous structure at the posterior of the tongue that folds over the opening of the trachea during swallowing.

episodic memory: see *memory*

Estuary English: The name given to the form(s) of English that are widely spoken in and around London and the southeast of England more generally. The term *Estuary* relates to the River Thames and its estuary.

Eustachian tube: A tube which links the middle ear to the nasopharynx. Ventilation of the middle ear is achieved through the opening of the Eustachian tube. The tensor veli palatini muscle is the most important muscle for opening the Eustachian tube.

evidence-based practice: The use of the best available evidence to inform decisions about a client's clinical care. Evidence-based practice underpins the clinical practice guidelines of bodies such as the American Speech-Language-Hearing Association and the Royal College of Speech and Language Therapists.

executive dysfunction: (also, executive function deficits) Executive functions are a group of cognitive skills that are essential to goal-directed behaviour (e.g. planning ability, mental flexibility) and that are believed to be mediated in large part by the brain's frontal lobes. Impairment of these cognitive skills is thought to be related to communication difficulties in clients who sustain a traumatic brain injury.

executive function: see *executive dysfunction*

expressive language disorder: see *language disorder*

external auditory meatus: see *ear canal*

facial expression: A vital component of non-verbal communication that can convey considerable information about a speaker's communicative intentions. For many children and adults, the use and interpretation of facial expressions is compromised (e.g. in autism spectrum disorder).

facial nerve: The name of the seventh paired cranial nerve (CN VII). The motor portion of the nerve supplies all the facial musculature including the buccinator, frontalis and orbicularis oris. CN VII also has a sensory portion.

false belief test: Also known as Sally-Anne experiments, false belief tests are a standard test of theory of mind. These tests typically involve deception of an actor in a scenario about the location of an object. The child or adult who can establish that the actor has a false belief about the location of the object passes the test. Normally developing children pass false belief tests for the first time between 3 and 4 years of age.

fasciculation: Fine, rapid, flickering and sometimes worm-like twitching of a portion of muscle. In the tongue, fasciculations may be observed as small movements on the tongue surface. Fasciculations can be observed in healthy persons and in clients with neurological disorders (e.g. motor neurone disease).

fibreoptic endoscopic evaluation of swallowing (FEES): This technique involves the transnasal insertion of a flexible nasendoscope to the level of the oropharynx or hypopharynx. FEES is used in order to evaluate laryngopharyngeal physiology, management of secretions and the ability to swallow food and fluids.

fibreoptic laryngoscopy: The use of a rigid or flexible fibreoptic laryngoscope to conduct a visual examination of the larynx and adjacent structures. In flexible fibreoptic laryngoscopy, the nasal passage may be numbed with a local anaesthetic spray and an anaesthetic lozenge or spray is administered to the back of the throat to suppress the gag reflex. A flexible fibreoptic endoscope is then passed along the floor of one of the nostrils. In rigid fibreoptic laryngoscopy, the anaesthetized patient is lying on his back with shoulders raised slightly and the neck extended. From a position behind the patient's head, the physician guides the laryngoscope towards the larynx.

figurative language: Metaphorical, idiomatic and other non-literal language in which the meaning of an utterance is not derivable from the sum of its component words. Figurative language is not confined to literary texts but occurs in everyday language use. See *idiom*, *irony* and *metaphor*.

final consonant deletion: Deletion of final consonants occurs when the final singleton consonant in a word or syllable is omitted (e.g. /bo/ for *boat* and /mɑ/ for *mop*). In typical development, final consonant deletion has usually been eliminated by approximately 3;3 years.

finger agnosia: An inability to distinguish or identify individual fingers of the hand. It is diagnosed by asking the patient to name individual fingers or point to fingers that are named by the examiner.

fistula: Oronasal fistulae (singular: fistula) are holes or openings that occur in the palate and link the oral and nasal cavities. Fistula formation is a common complication of primary palatoplasty in children with cleft palate. The most common locations for post-palatoplasty fistulae are on the hard palate and at the junction of the hard and soft palate. Fistulae may form when there is tissue breakdown due to tension at the site of wound closure, tension after maxillary orthodontics or on account of infection.

flaccid dysarthria: A form of dysarthria related to a lower motor neurone lesion. Flaccid dysarthria is a feature of many syndromes (e.g. Down syndrome, Prader-Willi syndrome) and may be caused by a CVA or neurodegenerative disease (e.g. motor neurone disease).

fluency: The production of speech in a rhythmic, smooth manner. Fluency is affected by aspects of speech production (e.g. good respiratory support for speech) and language (e.g. efficient lexical retrieval).

fluency disorder: Any anomaly in the flow of speech. Stuttering (or stammering) and cluttering are fluency disorders. However, fluency may also be compromised in clients with other conditions such as aphasia.

fluent aphasia: One of two main forms of aphasia in which there is fluent, effortless production of language. Spoken output contains jargon but exhibits normal suprasegmental features.

forensic impact: A communication disorder may result in antisocial behaviour such as damage to property and harm to individuals. The forensic impact of a communication disorder may bring a child or adult into contact with the criminal justice system.

formal thought disorder: see *thought disorder*

fragile X syndrome (FXS): The most common inherited form of intellectual disability which is caused by the fragile X mental retardation 1 (FMR1) gene on the X chromosome. It is more commonly seen in males.

frequency altered feedback: Frequency altered feedback increases or decreases the frequency of the acoustic signal, causing the speaker to hear his or her own speech at a lower-than-normal or higher-than-normal pitch. Frequency altered feedback is used alongside delayed auditory feedback in SpeechEasy™ to emulate choral speech and induce fluency in the person who stutters.

Friedreich's ataxia: A rare, inherited disease in which there is impaired muscle coordination (ataxia) that worsens over time. The spinal cord, peripheral nerves and cerebellum degenerate. Symptoms typically begin between the ages of 5 and 15 years. There is no impairment of cognitive functions (thinking and reasoning abilities). Dysarthria develops and can get progressively worse.

frontotemporal dementia: A form of dementia that includes a behavioural variant as well as language variants known as logopenic, semantic and agrammatic/non-fluent primary progressive aphasia.

frontotemporal lobar degeneration: see *frontotemporal dementia*

functional communication: Any form of behaviour that expresses an individual's needs, wants, feelings and preferences in a way that others can understand. Personalized movements, gestures, verbalizations, signs, pictures, words and output from AAC devices all contribute to functional communication.

functional dysphonia: see *functional voice disorder*

functional magnetic resonance imaging (fMRI): A technique for measuring and mapping brain activity. fMRI detects changes in blood oxygenation and flow that occurs in response to neural activity. The technique may be used to localize psychological functions to specific brain regions and to make diagnoses of diseases such as dementia.

functional voice disorder: A voice disorder that arises in the absence of an abnormal structural finding in the larynx or a systemic medical or neurological condition.

fundamental frequency: The physical correlate of pitch. Fundamental frequency (F_0) is the rate of vibration of the vocal folds measured in Hertz (Hz).

gag reflex: The gag reflex is a protective response that prevents foreign objects or noxious material from entering the pharynx, larynx or trachea. It is not elicited during a normal swallow but is routinely assessed during a dysphagia evaluation.

gastroenterologist: The medical specialist who practises gastroenterology. See *gastroenterology*.

gastroenterology: The medical specialty that is concerned with disorders and conditions of the gastrointestinal tract. Gastroenterologists assess and treat disorders of the oesophagus, stomach, small and large intestines, pancreas and liver.

gastroesophageal reflux disease: see *laryngopharyngeal reflux*

gender reassignment: The process undertaken by individuals who experience gender dysphoria. Gender reassignment is achieved through surgery, hormone treatments and voice therapy. Voice therapy is most often required in male-to-female transsexuals.

general practitioner: In the UK, a general practitioner or family doctor treats patients in the community and refers them to specialists or consultants for further evaluation. In the USA, general practitioners are known as primary care physicians.

generalization: A process in which a client is able to move from using linguistic forms and communication skills acquired in structured, formal situations such as a clinic to using these same forms and skills in real-life contexts.

genetic syndrome: Multiple anomalies or symptoms related to an underlying genetic or chromosomal defect. Three common genetic syndromes are Down syndrome (trisomy 21), fragile X syndrome (transcriptional silencing of FMR1 gene on X chromosome) and Williams syndrome (microdeletion of genes in chromosome 7).

genetics: The branch of biology that deals with heredity, especially mechanisms of hereditary transmission, and variation of inherited characteristics among similar or related organisms.

geriatrics: The branch of medicine that studies the medical conditions associated with older age.

gerontology: A multidisciplinary field that studies social, psychological and biological aspects of the ageing process.

gesture: The use of the hands and other parts of the body for communicative purposes. Gesture may be used alongside speech or in place of speech during communication.

glossectomy: Surgical removal of the tongue either in part (partial glossectomy) or in whole (total glossectomy). Glossectomy is usually necessitated by the presence of oral cancer and may be performed in isolation or alongside other procedures (e.g. laryngectomy). The intelligibility of post-glossectomy speech production is highly variable and is influenced by a range of factors including the extent and mobility of remaining tongue tissue.

Goldenhar syndrome: Also known as oculo-auriculo-vertebral dysplasia. This is a disorder of unknown aetiology in which there is unilateral malformation of craniofacial structures, including eye, oral and musculoskeletal anomalies. Ear anomalies include auricular appendages, atresia of the external auditory canals (causing conductive hearing loss), unilateral microtia and unilateral, posteriorly placed ear. Mental retardation is not common in this syndrome.

grammar: see *syntax*

grimace: Nasal grimace often occurs in children with cleft palate who have nasal air emissions. A child attempts to inhibit these emissions by constricting the nose. Nasal grimace can involve just the nostrils (nares) or may extend to the bridge of the nose or the forehead. Nasal grimace often resolves with the treatment of velopharyngeal incompetence.

hallucination: The perception of things that do not exist. Hallucinations may be visual or auditory in nature. Auditory hallucinations are most common in schizophrenia.

head and neck cancer: Cancers which usually originate in the squamous cells that line the mucosal surfaces inside the head and neck. This includes cancers of the oral cavity, pharynx, larynx, paranasal sinuses and nasal cavity, and salivary glands (although cells other than squamous cells may be involved in the latter).

hearing impairment: see *hearing loss*

hearing loss: Hearing may be impaired on account of anomalies in the external and middle ear (conductive hearing loss) or anomalies in the inner ear and auditory cortices of the brain (sensorineural hearing loss). Depending on the type and severity of hearing loss, different types of amplification (e.g. cochlear implants) may be required.

hemiplegia: A paralysis of one side of the body. Hemiplegia may be congenital in nature (e.g. in cerebral palsy) or may have its onset in adulthood (e.g. subsequent to a stroke). A less serious condition, hemiparesis, describes a weakness of one side of the body.

herpes simplex encephalitis: A cerebral infection that is caused by the herpes simplex virus. There are two types of herpes simplex virus (HSV-1 and HSV-2) and either can cause encephalitis.

histology: The branch of biology that studies tissues. Histologists conduct microscopic examinations of the cells that constitute tissues.

hoarseness: A term used to describe a vocal quality in which the voice is perceived to be rough, harsh or deep. Hoarseness may be an early sign of local disease or the manifestation of a systemic illness.

humour: A technical expression which is intended to cover all pre-theoretical notions of comical, ridiculous or laughable language. Humour is studied by pragmatists. The use and appreciation of humour are impaired in a range of clients with communication disorders.

hyoid bone: A horseshoe-shaped bone which is located in the mid-neck, above the thyroid cartilage and anterior to the trachea.

hyperactivity: Hyperactivity describes a set of behaviours which includes constant activity, distractibility, impulsiveness, inability to concentrate and aggressiveness. Hyperactive behaviours include fidgeting, talking too much and constant moving. Hyperactivity is a feature of ADHD but may also be associated with other conditions (e.g. hyperthyroidism).

hyperadduction: A laryngeal finding in which there is increased closing force, or adduction time, in the glottal cycle. Hyperadduction can occur as a primary problem which may then give rise to secondary pathology. Alternatively, it may serve as a compensatory behaviour in response to the presence of laryngeal pathology. The speaker who engages in hyperadduction may have a vocal presentation that ranges from complete aphonia to a mildly hoarse voice.

hyperfunctional voice disorder: A voice disorder characterized by excessive phonatory effort. The muscle groups involved in phonation, particularly the intrinsic laryngeal muscles, display excessive tension. Muscle tension dysphonia is a hyperfunctional voice disorder and is often used to refer to this group of voice disorders.

hypernasal resonance: see *hypernasality*

hypernasal speech: see *hypernasality*

hypernasality: Excessive nasal resonance in speech, which may be caused by velopharyngeal incompetence. Hypernasal speech is a feature of cleft palate speech and dysarthric speech.

hyperreflexia: Overactive or exaggerated reflexes. Hyperreflexia is indicative of upper motor neuron dysfunction, which may be caused by stroke, tumours and trauma.

hypertonia: Increased muscle tone. Hypertonia is a feature of some dysarthrias (e.g. spastic dysarthria) and neurodevelopmental disorders (e.g. cerebral palsy).

hypoglossal nerve: Cranial nerve XII. The hypoglossal nerve controls all tongue movements. Lower motor neuron (nuclear and infranuclear) lesions produce paralysis, atrophy and fasciculations of the tongue on the involved side. Upper motor neuron (supranuclear) lesions produce mild to moderate contralateral weakness that may be transient. On protrusion, the tongue deviates to the side opposite to the lesion.

hypokinetic dysarthria: A form of dysarthria that is associated with lesions of the basal ganglia and associated brainstem nuclei. Hypokinetic dysarthria is a feature of Parkinson's disease (PD). All aspects of speech production may be compromised in PD, although disturbances of prosody, phonation and articulation are most common.

hypomimia: A cardinal sign of Parkinson's disease, hypomimia is characterized by a marked diminution of expressive gestures of the face, including brow movements that accompany speech and emotional facial expressions. Hypomimia is often present in only one side of the face.

hypophonia: Reduced vocal volume and strength that develops when Parkinson's disease affects the muscles that control the vocal folds. Sometimes the folds can also become thinned. Hypophonia generally improves with anti-Parkinson's medications. It often co-exists with dysarthria.

idiom: A linguistic expression, the meaning of which cannot be based on the meanings of its individual words (i.e. the meaning of idiomatic expressions is non-compositional). Common idioms include *pop the question* and *let the cat out of the bag*. The understanding or comprehension of idioms is often compromised in clients with pragmatic disorders.

immittance audiometry: An objective technique that assesses middle ear function by means of three procedures: static immittance (measure of the contribution of the middle ear to acoustic impedance), tympanometry and the measurement of acoustic reflex threshold sensitivity. Immittance audiometry may be used to detect middle ear effusion.

impedance audiometry: see *immittance audiometry*

implicature: A type of implied or implicated meaning that goes beyond what is said by an utterance. Grice recognized the following types of implicature: generalized conversational implicatures (includes scalar implicatures), particularized conversational implicatures and conventional implicatures.

impulsivity: Impulsivity is broadly defined as action without foresight. It is a feature of many psychiatric conditions including ADHD, mania and substance abuse.

inattention: A state in which there is a lack of focused awareness on a subset of the perceptual information available in the environment. Inattention is a core symptom of ADHD and is found in clients with traumatic and other brain injuries and diseases.

incidence: The rate of occurrence of new cases of a disease or condition. Incidence is calculated by dividing the number of new cases of a disease or condition in a specified time period (usually a year) by the size of the population under consideration.

incomplete partition dysplasia: A congenital malformation of the cochlea. There are two types of incomplete partition dysplasia. In type I, the cochlea lacks the entire modiolus and cribriform area, resulting in a cystic appearance. There is an accompanying large cystic vestibule. In type II, the cochlea consists of 1.5 turns. There is a dilated vestibule and enlarged vestibular aqueduct.

incus: The second of three ossicles in the middle ear. The incus articulates with the head of the malleus anteromedially and the stapes inferomedially.

indirect speech act: A speech act can be performed directly (e.g. *Open the window!*) or indirectly (e.g. *Can you open the window?*). The choice of speech act is determined by politeness considerations among other factors. An indirect speech act is often produced by questioning one of the preparatory conditions on the performance of a speech act (in the case of the above directive, that the hearer *can* undertake the requested action).

inferencing: A cognitive process in which a conclusion is derived from premises. There are several different types of inferences that vary according to the strength of the warrant provided by the premises. Inferencing is vital for pragmatic language understanding, although the exact nature of the inferences involved (deductive, inductive, etc.) is uncertain.

inflectional morphology: A branch of morphology that examines bound morphological markers of grammatical categories and relations. For example, the inflectional suffixes in *walking* and *walks* indicate progressive aspect and present tense, respectively.

inflectional suffix: A type of bound morpheme that marks grammatical categories such a plural (e.g. dogs), progressive aspect (e.g. walking) and past tense (e.g. walked). Unlike derivational suffixes, inflectional suffixes never change a word from one grammatical class to another.

information management: Management of the amount and type of information that is conveyed during conversation and other forms of discourse is known as information management. It is a key discourse skill of language users. Problems with information management arise when a speaker is over-informative, under-informative or contributes information which is irrelevant.

informational encapsulation: A feature of cognitive modules as envisaged by Jerry Fodor. A module is informationally encapsulated to the extent that in the course of processing a given set of inputs, it cannot access information stored elsewhere. For example, a visual perception module can process only visual perceptual input data and does not have access to information that is stored in the mind's central system.

inner ear: The third gross division of the ear. The inner ear contains three semicircular canals, utricle and saccule, which serve the sense of equilibrium. It also contains the cochlea, which is responsible for producing an electrophysiological response to sound.

intellectual disability: A term used in the *Diagnostic and Statistical Manual of Mental Disorders* (DSM-5) to describe children and adults with an intelligence quotient (IQ) below 70. Intellectual disability is a feature of many syndromes (e.g. Down syndrome) and is found in other clinical conditions (e.g. autism spectrum disorder). In the UK, another term that is used to describe children and adults with intellectual disability is *learning disability*.

intelligibility: The ease with which a hearer can understand the spoken output of a speaker. Speech disorders such as dysarthria and apraxia of speech can compromise a speaker's intelligibility. A highly unintelligible speaker may need to use an alternative communication system.

intercostal muscle: Eleven internal intercostal muscles and eleven external intercostal muscles are located in the intercostal spaces on each side of the rib cage. Contraction of the internal intercostal muscles reduces the transverse dimension of the thoracic cavity during expiration. Contraction of the external intercostal muscles expands the transverse dimension of the thoracic cavity during inspiration.

intercostal nerve: Somatic nerves that rise from the anterior divisions of the thoracic spinal nerves from T1 to T11. These nerves supply the thoracic wall, pleura (membranous sac that encloses the lungs and lines the thoracic cavity) and peritoneum (a large serous membrane that forms a closed sac within the abdominal cavity).

International Classification of Functioning, Disability and Health (ICF): A framework published by the World Health Organization and used to measure health and disability at individual and population levels. The ICF belongs to the WHO family of international classifications which includes the *International Classification of Diseases – Eleventh Edition* (ICD-11). While the ICD-11 gives users an aetiological framework for the classification, by diagnosis, of diseases, disorders and other health conditions, the ICF classifies functioning and disability associated with health conditions.

inversion: A syntactic operation in which two elements in a sentence change position with each other. For example, in order to form a *yes–no* interrogative in English, a speaker must invert the subject noun or pronoun and auxiliary verb in a sentence, e.g. *You are going to the pub* → *Are you going to the pub?*

irony: In conversation and other forms of discourse, speakers and writers can produce utterances which it is clear from context they do not believe to be true in order to convey an ironic attitude towards a situation or event. For example, the speaker who utters *What delightful weather we're having!* in the middle of a thunderstorm is intending to be ironic.

jitter: An acoustic characteristic of voice signals that is quantified as the cycle-to-cycle variations of fundamental frequency.

lamina propria: The middle of three layers of the vocal folds. The lamina propria sits above the vocalis muscle and below the epithelium. It contains deep, intermediate and superficial layers that differ in terms of their histology.

language decoding: The stage in the human communication cycle in which linguistic rules are used to analyse the phonological and syntactic structure and semantic content of utterances.

language delay: This is where children fail to exhibit expressive and receptive language skills at specific ages. Language delay is associated with poor academic achievement and behavioural problems in children.

language development: The stages through which young children pass on their way to acquiring full mastery of their native language. Some aspects of language development occur earlier than others. For example, while most phonological development takes place between 1 year 6 months and 4 years, pragmatic development extends into adolescence and young adulthood.

language disorder: The term used to describe a breakdown in the formulation or production of language (expressive language disorder) and the comprehension or understanding of language (receptive language disorder). In clinical terms, a language disorder is distinct from a speech disorder in that only the former deals with symbolic aspects of communication.

language encoding: The stage in the human communication cycle in which phonological, syntactic and semantic elements are selected in order to give linguistic expression to a communicative intention.

laryngeal apraxia: Also known as apraxia of phonation, laryngeal apraxia is a motor programming impairment that is isolated to the larynx. Supralaryngeal and respiratory components of speech production are not disrupted. This is confirmed by the use of an electrolarynx. When the need to switch phonation on and off is removed – as it is when an electrolarynx is used – normal speech production can be achieved.

laryngeal cancer: A malignant neoplasm can develop on any of the tissues of the larynx, resulting in laryngeal cancer or carcinoma. Most laryngeal cancers are squamous cell carcinomas. Smoking, acid reflux and human papillomavirus are aetiological factors. Depending on the location, type and size of a tumour, a combination of surgery (partial or total laryngectomy), radiotherapy and chemotherapy may be used in treatment.

laryngectomy: Surgical removal of the larynx either in whole (total laryngectomy) or in part (partial laryngectomy). A laryngectomy is most often undertaken to treat laryngeal cancer. Surgeons aim to conserve as much of the structure and function of the larynx as possible. For example, a supraglottic laryngectomy is performed to remove a laryngeal tumour that originates from the epiglottis, aryepiglottic folds and false vocal cords while minimizing morbidity and maintaining the three functions of the larynx (airway protection, respiration and phonation).

laryngology: A branch of medicine that specializes in voice disorders and diseases and injuries of the larynx. Laryngology is a sub-discipline of otorhinolaryngology.

laryngomalacia: A congenital abnormality in which there is supraglottic collapse of laryngeal cartilage during the inspiratory phase of respiration. This causes intermittent upper airway obstruction and stridor.

laryngopharyngeal reflux: An extraoesophageal variant of gastroesophageal reflux disease (GERD) that affects the larynx and pharynx. The acidic contents of the stomach make their way to the top of the oesophagus and spill over into the larynx. Laryngopharyngeal reflux has been linked to a number of vocal fold pathologies including laryngeal carcinoma.

laryngoscopy: A technique used to examine the larynx. In mirror laryngoscopy, the examining physician uses gauze to hold the end of the client's tongue while a laryngeal mirror is positioned just below the back of the soft palate as the patient says 'ee'. In patients where this procedure elicits a strong gag reflex, fibreoptic laryngoscopy may be a more appropriate technique. A flexible endoscope is passed transnasally into a position above the larynx. Insertion of the scope may be made more tolerable by the use of a local anaesthetic spray.

larynx: A muscular and cartilaginous structure that is lined with mucus membrane. The larynx is composed of nine pieces of hyaline cartilage. Its functions are to hold the respiratory tract open, to guard the lower respiratory tract against particulate matter, and to produce voice during speech production.

learning disability: see *intellectual disability*

left hemisphere: The left side of the brain or cerebrum. The left cerebral hemisphere controls the right side of the body so that a stroke or other neurological injury of this hemisphere can impair movement of the right arm and leg. In 97% of the population, language is represented in the left hemisphere. Accordingly, stroke-induced lesions of the left hemisphere can result in aphasia.

levator veli palatini: The primary muscles responsible for velar elevation during speech. The levator veli palatini muscles are innervated by the vagus nerve (CN X) and the spinal accessory nerve (CN XI). These muscles are aberrant in children with cleft palate, leading to velopharyngeal incompetence.

levodopa: A dopamine precursor that is an effective dopamine replacement agent used to treat Parkinson's disease. The clinical use of levodopa may be limited by complications such as response fluctuations, dyskinesia (a motor disturbance) and psychiatric problems.

lexical diversity: At its most general, lexical diversity describes the number of different words in a sample of speech or writing of a set length. On some definitions of lexical diversity, the difficulty or relative rarity of words is also taken into account. Measures of lexical diversity are taken to indicate the extent of an individual's vocabulary development (in a child) or residual lexical abilities (in an adult with acquired brain injury).

lexical reiteration: A form of lexical cohesion in which sentences are linked to each other through the repetition of words (*man . . . man*), the use of synonyms or near-synonyms (*disease . . . illness*), the use of a superordinate term (*poodle . . . dog*) or the use of a general word (*table . . . thing*). In the following sentences, a superordinate term (*animal*) links the second sentence to the first sentence: *The dog narrowly avoided the bus. The frightened animal was comforted by pedestrians.*

lexical relations: Semantic relations between lexemes in the same language. Lexical relations include synonymy (*liberty – freedom*), antonymy (*rich – poor*), meronymy (*eye – retina*) and hyponymy (*tulip – flower*).

lexical retrieval: The retrieval of words from a speaker's mental lexicon. Lexical retrieval is often impaired in people with aphasia. It may manifest itself in the use of non-specific vocabulary (e.g. *thing*, *stuff*), the use of words that are semantically related to the target word (semantic paraphasias) or a tendency to 'talk around' a target word (circumlocution).

lexical semantics: The branch of semantics that studies word meaning and meaning relations between words.

lexical stress: In any English word with more than one syllable, the syllables differ in their relative salience. Lexical or word stress is accentuation of syllables within words (e.g. *elephant*, *investigation*). Some lexical stresses are picked out for sentential stress known as 'accent', e.g. *Albert went to the zoo*.

limb apraxia: A disorder of motor planning in the absence of impaired muscle control that affects voluntary positioning and sequencing of muscle movements of the limbs.

linguistic competence: A native speaker's intuitive knowledge of the grammar of language, where 'grammar' is understood to include phonology, syntax and semantics. Chomsky distinguishes linguistic competence from performance.

literacy: There is no standard definition of literacy. All definitions include the ability to read and write to an appropriate level of fluency. Additionally, some definitions also make reference to the ability to speak and listen well.

lower motor neuron: These are neurons that directly innervate skeletal muscle. The cell bodies of these neurons are located in the ventral horns of the spinal cord or the motor nuclei of the brainstem.

macroglossia: A large tongue, which is a feature of several syndromes including Beckwith-Wiedemann syndrome and Down syndrome.

magnetoencephalography (MEG): A non-invasive neurophysiological technique that measures the magnetic fields generated by neuronal activity of the brain.

Makaton: A language programme that uses signs and symbols to help children and adults to communicate. Makaton is designed to support spoken language, with signs and symbols used alongside speech in spoken word order. Makaton can be used with clients who have no speech and with clients whose speech is unintelligible.

mandibulectomy: Partial or complete surgical removal of the mandible or lower jaw, typically on account of cancer. A mandibulectomy may be performed on its own or in combination with other surgical procedures (e.g. glossectomy).

manner of articulation: The approximation or constriction made between the active and passive articulators and the type of sound – plosives, fricatives, etc. – that this produces. In the Appendix, different manners of articulation are indicated on the vertical axis of the IPA chart.

manometry: Manometry is measurement of pressure in various parts of the gastrointestinal tract. Oesophageal manometry meaures the pressure in the upper and lower oesophageal sphincters, determines the effectiveness and coordination of propulsive movements and detects abnormal contractions. It can be used to identify motility disorders such as achalasia and is an investigative technique in the diagnosis of oesophageal dysphagia.

mastication: A sensorimotor activity that is aimed at the preparation of food for swallowing. Mastication or chewing is a complex process that involves facial, elevator and suprahyoidal muscles along with the tongue.

mastoid bone: The posterior component of the temporal bone. The mastoid bone contains a network of air cells. This air cell system may become infected (mastoiditis) when untreated or inadequately treated acute otitis media spreads from the middle ear into the mastoid bone.

mastoidectomy: A surgical procedure that results in the exposure of the mastoid air cells, middle ear space and ossicles. It may be undertaken to eradicate chronic infections of the ear and to remove cholesteatoma.

maxillofacial surgery: Oral and maxillofacial surgery is the medical specialism that is concerned with the diagnosis and treatment of diseases affecting the mouth, jaws, face and neck. Oral and maxillofacial surgeons treat children with cleft palate and other congenital anomalies, adults with head and neck cancers, and individuals who sustain a range of traumatic injuries.

maxim: A proposal of Grice in which four maxims of quality, quantity, relation and manner are used to give effect to the cooperative principle. Maxims can be flouted or not observed in various ways often with a view to generating implied meanings (implicatures).

mean length of utterance (MLU): An index of grammatical development that is measured in words or morphemes. As children acquire new grammatical knowledge (e.g. the addition of obligatory morphemes), the MLU of their utterances increases.

memory: A higher-order cognitive function in which there is storage and recall of different types of information. Some forms of memory relate specifically to language (e.g. semantic memory), some are defined by temporal characteristics (e.g. short-term and long-term memory) and some contain personal life events (e.g. autobiographical memory). There are different definitions of memory. For some theorists, working memory is the attention-related aspects of short-term memory, while for other theorists working memory includes short-term memory and other processing mechanisms that help to make use of short-term memory (Cowan, 2008). Injury and disease can disrupt specific types of memory. For example, impairment of episodic memory (i.e. recall of specific events) is a feature of Alzheimer's disease in the mild to moderate stages.

Ménière's disease: An inner ear disorder in which the symptoms are tinnitus, vertigo and deafness. The sensorineural hearing loss is low frequency and fluctuates.

meningitis: A bacterial or viral infection in which there is inflammation of the meninges, the membranes that envelope the brain and spinal cord.

Meningitis is a significant cause of developmental and acquired speech, language and hearing disorders.

mental status: A range of cortical functions contribute to an individual's mental status and are assessed as part of a mental status examination. Among these cortical functions are receptive and expressive language, praxis, orientation, judgement and visual recognition.

metaphor: A pragmatic phenomenon in which a speaker intends to describe an attribute of X by relating X to prominent features or characteristics of Y. For example, in the utterance *The rugby players were lions on the field*, a speaker does not intend to say that the players were actual lions, merely that the players were courageous, strong and fearless during a game of rugby.

micrognathia: A small lower jaw or mandible. Micrognathia is a feature of a number of syndromes (e.g. Pierre Robin syndrome). Where the position of the jaw causes compression of the trachea, a tracheostomy needs to be performed in order to protect the airway.

microtia: A small external ear or pinna. There are different grades of microtia, from an ear which is smaller than normal but has normal anatomy for the most part to the complete absence of the external ear and ear canal (anotia).

middle ear: A bony, air-filled cavity between the tympanic membrane and the inner ear. The middle ear contains the ossicles – malleus, incus and stapes – that mechanically transmit and amplify vibrations from the tympanic membrane to the cochlea. It also communicates with the nasopharynx via the Eustachian tube.

middle ear cleft: This structure comprises the Eustachian tube, middle ear cavity and the mastoid air cell system.

mild cognitive impairment: A condition in which individuals have more memory or other cognitive problems for their age, but their symptoms do not affect functioning. Mild cognitive impairment can be, but is not always, a sign of progressive decline to dementia.

minimal pair: Two words that differ in meaning and also differ by a single segment, e.g. *light* [laɪt] and *like* [laɪk].

modularity: The view that a series of modules are responsible for cognitive functions such as language and perception. On some versions of modularity, modules are specialized to process one type of data (e.g. visual perceptual data), are innate and exhibit informational encapsulation, among a number of other features. The modularity of mind thesis was originally proposed by the philosopher of psychology, Jerry Fodor.

monoloudness: A lack of normal variation of vocal intensity during speech production. Monoloudness is a feature of hypokinetic dysarthria in Parkinson's disease.

monophthong: A single or simple vowel sound that forms the nucleus of a syllable. During articulation of a monophthong, the tongue is more or less static and the pitch of the sound is relatively constant.

monopitch: A lack of normal variation of fundamental frequency during speech production. Monopitch is a feature of hypokinetic dysarthria in Parkinson's disease.

morpheme: The smallest meaningful unit of a word. Free morphemes can occur on their own and are thus words (e.g. *fly*, *cat*). Bound morphemes cannot exist in isolation and must be attached to other morphemes (e.g. un*happy*, *agree*able).

morphology: The linguistic discipline that studies the internal structure of words and the patterns and principles that underlie their composition. The morpheme is the unit of analysis.

morphosyntax: The intersection between morphology and syntax. Morphosyntax is impaired in certain clients who are assessed and treated by speech and language therapists, e.g. children with specific language impairment.

motor development: The development of gross motor skills (e.g. walking) and fine motor skills (e.g. writing) in childhood. Motor development is delayed in children with a range of developmental disorders and syndromes. SLTs record information about motor development during the taking of a case history.

motor milestone: These are key landmarks in a child's development of gross and fine motor skills. They include achievements such as the ability to sit without support (gross motor milestone) and use the thumb and fingertips to grasp objects (fine motor milestone). Large-scale studies of normally developing children have established 'windows' in a child's development during which these milestones are achieved.

motor neurone disease: A progressive neurodegenerative disease in which there is a widespread and often rapid deterioration of upper and lower motor neurones. Motor neurone disease (MND) affects all aspects of speech production and eventually swallowing and feeding. There are three types of MND: amyotrophic lateral sclerosis; progressive bulbar palsy; and progressive muscular atrophy.

motor speech disorder: An impairment of speech production which may arise as a result of disruption in motor programming (apraxia of speech) and/or motor execution (dysarthria). Motor speech disorders may be developmental or acquired in nature and can result in mild to severe unintelligibility.

motor speech execution: The stage in the human communication cycle in which the muscles of the articulatory, resonatory, phonatory and respiratory mechanisms perform the movements that are required to produce speech.

motor speech programming: The stage in the human communication cycle in which there is planning of the movements of the articulatory, resonatory, phonatory and respiratory mechanisms for speech production.

multidisciplinary team: In healthcare, the multidisciplinary team is composed of individuals with specialized skills and expertise from different medical and health professions. These individuals work together to make treatment recommendations that facilitate high-quality patient care.

multilingualism: The use of more than two languages by an individual. Figures for the worldwide prevalence of multilingualism do not exist. Like bilingualism, multilingualism raises special issues in relation to language development and disorders and the recovery and treatment of language in conditions such as trilingual aphasia.

multiple negation: The use of two or more negative markers, e.g. *I didn't do nothing*. While single negation is a feature of Standard English (e.g. *I didn't do anything*), multiple negation is a feature of African American Vernacular English and other vernacular English dialects.

multiple sclerosis (MS): An autoimmune disease in which there is demyelination of neurones in the central nervous system. There are three forms of MS: primary progressive; secondary progressive; and relapsing-remitting. Dysarthria, dysphagia and cognitive impairment are present in a significant number of individuals with MS.

muscle tension dysphonia: A hyperfunctional voice disorder in which there is strained-strangled voice quality similar to that of adductor spasmodic dysphonia. There is the appearance of excessive tension in the neck area and associated laryngeal hyperfunction. The patient frequently reports vocal fatigue.

mutism: Speechlessness, which can have a neurological or behavioural aetiology. Mutism is a feature of many clinical conditions including childhood posterior fossa tumour, traumatic brain injury, dementia and Landau-Kleffner syndrome.

narrative discourse: A type of spoken or written discourse in which the events of a story are narrated to a listener or reader. The events so narrated are normally in the past and typically involve one or more actors.

nasal emission: Nasal (air) emission occurs when there is an attempt to build up intraoral air pressure for the production of consonants, but air escapes through the velopharyngeal port or oronasal fistulae. Nasal emission can be audible or inaudible, and can occur with hypernasality or with normal resonance.

nasal turbulence: Nasal turbulence is the most severe form of audible nasal emission. It is sometimes referred to as 'nasal rustle'. Nasal turbulence is associated with a smaller size of velopharyngeal gap compared to that in speakers with hypernasality. The smaller velopharyngeal gap results in increased friction as air is forced through it.

nasogastric tube: A plastic tubing device that allows delivery of nutritionally complete feed directly into the stomach or removal of stomach contents. A nasogastric tube is used for feeding purposes in babies, children and adults who have inadequate or unsafe oral intake.

nasometer: see *nasometry*

nasometry: An objective technique used to measure the acoustic correlate of nasality. The nasometer produces a score that represents the ratio of energy in oral and nasal acoustic sound signals. Nasometry can be used to supplement the perception of hypernasal resonance in clients with velopharyngeal insufficiency.

nasopharynx: The part of the pharynx that lies below the skull base and opens into the oropharynx. The pharyngeal tonsils are located in its posterior wall and the Eustachian tubes open into its side walls. The nasopharynx has a ciliated lining that moves mucous and debris downwards for swallowing.

nativism: The view that the capacity to acquire a first language is innate and hard-wired at birth. According to nativists, children are born with an ability to organize laws of language, and it is this ability that enables them for the most part to acquire their native language with ease.

near infrared spectroscopy (NIRS): A non-invasive technique for examining brain tissue function. Light in the near infrared frequency range can penetrate a centimetre or two into the typical adult brain. This technique can be used to measure cerebral blood flow.

neck stoma: An artificial opening in the neck through which a patient breathes following laryngectomy. Because the opening leads directly into the trachea, there are none of the defences provided by the oral and nasal cavities in the speaker with normal anatomy. For example, the nasal cavities normally filter air and add moisture to it. In their absence, potentially infectious agents may enter the stoma. Continual stoma care is needed to keep the stoma clean and free of infection. The stoma is occluded during tracheoesophageal voice production.

negative symptom: The loss or diminution of normal functions. The negative symptoms of schizophrenia include blunted affect, alogia (poverty of speech), asociality, avolition (lack of self-initiated and purposeful acts) and anhedonia (diminished capacity to experience pleasure). See *positive symptom*.

neurodevelopmental disorder: A disorder that arises on account of anomalies in the development of the central nervous system. Two common neurodevelopmental disorders are autism spectrum disorder and attention deficit hyperactivity disorder.

neurogenic communication disorder: Any communication disorder caused by neurological impairment, injury or disease. Dysarthria, apraxia of speech and aphasia are all neurogenic communication disorders.

neurogenic dysphagia: see *dysphagia*

neurogenic stuttering: The onset of dysfluency in adults as a result of neurological injury, typically caused by a cerebrovascular accident.

neurologist: The medical specialist who practises neurology. See *neurology*.

neurology: The branch of medicine concerned with the study, assessment and treatment of disorders of the nervous system.

neuropragmatics: A branch of neurolinguistics that examines the neural substrates of pragmatic phenomena such as irony and metaphor interpretation. The emergence of this discipline has been facilitated by recent advances in brain imaging techniques such as fMRI.

neuropsychologist: The professional who specializes in neuropsychology. See *neuropsychology*.

neuropsychology: The study of the relationship between brain structure and behaviour. Neuropsychology has experimental, cognitive and clinical sub-disciplines. One of the sub-disciplines most relevant to SLT – clinical neuropsychology – is concerned with the assessment and rehabilitation of individuals with impaired function following brain injury, illness or trauma.

neurosurgery: The medical specialism concerned with the diagnosis and surgical treatment of disorders of the central nervous system (CNS) and peripheral nervous system (PNS). These disorders include congenital anomalies, trauma, tumours, vascular disorders, infections and degenerative diseases of the CNS and PNS.

noise-induced hearing loss: A form of sensorineural hearing loss that is caused by exposure to noise, resulting in damage to the hair cells in the cochlea. On an audiogram, noise-induced hearing loss appears as an audiometric notch at 4 kHz, with better hearing at frequencies above and below this notch.

noise-to-harmonics ratio: The amplitude of noise relative to tonal components in speech. The noise-to-harmonics ratio is an acoustic measure that is used in an assessment of clients with dysphonia.

non-oral feeding: When oral feeding is assessed to be unsafe (e.g. a patient is at risk of aspiration), non-oral feeding may be instituted. This may be achieved through the use of a percutaneous endoscopic gastrostomy (PEG) feeding tube. A flexible feeding tube is placed through the abdominal wall and into the stomach. This allows nutrition, fluids and medications to enter the stomach directly, thus bypassing the mouth and oesophagus.

Noonan syndrome: A genetic disorder that occurs in approximately 1 in 1,000 to 2,500 people. Individuals with Noonan syndrome display mildly unusual facial characteristics, short stature, heart defects, bleeding problems and skeletal malformations among other problems. Most children with Noonan syndrome have normal intellectual abilities. However, a small number exhibit special educational needs and have intellectual disability.

norm-referenced test: A standardized test in which a client's performance is compared to the performance of another group of individuals known as the normative group. This group is a representative sample of individuals of the same age, sex, etc. as the client.

nosology: The branch of medical science that deals with the classification of diseases.

occupational impact: see *vocational impact*

occupational therapist: The health professional who assesses and treats clients with a range of conditions that limit their ability to engage in activities of daily living. These activities include an occupation as narrowly defined, but also a range of leisure activities and activities related to personal care.

oesophageal dysphagia: see *dysphagia*

oesophageal speech: A form of extralaryngeal communication used by clients following laryngectomy. Air is brought down into the oesophagus and released under control. As it passes through the upper oesophageal sphincter, the sphincter vibrates to produce a source of voice for speech production. Oesophageal speech may be used as the only method of communication or alongside other forms of extralaryngeal communication (e.g. an electrolarynx).

oesophagectomy: Surgical removal of all or part of the oesophagus, usually in order to treat oesophageal cancer. The top of the stomach is connected to the remaining part of the oesophagus, either directly or with a section of intestine serving as a bridge between the two. Oesophagectomy may be performed in isolation or alongside other procedures such as glossectomy and laryngectomy.

oesophagitis: An inflammation of the lining of the oesophagus that may be caused by infections (e.g. candida albicans), gastroesophageal reflux disease (GERD), drugs (e.g. aspirin) and a high concentration of white blood cells related to allergic reactions (eosinophilic oesophagitis).

oesophagoscopy: A procedure in which a flexible endoscope is inserted through the mouth, or less commonly the nose, into the oesophagus.

oesophagus: A muscular tube that is 18 to 25cm long in adults from the upper sphincter to the lower sphincter. The oesophagus can distend to approximately 2 cm in the anterior-posterior dimension and up to 3cm laterally to accommodate a swallowed bolus. The wall of the oesophagus is composed of striated muscle in the upper part, smooth muscle in the lower part and both types of muscle in the middle.

olfaction: The sense of smell.

oncologist: The medical specialist who practises oncology. See *oncology*.

oncology: The branch of medicine that assesses, diagnoses and treats cancer. There are different sub-disciplines in oncology: medical oncology (the use of chemotherapy, hormone therapy and other drugs to treat cancer); radiation oncology (the use of radiation therapy to treat cancer); and surgical oncology (the use of surgery and other procedures to treat cancer).

oral apraxia: A disorder of the motor programming of movements required to produce non-speech, oral movements. Oral apraxia may occur in isolation or alongside apraxia of speech.

oral cancer: Any malignant neoplasm of the tongue, lips, palate, jaw and gums. Human papillomavirus, tobacco and alcohol consumption are aetiological factors in the development of oral cancer.

oral cavity: The oral cavity is bounded anteriorly by the lips, laterally by the cheeks, superiorly by the hard palate and inferiorly by the mucosa covering the superior surface of the tongue and the sheet of muscles attaching to the inner side of the mandible. The oral cavity has speech and vegetative (respiration and ingestion) functions.

oral feeding: The ingestion of food and liquid through the oral cavity and then onwards through the digestive tract. See *non-oral feeding*.

orbicularis oris: The sphincter muscle that encircles the upper and lower lips. Contraction of this muscle closes the mouth and puckers the lips as in whistling. The orbicularis oris is innervated by the facial nerve (CN VII).

organ of Corti: The receptor organ for hearing in the cochlea in the inner ear. The organ of Corti consists of hair cells that are displaced by the movement of fluid in the cochlea when the stapes footplate acts against the oval window. An electrophysiological response in the hair cells results in nervous impulse transmission to the auditory cortices of the brain via the vestibulocochlear nerve.

organic voice disorder: Any voice disorder that is caused by an abnormal structural finding in the larynx (e.g. laryngeal cancer) or a systemic medical or neurological condition (e.g. stroke-induced vocal fold paralysis).

oropharyngeal dysphagia: see *dysphagia*

orthodontics: The dental specialty concerned with facial growth, development of dentition and occlusion, and the assessment, diagnosis and treatment of malocclusions and facial irregularities.

orthography: The linguistic study of written language including letters, punctuation marks and spelling. Also, an orthography is a systematic, standardized writing system for a particular language.

ossicle: The ear ossicles are the malleus, incus and stapes in the middle ear. The ossicles are the smallest bones in the human body. They are responsible for the conversion of sound waves into mechanical vibrations which are transmitted to the oval window.

otitis media: A middle ear condition commonly known as 'glue ear'. Inadequate ventilation of the middle ear by the Eustachian tube results in the production of mucus. The build-up of mucus impedes movement of the ossicular chain, leading to a conductive hearing loss. Otitis media is a common ear problem in children with cleft palate.

otolaryngologist: The medical specialist who practises otolaryngology or ENT medicine.

otolaryngology: see *otorhinolaryngology*

otorhinolaryngology: The branch of medicine that assesses, diagnoses and treats diseases of the ears, nose and throat. This discipline is known as ENT medicine in the UK.

otosclerosis: A middle ear condition in which new bone growth on the anterior stapes footplate disrupts the functioning of the ossicular chain and causes conductive hearing loss. Otosclerosis can be treated through a surgical procedure known as stapedectomy.

paediatrician: The medical specialist who practises paediatric medicine. See *paediatrics*.

paediatrics: The medical specialty that is concerned with the physical, mental and social health of children from birth to young adulthood.

palatal lift: A prosthesis which is used in patients with velopharyngeal incompetence resulting from compromised motor control of the soft palate and related musculature in conditions such as cleft palate, cerebrovascular accidents and traumatic brain injuries. The appliance works by displacing the soft palate to the level of normal palatal elevation. This allows closure of the velopharyngeal port to be achieved by pharyngeal wall action.

palliative care: The active holistic care of patients with advanced progressive illnesses such as cancer and neurodegenerative diseases (e.g. motor neurone disease). The management of symptoms (e.g. pain) and the provision of psychological and other support are central to this care.

Parkinson's disease: A neurodegenerative disease caused by the loss of cells that produce dopamine (a neurotransmitter substance) in the substantia nigra of the brain. There are four forms of parkinsonism: idiopathic Parkinson's; multiple system atrophy; progressive supranuclear palsy; and drug-induced parkinsonism. Dysarthria is commonly seen in Parkinson's disease with reduced vocal intensity a common and early feature of the disorder.

partial cricotracheal resection: A surgical procedure that is used to treat subglottic stenosis, a common laryngeal anomaly in children. During this procedure, the whole diseased segment of the airway is resected.

particularization: According to generative grammar, particularization is the process whereby a child's in-built theory of universal grammar comes to reflect the grammar of the language of the speech community in which the child lives.

passive articulator: An articulator that makes little or no movement during the production of speech sounds. Passive articulators are largely immobile because they are connected to the skull. They include the upper lip, upper teeth, upper surface of the oral cavity and back wall of the pharynx.

pathogenesis: The origin and development of a disease.

perception: The process by means of which sensory stimuli are recognized or interpreted. Agnosias occur when perception is disrupted. For example, auditory verbal agnosia – the inability to recognize the spoken form of words – occurs in Landau-Kleffner syndrome.

percutaneous endoscopic gastrostomy (PEG): A procedure in which endoscopy is used to guide the insertion of a tube into the stomach via the abdominal wall. A PEG tube provides enteral feeding to patients who have functionally normal gastrointestinal tracts but who cannot meet their nutritional needs because of inadequate oral intake.

performative verb: A verb that indicates the illocutionary force of an utterance. For example, the performative verb 'bet' in the utterance *I bet you ten* *pounds that Golden Star will win* indicates that this utterance has the illocutionary force of a bet.

peripheral nervous system: The part of the nervous system that consists of the nerves that branch out from the brain and spinal cord. The peripheral nervous system is further subdivided into the somatic nervous system (nerves that go to the skin and muscles and that mediate conscious activities) and the autonomic nervous system (nerves that connect the central nervous system to visceral organs such as the heart and that mediate unconscious activities).

pharyngectomy: Surgical removal of all or part of the pharynx to treat pharyngeal cancer. Malignant neoplasms may arise in the nasopharynx (e.g. adenoids), oropharynx or hypopharynx (e.g. pyriform sinuses). Pharyngectomy may be performed in isolation or alongside other procedures, e.g. laryngectomy.

pharynx: The pharynx is the space shared by the respiratory system and digestive tract. It is divided into three areas: the nasopharynx, the oropharynx and the hypopharynx. The nasopharynx is located behind the nasal cavities and belongs entirely to the respiratory tract. The oropharynx opens into the oral cavity anteriorly and into the hypopharynx inferiorly. The hypopharynx extends from the base of the tongue to the apex of the pyriform sinuses.

phenotype: The observable traits of an individual such as blood type, height and eye colour. The physical characteristics associated with the expression of genes.

phonation: The production of voice by the larynx. Phonation is a speech production subsystem which may be impaired in speech and voice disorders.

phonetics: The study of human speech sounds according to how they are made (articulatory phonetics), their physical properties (acoustic phonetics) and how they are perceived (speech perception).

phonological awareness: The ability to conceive of spoken words as sequences of sound segments that correspond to written units and to access and manipulate those segments. Phonological awareness is a metalinguistic ability that requires knowledge of different sizes of phonological segments of spoken words (e.g. phonemes, syllables) as well as the conscious ability to manipulate (blend, segment, etc.) those phonological units.

phonological development: The stage in language development during which a child establishes the sound system of his or her native language. In normally developing children, most phonological development occurs between 1 year 6 months and 4 years.

phonological disorder: see *developmental phonological disorder*

phonological feature: Phonemes or segments are not indivisible units but are composed of phonological features. These features distinguish phonemes. For example, /t/ and /d/ share the features [− continuant] [− sonorant] and

[+ coronal]. They differ in the feature [voiced] with /t/ [− voiced] and /d/ [+ voiced].

phonological process: Sound and syllable simplification processes that are a feature of the speech of normally developing children and children with speech sound disorders. Examples of phonological processes are stopping (e.g. *five* [paɪb]), fronting (e.g. *cake* [teɪk]) and consonant cluster reduction (e.g. *green* [gin]).

phonology: The study of the organization of speech sounds into systems. Phonologists examine how particular sounds are used to distinguish between words (e.g. *pat – bat*). The phoneme is the unit of analysis.

phrenic nerve: These nerves arise from the ventral rami of C3, C4 and C5. They course through the neck and thorax to provide motor innervation to the diaphragm and sensory innervation to the diaphragmatic pleura, pericardium (membrane around the heart) and subdiaphragmatic pleura.

physiology: The study of how cells, tissues and organisms function. Along with anatomy, physiology is an essential biological discipline for study by SLTs.

physiotherapist: The health professional who assesses, diagnoses and treats individuals who experience movement disorders as a result of illness, injury or disability. Through movement and exercise, manual therapy, education and advice, physiotherapists can help clients with these disorders maintain independence and improve their quality of life.

Piaget, Jean: A Swiss psychologist (1896–1980) who undertook the first systematic study of cognitive development in children. The four stages in this development are the sensorimotor stage (birth to 2 years), the preoperational stage (2 to 6 or 7 years), the concrete operational stage (7 to 11 or 12 years) and the formal operational stage (12 years into adulthood).

Pierre Robin syndrome: This syndrome is characterized by micrognathia (severe underdevelopment of the mandible) and glossoptosis (falling back of the tongue) that causes airway obstruction and respiratory distress. Approximately half of children with this syndrome can present with an incomplete cleft of the palate.

pitch: The perceptual correlate of fundamental frequency. Vocal pitch is a feature of prosody. Monopitch is a prosodic disturbance in hypokinetic and flaccid dysarthria.

place of articulation: The location in the vocal tract where there is a primary obstruction to the airstream, e.g. [p] bilabial, [t] alveolar, [k] velar and [ʔ] glottal. In the Appendix, different places of articulation are indicated on the horizontal axis of the IPA chart.

positive symptom: The presence of abnormal behaviour in schizophrenia. Positive symptoms include delusions (the holding of false and bizarre beliefs), hallucinations (the perception of things that do not exist) and disorganized speech or thought disorder. Auditory hallucinations are more common than visual hallucinations in individuals with schizophrenia. See *negative symptom*.

positron emission tomography (PET): A specialized radiology procedure that uses a radioactive substance (a radionuclide) to evaluate the metabolism of a particular organ or tissue. PET is most commonly used in the fields of neurology, oncology and cardiology.

poverty of speech: Also known as alogia. Poverty of speech describes the substantially reduced verbal output that is a negative symptom of schizophrenia.

pragmatic development: The developmental stages through which children pass on their way to acquiring full mastery of pragmatic aspects of language such as speech acts, deixis and implicatures. Pragmatic development extends well beyond the point at which rule-based or structural aspects of the language system (e.g. syntax) are established.

pragmatic language impairment: A successor to the term *semantic-pragmatic disorder*. Pragmatic language impairment describes a subgroup of children with specific language impairment in which there are marked difficulties with the pragmatics of language. The label 'social (pragmatic) communication disorder' is used in DSM-5 to describe individuals with pragmatic language impairment. See *social (pragmatic) communication disorder*.

pragmatics: The study of language use and aspects of meaning that are dependent on context. Pragmatic meaning is variously referred to as speaker meaning, implied meaning, non-literal meaning and non-truth-conditional meaning.

prefixation: A word-formation process in which a bound lexical morpheme is attached to the front of a base (e.g. dishonour, unreal).

presbycusis: Sensorineural hearing loss that results from the deterioration of the cochlea and auditory nerve as a consequence of the natural ageing process. The hearing loss is mostly high frequency in nature.

presbylarynx: Literally 'old larynx', a voice disorder that is the result of degenerative, age-related changes in the larynx. In presbylarynx, the vocal folds close at the front and back but fail to adduct in the middle. This leads to a rapid loss of air through the glottis during phonation with consequent reduction of phonation time. Other glottic characteristics of presbylarynx include prominence of the vocal processes and a spindle-shaped glottic chink.

presupposition: This describes information that is assumed, taken for granted or in the background of an utterance. Presuppositions reduce the amount of information that a speaker must explicitly state. They are triggered by certain lexical items (e.g. factive verbs *She realised the situation was hopeless*) and constructions (e.g. cleft construction *It was the boy who broke the window*).

prevalence: The total number of individuals in a population who have a disease or health condition at a specific period of time. Prevalence is usually expressed as a percentage of the population.

primary CNS lymphoma: A non-Hodgkin's lymphoma that arises within, and is restricted to, the nervous system. Although it may involve the leptomeninges (arachnoid membrane and pia mater), eyes, spinal cord, or any combination of these sites, it usually presents as a brain tumour.

primary motor cortex: Located in the precentral gyrus (Brodmann's area 4), the primary motor cortex is essential for the voluntary control of movement. It is a major source of descending projections to motor neurones in the spinal cord and cranial nerve nuclei.

primary progressive aphasia: A slowly progressive aphasia that occurs initially in the absence of generalized dementia. As speech and language impairments in primary progressive aphasia (PPA) worsen over time, patients begin to exhibit more of the classical symptoms of dementia. PPA is associated with a number of neuropathologies including Alzheimer's disease, frontotemporal dementia, Lewy body dementia and vascular dementia. Three subtypes of PPA are recognized: non-fluent/agrammatic, logopenic and semantic PPA. The non-fluent/agrammatic variant of primary progressive aphasia is also known as progressive non-fluent aphasia.

problem-solving: A cognitive skill that involves the identification and resolution of problems. Problem-solving is an executive function. As such, it is often impaired in clients with executive dysfunction.

professional voice user: Any individual who uses their voice professionally. Professional voice users include singers, actors, public speakers, fitness instructors, teachers and lecturers. Because of the high professional demands on their speaking and singing voices, these occupational groups are at risk of developing laryngeal pathologies such as vocal nodules.

prognosis: The probability or risk of an individual developing a particular state of health (an outcome) over a specific period of time given that individual's clinical and non-clinical profile. An outcome may include an event such as death or a quantity such as disease progression.

progressive nonfluent aphasia: see *primary progressive aphasia*

prolongation: see *stuttering*

prolonged speech: A speech pattern that is learned in fluency-shaping stuttering therapies. The main features of prolonged speech are syllable prolongations, gentle voice onsets, smooth sound transitions and light articulatory contacts.

prosody: The study of the suprasegmental features of speech such as stress and intonation. Prosody can be divided into linguistic prosody, which is the means by which speakers can clarify potentially ambiguous syntax, and affective or emotional prosody, which allows speakers to express attitudes and emotions.

proximal aetiology: Aetiological factors that are the most immediate cause of a disease or disorder. For example, intellectual disability is a proximal aetiology of language disorder in children with genetic syndromes such as fragile X syndrome (FXS). The genetic anomalies that cause these syndromes – in the case of FXS, the fragile X mental retardation 1 gene on the X chromosome – are the distal aetiology of language disorder.

psychiatrist: The medical specialist who practises psychiatry. see *psychiatry*.

psychiatry: The medical specialty that assesses, diagnoses and treats mental, emotional and behavioural disorders.

psychogenic dysphonia: The loss of voice in the absence of apparent structural or neurological pathology. Psychogenic dysphonias such as conversion aphonia are usually associated with traumatic life events and emotional difficulties.

psychogenic stuttering: The onset of dysfluency in adulthood subsequent to a traumatic event or other psychological stressor.

psychological impact: Communication and swallowing disorders can have adverse consequences for an individual's mental health and psychological well-being. The psychological impact of these disorders may include depression, anxiety and low self-esteem.

psychometric test: A formal, standardized test that is designed to measure an aspect of mental performance. This may be memory, perception, reasoning and problem-solving skills. Psychometric tests are also used to assess personality attributes.

psychopathology: This term describes the origin of mental disorders, how they develop and their symptoms. A range of professionals, including psychiatrists, psychologists and counsellors, are interested in the study and management of psychopathology.

psychotherapy: A general term to describe a number of treatments for mental health problems by talking to a psychiatrist, psychologist or other mental health professional.

puberphonia: Also known as mutational falsetto, this voice disorder is typically seen in adolescent males who continue to speak with a pre-pubescent voice beyond the point at which voice mutation occurs.

pure tone audiometry: The most commonly performed hearing test, this pure tone air conduction procedure gives a record of hearing level by frequency (125–8 k Hz). Sound is delivered to the ear canal via headphones or ear inserts, and results are graphed on an audiogram.

pyramidal system: The motor system that controls all voluntary movements. The pyramidal tract consists of two types of neurone: upper motor neurones and lower motor neurones. The upper motor neurones extend from the primary motor cortex to the spinal cord. The lower motor neurones extend from the anterior horn of the spinal cord to the skeletal muscles.

pyriform sinus: The pyriform sinus is part of the hypopharynx. It is a funnel-shaped structure that begins superiorly at the glossoepiglottic fold and extends inferiorly with its apex at the level of the cricopharyngeus. It is bounded laterally by the thyroid lamina and posteriorly by the lateral wall of the hypopharynx. Its medial boundary is the lateral surface of the arytenoid.

quality of life: The World Health Organization defines 'quality of life' as individuals' perception of their position in life in the context of the culture and value systems in which they live and in relation to their goals, expectations, standards and concerns. It is a broad-ranging concept affected in a complex way by the person's physical health, psychological state, level of independence, social relationships, personal beliefs and their relationship to salient features of their environment (WHO, 1997).

radiotherapy: The use of high-energy radiation to shrink tumours and kill cancer cells. X-rays, gamma rays and charged particles are types of radiation that are used in radiotherapy. A machine outside the body may deliver the radiation (external-beam radiation therapy). Alternatively, it may be delivered from radioactive material that is placed in the body (internal radiation therapy or brachytherapy).

randomized controlled trial: A study design in which participants are randomly assigned to an experimental group or a control group. Because the groups are treated in exactly the same way with the exception of the experimental treatment that is under investigation, any difference in the outcomes of the two groups can be attributed to the intervention.

reasoning: A higher-order cognitive function in which individuals draw specific conclusions from general principles or premises (deductive reasoning) or general principles from specific instances (inductive reasoning). Aside from deduction and induction, there are also presumptive or plausible forms of reasoning.

receptive language disorder: see *language disorder*

receptive syntax: see *syntax*

receptive vocabulary: see *vocabulary*

recruitment: The abnormally rapid growth of perceived loudness as intensity of sound increases. Recruitment is thought to be a hallmark of cochlear dysfunction and is a feature of a number of disorders including presbycusis and Ménière's disease.

recurrent laryngeal nerve: A branch of the vagus nerve (CN X) that supplies all the intrinsic muscles of the larynx with the exception of the cricothyroid muscles.

reference: The use of a linguistic expression to identify things in the external world. Reference is an important concept in a semantic account of meaning (hence, the term *referential meaning*).

referent: The object or event in the external world that is identified by an act of reference.

reflux laryngitis: Inflammation of laryngeal mucosa and presence of dysphonia related to acid reflux from the oesophagus entering the larynx.

register: Also known as *register variation*, register describes how language can vary to reflect changes in situation or context. On some definitions, register is used to capture variation based on aspects of people's identities that are not permanent, such as occupations (use of legalese by lawyers) and temporary roles (use of baby-talk by an adult who is interacting with a child).

reliability: An attribute of a test or assessment that captures its consistency across repeated measures of the same phenomenon. A reliable test is one in which the results obtained are replicable, i.e. different examiners report similar scores for the same individuals.

repetition: see *stuttering*

respiration: Inhalation and exhalation during breathing. Respiration is one of the speech production subsystems. Impairments of respiration can lead to reduced breath support for speech in neurodegenerative diseases (e.g. motor neurone disease) and other conditions (e.g. cerebral palsy).

respiratory therapist: A healthcare practitioner who assesses, diagnoses, monitors and treats patients who suffer from dysfunctions of the cardiopulmonary system, including any disease or disorder that has a negative impact on breathing and lung capacity.

response inhibition: The suppression of actions that are inappropriate in a given context and interfere with goal-directed behaviour. Executive control processes are critical to response inhibition. When these processes are impaired (e.g. in clients with traumatic brain injury), response inhibition is poor as a result.

Rett syndrome: A neurodevelopmental disorder caused by a mutation in the MECP2 gene. It affects girls almost exclusively. Normal early growth and development is followed by a slowing of development, loss of purposeful use of the hands and distinctive hand movements. There is slowed brain and head growth, problems with walking, seizures and intellectual disability.

right hemisphere: The right cerebral hemisphere of the brain. Damage to the right cerebral hemisphere can (occasionally) cause aphasia and may result in deficits in pragmatic and discourse skills. The right hemisphere also plays an important role in prosody and processing of emotions.

right-hemisphere damage: see *right-hemisphere language disorder*

right-hemisphere language disorder: Stroke-induced and other lesions in the right hemisphere of the brain produce a different pattern of language impairment from that which occurs in left-hemisphere damage. Structural language is often intact. However, significant impairments in pragmatics and discourse can compromise many aspects of communication.

sarcasm: see *irony*

scala tympani: The perilymph-filled lower chamber in the cochlea of the inner ear. The scala tympani connects to the scala vestibuli by means of an opening called the helicotrema at the apex of the cochlea.

schizophrenia: A serious mental illness that is diagnosed on the basis of positive and negative symptoms. Positive symptoms include thought disorder, delusions and hallucinations (mostly auditory). Negative symptoms include affective flattening, poverty of speech, apathy, avolition and social withdrawal.

selective attention: see *attention*

self-esteem: A person's overall subjective emotional evaluation of his or her own worth. Poor self-esteem is a feature of many primary communication disorders (e.g. specific language impairment) and conditions that can cause communication disorders (e.g. traumatic brain injury and stroke).

semantic component: The approach of componential analysis in semantics aims to analyse word meaning in terms of a number of semantic components or primitives. For example, the word *bachelor* may be analysed in terms of three components [UNMARRIED] [ADULT] [MALE].

semantic dementia: A form of frontotemporal dementia in which there is progressive bilateral degeneration of the temporal lobes. The most pronounced feature of this form of dementia is degradation of semantic knowledge, which is evident across all modalities (e.g. written and spoken language) and modes of input and output (e.g. comprehension and expression).

semantic development: The acquisition of word and sentence meaning by young children. Children's first words relate to objects and people in their immediate environment. There are different theories of lexical acquisition according to which children learn words by identifying what objects they refer to (associationism) or by reading the referential intentions of speakers when they use words (theory of mind). Children first begin to express aspects of sentence semantics in the two-word stage of language development when utterances such as *spoon dirty* are used to express the semantic relation entity + attribute.

semantic memory: A store of knowledge about people, objects, actions, relations, self and culture that is acquired through experience. We draw on semantic memory when we state that a dog is a mammal with four legs and a tail. Semantic memory is degraded in adults with semantic dementia, the temporal lobe variant of frontotemporal dementia.

semantic network: Used to represent simple knowledge about animals, people and objects and the relations between them. These relations may be one of subclass (e.g. mammal is a subclass of animal), instance (e.g. Moby is an instance of guppy) and property (e.g. fin is a property of fish). These relations permit certain inferences to be drawn. For example, we can infer that Moby has fins. This is because Moby is a guppy which is a subclass of fish and fish have fins as a property.

semantic paraphasia: A language error in which a word that is semantically related to the target form is produced (e.g. 'ear' for *eye*). Semantic paraphasias are a feature of aphasia in adults.

semantic relation: The emergence of two-word utterances during language development permits the expression of semantic relations by children for the first time. These relations include agent + action (*Mummy sleep*), possessor + possession (*Daddy coat*) and action + affected (*drop teddy*).

Children with intellectual disability also express these same semantic relations but at a delayed rate.

semantic role: Semantic roles describe different entities in a situation and are associated with the argument structure of verbs, e.g. The flash of lightning$_{STIMULUS}$ blinded the onlookers$_{EXPERIENCER}$. Some semantic roles are obligatory in the argument structure of verbs (e.g. agent), while others are optional (e.g. instrument).

semantics: The study of the linguistic meaning of words (lexical semantics) and sentences.

semicircular canal: The inner ear organ that senses head rotations. There are three semicircular canals. Each has a bulbous expansion called the ampulla that contains the crista, hair bundles and cupula. When the head rotates, the cupula is distorted by the fluid in the canal.

sense: The sense of an expression is its place in a system of semantic relationships with other expressions in a language. Many words have multiple senses. When these senses are related, they are known as polysemous senses (e.g. *arm* 'part of body' versus 'part of chair'). When these senses are unrelated, they are known as homonymous senses (e.g. *bark* 'cry of a dog' versus 'outer layer of tree'). Polysemy and homonymy are the basis of lexical ambiguity, e.g. *The arm was broken in two places* (human arm or arm of chair was broken in two places).

sensorineural hearing loss: Hearing loss that is related to cochlear damage, impairment of the auditory pathway to the brain and damage of the auditory cortices in the brain. Possible causes of sensorineural hearing loss include infections such as meningitis, trauma and cerebrovascular accidents.

sexual dimorphism: The existence of physical differences between males and females of the same species beyond the differences in sex organs.

shimmer: An acoustic perturbation parameter that indicates the irregularity of voice intensity from one acoustic wave to the next. Shimmer is often used in the description of pathological voice quality.

silent aspiration: see *aspiration*

single-photon emission computed tomography (SPECT): A nuclear imaging test that allows clinicians to observe how blood flows through arteries and veins in the brain. SPECT uses computed tomography and a radioactive material known as a tracer.

social (pragmatic) communication disorder: A new diagnostic category contained for the first time in the fifth edition of the *Diagnostic and Statistical Manual of Mental Disorders*. For a diagnosis of social communication disorder to be made, there must be persistent difficulties in the social use of verbal and non-verbal communication. Deficits must result in functional limitations in effective communication, social participation, social relationships, academic achievement or occupational performance. Symptoms must have their onset in the early developmental period and should not be attributable to another medical or neurological condition or to low abilities in word structure and grammar. Symptoms must also not be better explained by ASD, intellectual disability, global developmental delay or another mental disorder. See *pragmatic language impairment*.

social communication skill: The use of verbal and non-verbal communicative skills to forge social relationships and achieve social integration. Social communication skills are disrupted in a range of clients who are assessed and treated by SLTs, including children and adults with autism spectrum disorder and adults who sustain a traumatic brain injury. Poor social communication skills are associated with psychological difficulties such as depression, and reduced vocational opportunities and academic achievement.

social functioning: The ability of a child or adult to fulfil certain social roles normally expected of individuals of the same age. Social functioning is compromised in many clients who are assessed and treated by SLTs (e.g. adults with schizophrenia). Impairments of social functioning may be seen in adults with traumatic brain injury who have experienced reduced social integration since injury, and in children with autism spectrum disorder who struggle to forge friendships.

social impact: Communication and swallowing disorders can have adverse consequences for an individual's social functioning. The social impact of these disorders may include social withdrawal, poor social reintegration after illness or injury and reduced friendship networks.

social interactionism: A theoretical approach to child language acquisition that emphasizes the importance of a child's interaction with parents and other caregivers. The requisite experience for language acquisition is social interaction with other speakers. There are different proponents of a social interactionist approach. According to Bruner, the involvement of the child in interaction provides her with a Language Acquisition Support System. Vygotsky argues that linguistic and communicative abilities are initially possessed by the dyad/infant-mother system and only later by the individual.

social worker: The professional who works with vulnerable children and adults to protect them from abuse, neglect or self-harm, and to help them enhance their well-being and quality of life.

socioeconomic status: The social standing or class of an individual or group that is often measured as a combination of education, income and occupation.

soft palate: A mobile, fibromuscular fold that is suspended from the hard palate posteriorly and ends in the uvula. It separates partially the nasopharynx and oropharynx and aids in closing the pharyngeal isthmus in swallowing and speech.

spastic dysarthria: A form of dysarthria caused by upper motor neurone (UMN) damage. The clinical signs of UMN damage may be seen in spastic dysarthria. These include spastic paralysis or paresis of the speech musculature, hyperreflexia (e.g. hyperactive jaw-jerk), the presence of pathological reflexes (e.g. sucking reflex) and little or no muscle atrophy.

spasticity: Abnormal increase in muscle tone or stiffness of muscle, which can compromise speech production and other movements. Spasticity is associated with upper motor neurone damage and is a feature of many conditions including cerebral palsy, multiple sclerosis and stroke.

specific language impairment (SLI): A severe developmental language disorder. Specific language impairment has been described as a diagnosis by exclusion, as language impairment occurs in the absence of hearing loss, craniofacial anomaly, intellectual disability, psychiatric disturbance and other factors that are known to cause language disorder.

speech act: A term used by Austin and later Searle to describe utterances that perform acts or actions. Both Austin and Searle recognized different types of speech acts such as assertives (e.g. statements) and directives (e.g. requests).

speech and language therapy (SLT): The profession that assesses, diagnoses and treats children and adults with communication and swallowing disorders. Speech and language therapy is known as *speech-language pathology* in the USA and *logopaedics* in some European countries.

speech audiometry: A key component of audiological assessment, speech audiometry can reveal more about how a hearing disorder impacts on communication in daily life than pure tone audiometry. One of the tests performed in speech audiometry is word-recognition testing. A subject repeats words that are presented through earphones, and a percentage correct score is calculated.

speech sound disorder: Difficulty with and/or delayed development of a child's speech. Speech sound disorder is an umbrella term for several categories of disorder including articulation disorder, phonological disorder and childhood apraxia of speech.

speech-language pathologist (SLP): (also, speech and language therapist) The health professional who practises speech-language pathology. See *speech and language therapy*.

spinal nerve: A set of 31 pairs of nerves. The motor and sensory fibres of these nerves exit the spinal column through the intervertebral foramina and pass through the meninges before joining to form the spinal nerves. The roots of the motor and sensory fibres are in the anterior horns and posterior root ganglia of the spinal cord, respectively.

spirometer: Spirometers are used to evaluate respiratory volumes. There are 'wet' and 'dry' types of spirometer. A wet spirometer consists of an air-collecting bell inverted in a vessel of water. Exhaled air from a subject displaces water in the bell, causing it to float. The change in the bell's position is directly proportional to the air inspired/expired by the subject. Dry or hand-held spirometers can be mechanical or electronic. In mechanical devices, exhaled air drives a small turbine, which moves a pointer on a dial. In electronic devices, the volume of air exhaled by a subject is displayed on a digital readout.

stammering: see *stuttering*

standardized test: Any test that is administered and scored in a predetermined, standard manner. Because the test is administered and scored in exactly the same way on each occasion of use, it is possible to attribute the results to the performance of the individual being tested and not to differences in how the test was conducted.

stapedectomy: Surgical removal of the stapes, one of the middle ear ossicles. The stapes is replaced by a prosthesis. Stapedectomy is the treatment of choice for otosclerosis.

stapedius muscle: The smallest skeletal muscle in the human body. The stapedius muscle attaches to the posterior aspect of the neck of the stapes. When contracted, it dampens vibrations of the ossicular chain, which are transmitted via the oval window to the cochlea.

stimulability: Stimulability refers to an individual's ability to produce a correct or improved production of a misarticulated sound when given oral and visual modelling.

stopping: A simplification process found in the speech of normally developing children and children with speech sound disorders. A fricative sound is replaced by a plosive, or stop sound. This can occur in any word position, e.g. in *five* [paIv] the substitution occurs in word-initial position.

story grammar: The structural components or elements that constitute a well-formed story, the way in which these components are arranged and the relationships among them. Most story grammars consist of an episode in a setting. The episode contains an event that brings about a reaction from the main character. This reaction leads the character to formulate a goal, make an attempt to reach the goal, achieve an outcome and arrive at an ending.

stria vascularis: Located in the lateral wall of the cochlea, the stria vascularis maintains the endocochlear potential of the cochlear endolymph. This potential is integral to hair cell transduction.

stridor: A harsh, vibratory sound of variable pitch caused by partial obstruction of the respiratory passages. Inspiratory stridor indicates obstruction of the airway above the glottis and is a symptom of many vocal fold pathologies. Expiratory stridor indicates obstruction in the lower trachea.

stroboscopy: see *strobovideolaryngoscopy*

strobovideolaryngoscopy: A technique which uses a laryngeal microphone to trigger a stroboscope that illuminates the vocal folds. This allows the otolaryngologist to examine the vocal folds in slow motion, and particularly the vibratory margin of the folds. Strobovideolaryngoscopy permits the visualization of small masses, vibratory asymmetries and adynamic segments due to scar tissue or early cancer.

stroke: see *cerebrovascular accident*

struggle behaviour: A type of behaviour in people who stutter in which there is visible tension or struggle in the face, articulators or other parts of the body during moments of stuttering.

stuttering: Also known as stammering, stuttering is a fluency disorder characterized by word- and syllable-initial iterations (repetitions) and perseverations (prolongations). Iterations can involve a single speech sound (e.g. s-s-s-soap) or more than one speech sound, the latter sound typically a schwa vowel (e.g. sə-sə-sə-side). Protractions or perseverations are always single speech sounds (e.g. s::::soap). Stuttering occurs in developmental, acquired (mostly neurogenic) and psychogenic forms.

style: Intra-speaker language variation. Speakers can alter their style as they pay greater attention to speech or try to become more like the audience they are addressing.

subdural haematoma: The collection of blood between the inner layer of the dura but external to the brain and arachnoid membrane. A subdural haematoma is commonly caused by a traumatic brain injury.

subglottic stenosis: A congenital or acquired narrowing (stenosis) of the subglottic airway, which is housed in the cricoid cartilage. Subglottic stenosis may be caused by intubation, trauma and autoimmune disorders such as Wegener's granulomatosis. It may also be idiopathic.

submucous cleft palate: see *cleft lip and palate*

substitution: A type of grammatical cohesion in which one item is replaced by another item that has the same structural function. For example, in the following sentences, the substitute term 'one' replaces 'house' and has the function of a noun: *John bought a new house. It was the one next to the church.*

suck reflex: A primitive reflex in infants that consists of sucking movements by the lips when they are stroked or touched.

suffixation: A morphemic word-formation process in which a bound lexical morpheme is added to the end of a base (e.g. *wonderful*). Suffixation is a word-class-changing morphological process. For example, *wonder* → *wonderful* is a change from noun to adjective.

sulcus vocalis: A linear depression or groove in the vocal fold mucosa which runs parallel to the free border and is usually bilateral and symmetrical. The glottic dysfunction in sulcus is complex, consisting of both glottal leakage (causing breathy voice) and stiffness of the free edge of the folds (causing rough voice).

supraglottic laryngectomy: see *laryngectomy*

supraglottoplasty: A surgical procedure which alleviates the obstruction during inspiration in children with laryngomalacia by widening the supraglottis.

surgical voice restoration: The use of a valve (voice prosthesis) to produce voice in clients with a laryngectomy. The prosthesis is fitted, often at the time of laryngectomy, to permit the passage of the pulmonary airstream into the upper region of the oesophagus. When the client blocks the stoma, the pulmonary airstream is directed through the valve and into the upper oesophagus where oesophageal voice is then achieved.

syntactic development: The stages through which young children pass on their way to acquiring the syntax of their native language. Syntactic development includes the acquisition of *yes–no* and *wh*-interrogatives as well as a range of phrases (e.g. noun phrases) and clause types (e.g. subordinate clauses). See *mean length of utterance*.

syntax: The study of sentence structure. The aim of a syntactic analysis of a language is to produce a precise and rigorous description of the rules that characterize the phrases and sentences of that language. The ability to produce and understand syntactically well-formed sentences – expressive and receptive syntax, respectively – may be impaired in children and adults with language disorder.

systematic review: A review of all research studies and their findings relating to a particular question. The purpose of a systematic review is to identify all published and unpublished studies in an area, select those studies that satisfy certain criteria for inclusion, assess the quality of the studies and the evidence that they produce, synthesize their findings and arrive at a balanced and impartial interpretation of their significance.

telerehabilitation: The use of information and communication technologies to provide rehabilitation services to people remotely in their homes or other environments.

thematic role: see *semantic role*

theory of mind (ToM): The ability to attribute cognitive and affective mental states (e.g. beliefs, happiness) both to one's own mind and to the minds of others. Deficits in theory of mind are a feature of many disorders in which there are significant communication problems including autism spectrum disorder and schizophrenia.

thought disorder: Also known as disorganized speech or formal thought disorder. Thought disorder is characterized as disorganized, illogical thinking or incoherent, tangential language in which there are frequent derailments (the patient slips off one track onto an unrelated or obliquely related track). Thought disorder is a positive symptom of schizophrenia. It may also be found in other psychiatric conditions (e.g. mania).

thyroid cartilage: The largest of the nine cartilages that make up the structure of the larynx. The thyroid cartilage is composed of hyaline cartilage and is palpable a half-inch below the body of the hyoid bone. It is composed of two rectangular laminae that are fused anteriorly in the midline.

thyroidectomy: Surgical removal of all or part of the thyroid gland. This procedure may result in damage to the recurrent laryngeal nerve, leading to vocal fold dysfunction.

tic disorder: An involuntary, rapid, recurrent, non-rhythmic motor movement or vocal production that is of sudden onset and serves no apparent purpose. Common motor tics are eye-blinking and hitting oneself. Vocal tics include throat-clearing and the use of socially unacceptable (often obscene) words (coprolalia).

tinnitus: A roaring, buzzing or ringing sound in the ears, which can impact on the mental health of affected individuals. Tinnitus is a symptom of many disorders including presbycusis, noise-induced hearing loss, ototoxicity related to the taking of aspirin and aminoglycoside antibiotics, Ménière's disease and acoustic neuroma.

top-down processing: Background knowledge and expectations can influence the processing of perceptual and linguistic data. Top-down processing is evident during constructive comprehension of language. This is where hearers 'fill in' details that they have not been explicitly given but can assume to be the case based on their background knowledge.

topic: There are both syntactic and pragmatic definitions of topic in linguistics. An intuitive characterization of topic is that it is what a sentence, conversation or narrative is about.

topic management: The selection, introduction, development and termination of a topic in conversation or other form of discourse. Topic management is disrupted in a range of clients with communication disorders, including individuals with ASD, schizophrenia, traumatic brain injury and dementia.

total communication: An approach to communication in which writing, gestures, body language, signs, symbols, photographs, objects of reference and electronic aids may be used in a consistent manner to support speech or as an alternative to speech.

tracheostomy: see *tracheotomy*

tracheotomy: A surgical procedure in which a transverse or vertical incision is made into the trachea through the tissues of the neck in order to create a temporary or permanent opening (known as *tracheostomy*) for respiration. The procedure has a number of clinical applications including the long-term mechanical ventilation of patients.

transcranial magnetic stimulation: A non-invasive neurophysiological technique during which a stimulation coil placed directly above the scalp creates a strong focal magnetic pulse directed at cortical areas. The brief change in magnetic field induces a corresponding electrical potential change in the affected cortex. This results in rapid neuronal depolarization and the generation of action potentials.

traumatic brain injury (TBI): There are two forms of traumatic brain injury. In an open or penetrating head injury, the skull is fractured or otherwise breached by a missile. In a closed head injury, the brain is damaged while the skull remains intact.

Treacher Collins syndrome: A craniofacial syndrome in which there is hypoplasia of the zygomatic (cheek) bones and mandible (micrognathia), external ear abnormalities, notching of the lower eyelid and absence of lower eyelashes. Less commonly, cleft palate with or without cleft lip is present. Approximately half of individuals have a conductive hearing loss that is related to malformation of the ossicles and hypoplasia of the middle ear cavities.

trisomy 21: The presence of three copies of chromosome 21 in Down syndrome. Trisomy 21 is found in more than 90% of Down syndrome cases. In mosaic trisomy 21, which occurs in less than 2% of Down syndrome cases, the presence of an additional chromosome 21 is found in some, but not all, cells of the individual. In 3–4% of Down syndrome cases, translocation trisomy 21 occurs. This is where part of chromosome 21 becomes attached to another chromosome, usually the 13th, 14th or 15th chromosome. See *Down syndrome*.

T-unit: A T-unit (or minimal terminable unit) contains one independent clause and its dependent clauses. Originally designed to assess syntactic development in the written work of children learning their first language, the T-unit is now widely used in measures of normal and disordered discourse.

turn-taking: The interactional nature of conversation is reflected in the exchange of turns between speaker and hearer. This two-way exchange of turns is known as turn-taking. Turn-taking is governed by rules about when it is appropriate to assume one's turn and relinquish it to another speaker.

tympanic membrane: Also known as the eardrum, the tympanic membrane is the lateral boundary of the middle ear. The manubrium of the malleus bone is attached to the medial surface of this membrane. The function of the tympanic membrane is to convert sound waves into mechanical vibrations of the ossicles. The tympanic membrane can be perforated during a middle ear infection (acute otitis media).

tympanometry: An objective technique for measuring the mobility or compliance of the tympanic membrane as a function of changing air pressures in the external auditory canal. This technique can be used to establish middle ear pressure through the measurement of the amount of air pressure in the external auditory canal that is needed to achieve maximum mobility of the eardrum.

ultrasound: Diagnostic ultrasound or sonography is an imaging method that uses high-frequency sound waves to produce images of structures within the body. This technique has a number of applications in SLT, including the assessment of oropharyngeal swallowing function and the treatment of speech disorders.

universal grammar: A set of principles which Chomsky believes to be innate or hard-wired into the brains of young children. These principles are general constraints on the structure of language, which are then particularized to the grammar of the language that children are acquiring. See *particularization*.

upper motor neuron: A neurone that originates in the motor cortex and synapses with lower motor neurones in the brainstem and spinal cord. An upper motor neurone that descends from the motor cortex to the brainstem is part of the corticobulbar tract. An upper motor neurone that descends from the motor cortex to the spinal cord is part of the corticospinal tract.

upper oesophageal sphincter: Also known as the inferior pharyngeal sphincter, the upper oesophageal sphincter is located at the lower end of the pharynx and guards the entrance into the oesophagus. Its functions are to prevent air from entering the oesophagus during breathing and to prevent reflux of oesophageal contents into the pharynx and airway aspiration.

VACTERL/VATER association: A disorder that is characterized by the presence of at least three of the following congenital abnormalities: vertebral (V) defects; anal (A) atresia; cardiac (C) defects; tracheo-oesophageal (TE) fistula; renal (R) anomalies; and limb (L) abnormalities. VACTERL association has an estimated incidence of 1 in 10,000 to 1 in 40,000 live births.

vagus nerve: The tenth cranial nerve (CN X). The vagus nerve courses from the medulla to the neck, chest and abdomen, where it provides parasympathetic input to the gastrointestinal system and to the heart. It also contains sensory and motor fibres. Lesions of the vagus nerve are relevant to speech-language pathologists as they result in palatal, pharyngeal and laryngeal paralysis and abnormalities of oesophageal motility.

validity: The extent to which a test or assessment measures what it is constructed to measure. Validity reflects the truthfulness of a measure.

vallecula: A wedge-shaped space formed between the base of the tongue and epiglottis. The valleculae and pyriform sinuses are known as the pharyngeal recesses or side pockets. Food may fall into and reside in these recesses before or after the swallowing reflex triggers.

velopharyngeal incompetence: The failure of the velopharyngeal port to close adequately during speech production. Velopharyngeal incompetence can be caused by structural anomalies (e.g. a short velum or excessively capacious pharynx) or by neurological impairment (e.g. an immobile velum after a stroke).

velopharyngeal insufficiency: see *velopharyngeal incompetence*

velopharyngeal port: The area between the velum and the lateral and posterior pharyngeal walls. In a client with velopharyngeal incompetence, this port is not fully closed by elevation of the velum and contraction of the pharyngeal walls. The result is hypernasal speech.

velum: see *soft palate*

vernacular: The native variety of a particular speech community that is learned orally in early childhood. Vernaculars exhibit linguistic features that are suppressed in standard languages. They often have less prestige than standard languages for this reason.

vestibule: The central part of the membranous labyrinth that is contained in the cavity of the bony labyrinth in the inner ear. The vestibule is situated behind the cochlea and in front of the semicircular canals. It contains the utricle and saccule, which are gravity receptors.

vestibulocochlear nerve: The eighth cranial nerve (CN VIII). This nerve has two roles. It provides innervation to the cochlea for hearing. It also provides innervation to the vestibule, which senses head position changes relative to gravity.

videoendoscopy: see *fibreoptic endoscopic evaluation of swallowing*

videofluoroscopy: A radiological investigation in which fluoroscopic images appear on the monitor of an X-ray machine while a patient is swallowing a radio-opaque bolus. This procedure is used extensively in the assessment of swallowing and dysphagia but may also be employed to understand aspects of articulation (e.g. velopharyngeal function).

visual agnosia: A deficit in object recognition that is confined to the visual modality. Elementary visual processes are intact and the deficit is not related to problems in language, memory or intellectual functioning.

vocabulary: The words of a language, sometimes called the lexicon. Lexicology is the branch of linguistics that studies the vocabulary of a language. A speaker's expressive vocabulary is the words that he can produce. Receptive vocabulary describes the words that a speaker can understand. Expressive and receptive vocabulary may be compromised in children and adults with language disorders.

vocal abuse and misuse: An expression used to describe the many ways in which voice users can engage in phonatory behaviours (e.g. hyperadduction of vocal folds) and other practices (e.g. excessive occupational voice use) that put them at risk of developing a voice disorder.

vocal fold haemorrhage: Vocal folds may bleed or haemorrhage, causing tiny, visible capillaries (varices or capillary ectasias) or larger perfusions of blood into the tissue of the folds. Risk factors for vocal fold haemorrhage include phonotrauma, laryngeal trauma, aspirin, non-steroidal anti-inflammatories and hormonal imbalances.

vocal fold paralysis: A significant cause of neurogenic voice disorder. In vocal fold paralysis and paresis (VFPP), the vocal folds do not adduct, abduct or elongate normally as a result of damage to one or more of the nerves that innervate them. Bilateral VFPP compromises the airway and necessitates a tracheotomy.

vocal hygiene: Vocal hygiene can be both a preventive strategy designed to avoid voice disorders and a management technique for individuals with voice disorders. A vocal hygiene programme makes clients aware of the impact of factors such as hydration, laryngopharyngeal/gastroesophageal reflux, tobacco smoke and alcohol on the laryngeal mechanism. Clients are also made aware of the effect of repeated throat clearing on the voice and of the need for mucous management to reduce clearing.

vocal intensity: The physical correlate of loudness, which is typically measured in decibels (dB). Vocal intensity is primarily modulated by subglottal pressure, amplitude of vibration and duration of the closed phase of the glottal cycle.

vocal nodule: Small, benign growths that occur along the margins of the vocal folds mostly at the junction of the anterior and middle third of the fold.

Nodules are the most common cause of voice disorders in school-age children and are often associated with professional voice users (e.g. singers). These growths are the result of vocal abuse and misuse.

vocal polyp: A benign growth of the vocal fold, which is larger than a vocal nodule. Polyps are fluid-filled and may have their own blood supply. Smoking, hypothyroidism, gastroesophageal reflux and vocal misuse are causes of polyps.

vocal tract: The air passages above the larynx are known as the vocal tract. The vocal tract can be divided into the oral tract (the mouth and pharynx) and the nasal tract (within the nose). From the larynx to the lips/nostrils, the vocal tract is some 17 cm in men.

vocational impact: Communication and swallowing disorders can have adverse consequences for an individual's vocational or occupational functioning. This may arise directly in the case where an individual does not have the requisite communication skills to assume a particular vocational role. It may also arise indirectly in the case where a communication disorder leads to poor academic achievement, which in turn limits the vocational roles that an individual can pursue.

voice disorder: see *dysphonia*

voice mutation: The changes that occur in the human voice during puberty. During voice mutation in girls, the vocal folds become 3–4 mm longer and voicing fundamental frequency drops by a third of an octave. In boys, vocal folds lengthen by up to 10 mm, and the fundamental frequency of the voice drops by approximately 1 octave.

voice onset time: This is the amount of time it takes for voicing to commence when a voiced sound occurs immediately after a voiceless consonant.

voice prosthesis: see *surgical voice restoration*

voice quality: The quality of a speaker's voice is a multidimensional concept that has perceptual, acoustic and physiological components. Voice quality is often captured by terms like 'breathy', 'hoarse' and 'strained-strangled'.

voice therapy: The full range of direct methods (e.g. vocal function exercises) and indirect methods (e.g. vocal hygiene) that can be used to treat voice disorders in children and adults.

voicing: The use of vocal fold vibration during the production of speech sounds. Sounds that require voicing for their production are called voiced sounds (e.g. [d] [v]). Sounds that do not require voicing for their production are called voiceless sounds (e.g. [t] [f]).

Wernicke's aphasia: A form of aphasia in which there is a severe impairment of auditory verbal comprehension in the presence of effortless, fluent speech. Expressive language is often incoherent on account of the presence of jargon (hence, the use of the term *jargon aphasia* to describe this type of aphasia). See *aphasia*.

Wernicke's area: A neuroanatomical landmark that is located on the superior temporal gyrus in the superior portion of Brodmann's area 22. Damage to this area is associated with Wernicke's aphasia, the key features of which are fluent, effortless but incoherent speech and poor auditory verbal comprehension.

Williams syndrome: A rare genetic disorder in which there is a deletion of 26 contiguous genes on chromosome 7q11.23. This genetic defect gives rise to intellectual disability and physical anomalies including dysmorphic facial features, elastin arteriopathy, short stature, connective tissue abnormalities and infantile hypercalcemia. The full-scale intelligence quotient is usually in the 50s to 60s with a range of 40–85.

word retrieval: see *lexical retrieval*

word-finding difficulty: see *anomia*

word-formation: A group of morphemic and non-morphemic processes that create new lexemes from existing morphemes and lexemes. Morphemic word-formation processes include prefixation (e.g. *disorganised*) and suffixation (e.g. *meaningful*). Non-morphemic word-formation processes include blending (e.g. *breakfast + lunch → brunch*), clipping (e.g. *influenza → flu*), acronym-formation (e.g. *North Atlantic Treaty Organization → NATO*) and reduplication (e.g. *walkie-talkie*).

working memory: see *memory*

Bibliography

Ackley, R. S. 2014. 'Hearing disorders', in L. Cummings (ed.), *Cambridge handbook of communication disorders*, Cambridge: Cambridge University Press, 359–80.

Ada, M., Isildak, H. and Saritzali, G. 2010. 'Congenital vocal cord paralysis', *Journal of Craniofacial Surgery* **21**:1, 273–4.

Ahlsén, E. 2006. *Introduction to neurolinguistics*, Amsterdam and Philadelphia: John Benjamins Publishing Company.

Aithal, S., Aithal, V., Kei, J. and Driscoll, C. 2012. 'Conductive hearing loss and middle ear pathology in young infants referred through a newborn universal hearing screening program in Australia', *Journal of the American Academy of Audiology* **23**:9, 673–85.

American Psychiatric Association 2013. *Diagnostic and statistical manual of mental disorders – Fifth edition*, Washington, DC: American Psychiatric Association.

2016a. *Understanding educational psychology*. Available online: www.apa.org/action/science/teaching-learning/index.aspx. Accessed 21 March 2016.

2016b. *Clinical psychology*. Available online: www.apa.org/ed/graduate/specialize/clinical.aspx. Accessed 12 April 2016.

American Speech-Language-Hearing Association (ASHA) 1998. *The roles of otolaryngologists and speech-language pathologists in the performance and interpretation of strobovideolaryngoscopy*. Available online: www.asha.org/policy/RP1998-00132.htm. Accessed 16 June 2016.

2013. *SLP health care survey 2013. Survey summary report: number and type of responses*, Rockville, MD: Author. Available online: www.asha.org/uploadedFiles/2013-SLP-Health-Care-Survey-Summary-Report.pdf. Accessed 16 June 2016.

2014. *2014 schools survey. Survey summary report: number and type of responses, SLP*, Rockville, MD: ASHA. Available online: www.asha.org/uploadedFiles/2014-Schools-Survey-SLP-Frequency-Report.pdf. Accessed 24 August 2015.

2015a. *2015 SLP health care survey summary report: number and type of responses*, Rockville, MD: ASHA. Available online: www.asha.org/uploadedFiles/2015-SLP-Health-Care-Survey-Summary.pdf. Accessed 24 August 2015.

2015b. *SLP health care survey 2015. Caseload characteristics*, Rockville, MD: Author. Available online: www.asha.org/uploadedFiles/2015-SLP-Health-Care-Survey-Caseload.pdf. Accessed 17 June 2016.

2016a. *Scope of practice in speech-language pathology*, Rockville, MD: Author.

2016b. *2016 schools survey. Survey summary report: numbers and types of responses, SLPs*, Rockville, MD: Author.

2016c. *Bilingual service delivery* (Practice Portal). Available online: www.asha.org/Practice-Portal/Professional-Issues/Bilingual-Service-Delivery. Accessed 5 August 2016.

2016d. *Blueprint for action: 2016 public policy agenda*. Available online: www.asha.org/Advocacy/2016-ASHA-Public-Policy-Agenda.htm. Accessed 11 August 2016.

Andreu, L., Sanz-Torrent, M., Olmos, J. G. and Macwhinney, B. 2013. 'The formulation of argument structure in SLI: an eye-movement study', *Clinical Linguistics & Phonetics* **27**:2, 111–33.

Arbuthnott, K. and Frank, J. 2000. 'Trail making test, part B as a measure of executive control: validation using a set-switching paradigm', *Journal of Clinical and Experimental Neuropsychology* **22**:4, 518–28.

Arslan, S., Işik, A. U., Imamoğlu, M., Topbaş, M., Aslan, Y. and Ural, A. 2013. 'Universal newborn hearing screening: automated transient evoked otoacoustic emissions', *B-ENT* **9**:2, 122–31.

Arvin, B., Prepageran, N. and Raman, R. 2013. 'High frequency presbycusis: is there an earlier onset?', *Indian Journal of Otolaryngology and Head & Neck Surgery* **65**:(Suppl. 3), 480–4.

Ashford, J., McCabe, D., Wheeler-Hegland, K., Frymark, T., Mullen, R., Musson, N., Schooling, T. and Hammond, C. S. 2009. 'Evidence-based systematic review: oropharyngeal dysphagia behavioral treatments: Part III – Impact of dysphagia treatments on populations with neurological disorders', *Journal of Rehabilitation Research and Development* **46**:2, 195–204.

Attaway, J., Stone, C. L., Sendor, C. and Rosario, E. R. 2015. 'Effect of amplification on speech and language in children with aural atresia', *American Journal of Audiology* **24**:3, 354–9.

Bacsfalvi, P. and Bernhardt, B. M. 2011. 'Long-term outcomes of speech therapy for seven adolescents with visual feedback technologies: ultrasound and electropalatography', *Clinical Linguistics & Phonetics* **25**:11–12, 1034–43.

Baker, J. 2003. 'Psychogenic voice disorders and traumatic stress experience: a discussion paper with two case reports', *Journal of Voice* **17**:3, 308–18.

Bakker, K. and Myers, F. 2011. *Instructional manual for the cluttering severity instrument*. Available at: http://associations.missouristate.edu/ica/Resources/Resources%20and%20Links%20pages/CSI%20software%20ALL/CSI%20Manual_EN.pdf. Accessed 13 May 2016.

Ball, M. J. [1984] 2014. 'Phonological development and assessment', in N. Miller (ed.), *Bilingualism and language disability: assessment & remediation*, London and New York: Psychology Press, 115–30.

2012. 'Vowels and consonants of the world's languages', in S. McLeod and B. A. Goldstein (eds.), *Multilingual aspects of speech sound disorders in children*, Bristol, Buffalo and Toronto: Multilingual Matters, 32–41.

Ballard, K. J., Wambaugh, J. L., Duffy, J. R., Layfield, C., Maas, E., Mauszycki, S. and McNeil, M. R. 2015. 'Treatment for acquired apraxia of speech: a systematic review of intervention research between 2004 and 2012', *American Journal of Speech-Language Pathology* **24**:2, 316–37.

Bao, L., Brownlie, E. B. and Beitchman, J. H. 2016. 'Mental health trajectories from adolescence to adulthood: language disorder and other childhood and adolescent risk factors', *Development and Psychopathology* **28**:2, 489–504.

Barker-Collo, S., Jones, A., Jones, K., Theadom, A., Dowell, A., Starkey, N. and Feigin, V. L. 2015. 'Prevalence, natural course and predictors of depression 1 year following traumatic brain injury from a population-based study in New Zealand', *Brain Injury* **29**:7–8, 859–65.

Baron-Cohen, S., Leslie, A. M. and Frith, U. 1985. 'Does the autistic child have a "theory of mind"?', *Cognition* **21**:1, 37–46.

Barr, W. B., Bilder, R. M., Goldberg, E., Kaplan, E. and Mukherjee, S. 1989. 'The neuropsychology of schizophrenic speech', *Journal of Communication Disorders* **22**:5, 327–49.

Bate, S., Kay, J., Code, C., Haslam, C. and Hallowell, B. 2010. 'Eighteen years on: what next for the PALPA', *International Journal of Speech-Language Pathology* **12**:3, 190–202.

Bauer, V., Aleric, Z. and Jancic, E. 2015. 'Comparing voice self-assessment with auditory perceptual analysis in patients with multiple sclerosis', *International Archives of Otorhinolaryngology* **19**:2, 100–5.

Baxter, S., Enderby, P., Evans, P. and Judge, S. 2012. 'Barriers and facilitators to the use of high-technology augmentative and alternative communication devices: a systematic review and qualitative synthesis', *International Journal of Language & Communication Disorders* **47**:2, 115–29.

Beal, J. C. 2010. *An introduction to regional Englishes: dialect variation in England*, Edinburgh: Edinburgh University Press.

Beck, A. T., Ward, C. H., Mendelson, M., Mock, J. and Erbaugh, J. 1961. 'An inventory for measuring depression', *Archives of General Psychiatry* **4**:6, 561–71.

Beech, T. J., Campbell, G., McDermott, A. L. and Batch, A. J. 2013. 'The effect of anti-reflux treatment on subjective voice measurements of patients with laryngopharyngeal reflux', *Journal of Laryngology and Otology* **127**:6, 590–4.

Beeke, S., Wilkinson, R. and Maxim, J. 2007. 'Individual variation in agrammatism: a single case study of the influence of interaction', *International Journal of Language & Communication Disorders* **42**:6, 629–47.

Behrman, A. 2005. 'Common practices of voice therapists in the evaluation of patients', *Journal of Voice* **19**:3, 454–69.

Beitchman, J. H., Brownlie, E. B. and Bao, L. 2014. 'Age 31 mental health outcomes of childhood language and speech disorders', *Journal of the American Academy of Child and Adolescent Psychiatry* **53**:10, 1102–10.

Belafsky, P. C. and Kuhn, M. A. 2014. *The clinician's guide to swallowing fluoroscopy*, New York: Springer Science + Business Media.

Bell, A. 1984. 'Language style as audience design', *Language in Society* **13**:2, 145–204.

Bell, N. 1987. *Visualizing and verbalizing for language comprehension and thinking*, Paso Robles, CA: Academy of Reading Publications.

Ben-David, B. M., Nguyen, L. L. and van Lieshout, P. H. 2011. 'Stroop effects in persons with traumatic brain injury: selective attention, speed of processing, or color-naming? A meta-analysis', *Journal of the International Neuropsychological Society* **17**:2, 354–63.

Bercow, J. 2008. *The Bercow report: a review of services for children and young people with speech, language, and communication needs*, Nottingham: DCSF Publications.

Bergström, L., Ward, E. C. and Finizia, C. 2016. 'Voice rehabilitation for laryngeal cancer patients: functional outcomes and patient perceptions', *Laryngoscope* **126**:9, 2029–35.

Berk, S. and Lillo-Martin, D. 2012. 'The two-word stage: motivated by linguistic or cognitive constraints?', *Cognitive Psychology* **65**:1, 118–40.

Bernhardt, B. H. 1992. 'The application of nonlinear phonological theory to intervention with one phonologically disordered child', *Clinical Linguistics & Phonetics* **6**:4, 283–316.

Bernhardt, B. H. and Stemberger, J. P. 1998. *Handbook of phonological development from the perspective of constraint-based nonlinear phonology*, San Diego: Academic Press.

Bernhardt, B. H. and Stoel-Gammon, C. 1994. 'Nonlinear phonology: introduction and clinical application', *Journal of Speech and Hearing Research* **37**:1, 123–43.

Best, W., Greenwood, A., Grassly, J., Herbert, R., Hickin, J. and Howard, D. 2013. 'Aphasia rehabilitation: does generalisation from anomia therapy occur and is it predictable? A case series study', *Cortex* **49**:9, 2345–57.

Best, W., Greenwood, A., Grassly, J. and Hickin, J. 2008. 'Bridging the gap: can impairment-based therapy for anomia have an impact at the psycho-social level?', *International Journal of Language & Communication Disorders* **43**:4, 390–407.

Bishop, D. V. M. 2003a. *Children's communication checklist – Second Edition*, London: Psychological Corporation.

2003b. *Test for Reception of Grammar – Version 2 (TROG-2)*, Oxford: Pearson Assessment.

Blanton, M. G. and Blanton, S. 1920. *Speech training for children: the hygiene of speech*, New York: The Century Co.

Bleile, K. M., Ireland, L. and Kiel, T. 2006. 'The professions around the world: new web-based directory goes global', *The ASHA Leader* **11**:7, 8–27.

Bliss, L. S., McCabe, A. and Miranda, A. E. 1998. 'Narrative assessment profile: discourse analysis for school-age children', *Journal of Communication Disorders* **31**:4, 347–63.

Blomgren, M. 2013. 'Behavioral treatments for children and adults who stutter: a review', *Psychology Research and Behavior Management* **6**, 9–19.

Bodén, K., Hallgren, Å. and Hedström, H. W. 2006. 'Effects of three different swallow maneuvers analysed by videomanometry', *Acta Radiologica* **47**:7, 628–33.

Bonner, M. F., Vesely, L., Price, C., Anderson, C., Richmond, L., Farag, C., Avants, B. and Grossman, M. 2009. 'Reversal of the concreteness effect in semantic dementia', *Neuropsychology* **26**:6, 568–79.

Boothroyd, A. 2007. 'Adult aural rehabilitation: what is it and does it work?', *Trends in Amplification* **11**:2, 63–71.

Boseley, M. E., Cunningham, M. J., Volk, M. S. and Hartnick, C. J. 2006. 'Validation of the pediatric voice-related quality-of-life survey', *Archives of Otolaryngology-Head & Neck Surgery* **132**:7, 717–20.

Bowen, C. 2016. *Speech-language pathology in East Africa*. Available online: www.speech-language-therapy.com/index.php?option=com_content&view=article&id=58: east&catid=13. Accessed 7 August 2016.

Brebner, C., McCormack, P. and Rickard Liow, S. 2016. 'Marking of verb tense in the English of preschool English-Mandarin bilingual children: evidence from language development profiles within subgroups on the Singapore English Action Picture Test', *International Journal of Language & Communication Disorders* **51**:1, 31–43.

Brown, R. 1973. *A first language: the early stages*, Cambridge, MA: Harvard University Press.

Bryan, K., Freer, J. and Furlong, C. 2007. 'Language and communication difficulties in juvenile offenders', *International Journal of Language & Communication Disorders* **42**:5, 505–20.

Buckingham, H. W. and Rekart, D. M. 1979. 'Semantic paraphasia', *Journal of Communication Disorders* **12**:3, 197–209.

Bushe, C. J., Falk, D., Anand, E., Casillas, M., Perrin, E., Chhabra-Khanna, R. and Detke, H. C. 2015. 'Olanzapine long-acting injection: a review of first experiences of post-injection delirium/sedation syndrome in routine clinical practice', *BMC Psychiatry* **15**, 65.

Busis, S. N. 2006. 'Presbycusis', in K. H. Calhoun and D. E. Eibling (eds.), *Geriatric otolaryngology*, New York: Taylor & Francis, 77–90.

Butcher, P., Elias, A. and Cavalli, L. 2007. *Understanding and treating psychogenic voice disorder: a CBT framework*, Chichester, West Sussex: John Wiley & Sons.

Byles, J. 2005. 'The epidemiology of communication and swallowing disorders', *Advances in Speech Language Pathology* **7**:1, 1–7.

Campbell, T. F. 1999. 'Functional treatment outcomes in young children with motor speech disorders', in A. J. Caruso and E. A. Strand (eds.), *Clinical management of motor speech disorders in children*, New York: Thieme Medical Publishers Inc., 385–96.

Campisi, P. and Busato, G.-M. 2015. 'Embryology of congenital airway disorders', in J. Lioy and S. E. Sobol (eds.), *Disorders of the neonatal airway: fundamentals for practice*, New York: Springer, 3–14.

Campisi, P., Tewfik, T. L., Manoukian, J. J. and Schloss, M. D. 2002. 'Computer-assisted voice analysis: establishing a pediatric database', *Archives of Otolaryngology – Head & Neck Surgery* **128**:2, 156–60.

Carding, P., Deary, V. and Miller, T. 2013. 'Cognitive behavioural therapy in the treatment of functional dysphonia in the United Kingdom', in E. M.-L. Yiu (ed.), *International perspectives on voice disorders*, Bristol, Buffalo and Toronto: Multilingual Matters, 133–48.

Carlson, H. L., Jadavji, Z., Mineyko, A., Damji, O., Hodge, J., Saunders, J., Hererro, M., Nowak, M., Patzelt, R., Mazur-Mosiewicz, A., MacMaster, F. P. and Kirton, A. 2016. 'Treatment of dysphasia with rTMS and language therapy after childhood stroke: multimodal imaging of plastic change', *Brain and Language* **159**, 23–34.

Casselman, J. W., Delanote, J., Kuhweide, R., van Dinther, J., De Foer, B. and Offeciers, E. F. 2015. 'Congenital malformations of the temporal bone', in M. Lemmerling and B. De Foer (eds.), *Temporal bone imaging*, Berlin and Heidelberg: Springer-Verlag, 119–54.

Centers for Disease Control and Prevention 2012. *What are developmental disabilities?* Available online: www.cdc.gov/ncbddd/developmental disabilities/features/birthdefects-dd-keyfindings.html. Accessed 23 August 2015.

Centre for Workforce Intelligence 2014. *Securing the future workforce supply: speech and language therapy stocktake*, London: Author.

Chae, S. W., Choi, G., Kang, H. J., Choi, J. O. and Jin, S. M. 2001. 'Clinical analysis of voice change as a parameter of premenstrual syndrome', *Journal of Voice* **15**:2, 278–83.

Chaika, E. 1982. 'A unified explanation for the diverse structural deviations reported for adult schizophrenics with disrupted speech', *Journal of Communication Disorders* **15**:3, 167–89.

Chan, D. W., Ho, C., Tsang, S.-M. and Chung, K. K. H. 2008. 'Estimating incidence of developmental dyslexia in Hong Kong: what differences do different criteria make?', *Australian Journal of Learning Difficulties* **13**:1, 1–16.

Chapman, S. B., Highley, A. P. and Thompson, J. L. 1998. 'Discourse in fluent aphasia and Alzheimer's disease: linguistic and pragmatic considerations', *Journal of Neurolinguistics* **11**:1–2, 55–78.

Charlton, R. A., Barrick, T. R., Markus, H. S. and Morris, R. G. 2009. 'Theory of mind associations with other cognitive functions and brain imaging in normal aging', *Psychology and Aging* **24**:2, 338–48.

Cherney, L. R. and van Vuuren, S. 2012. 'Telerehabilitation, virtual therapists, and acquired neurologic speech and language disorders', *Seminars in Speech and Language* **33**:3, 243–57.

Cheshire, J. 2004. 'Age- and generation-specific use of language', in U. Ammon, N. Dittmar, K. J. Mattheier and P. Trugill (eds.), *Sociolinguistics: international handbook of the science of language and society*, 2nd edn, Berlin: Mouton de Gruyter, 1552–63.

Chio, A., Logroscino, G., Hardiman, O., Swingler, R., Mitchell, D., Beghi, E. and Traynor, B. G. 2009. 'Prognostic factors in ALS: a critical review', *Amyotrophic Lateral Sclerosis* **10**:5–6, 310–23.

Choi, Y. H., Park, H. K. and Paik, N. J. 2016. 'A telerehabilitation approach for chronic aphasia following stroke', *Telemedicine Journal and E-Health* **22**:5, 434–40.

Chole, R. A. and Nason, R. 2009. 'Chronic otitis media and cholesteatoma', in J. B. Snow and P. A. Wackym (eds.), *Ballenger's otorhinolaryngology: head and neck surgery*, Shelton, CT: People's Medical Publishing House, 217–28.

Choo, A. L., Burnham, E., Hicks, K. and Chang, S. E. 2016. 'Dissociations among linguistic, cognitive, and auditory-motor neuroanatomical domains in children who stutter', *Journal of Communication Disorders* **61**, 29–47.

Christou, N. and Mathonnet, M. 2013. 'Complications after total thyroidectomy', *Journal of Visceral Surgery* **150**:4, 249–56.

Clark, C. E., Conture, E. G., Frankel, C. B. and Walden, T. A. 2012. 'Communicative and psychological dimensions of the KiddyCAT', *Journal of Communication Disorders* **45**:3, 223–34.

Clegg, J., Brumfitt, S., Parks, R. W. and Woodruff, P. W. R. 2007. 'Speech and language therapy intervention in schizophrenia: a case study', *International Journal of Language & Communication Disorders* **42**:S1, 81–101.

Cobo-Lewis, A. B., Oller, D. K., Lynch, M. P. and Levine, S. L. 1996. 'Relations of motor and vocal milestones in typically developing infants and infants with Down syndrome', *American Journal of Mental Retardation* **100**:5, 456–67.

Coelho, C., Ylvisaker, M. and Turkstra, L. S. 2005. 'Nonstandardized assessment approaches for individuals with traumatic brain injuries', *Seminars in Speech and Language* **26**:4, 223–41.

Coggins, T. E. 1979. 'Relational meaning encoded in the two-word utterances of stage 1 Down's syndrome children', *Journal of Speech and Hearing Research* **22**:1, 166–78.

Cohen, S. M., Dupont, W. D. and Courey, M. S. 2006. 'Quality-of-life impact of non-neoplastic voice disorders: a meta-analysis', *Annals of Otology, Rhinology, and Laryngology* **115**:2, 128–34.

Cohen, S. M., Jacobson, B. H., Garrett, C. G., Noordzij, J. P., Stewart, M. G., Attia, A., Ossoff, R. H. and Cleveland, T. F. 2007. 'Creation and validation of the singing voice handicap index', *Annals of Otology, Rhinology, and Laryngology* **116**:6, 402–6.

Colle, L., Angeleri, R., Vallana, M., Sacco, K., Bara, B. G. and Bosco, F. M. 2013. 'Understanding the communicative impairments in schizophrenia: a preliminary study', *Journal of Communication Disorders* **46**:3, 294–308.

Connor, N. P. and Bless, D. M. 2014. 'Functional and organic voice disorders', in L. Cummings (ed.), *Cambridge handbook of communication disorders*, Cambridge: Cambridge University Press, 321–40.

Cook, I. J. 2008. 'Diagnostic evaluation of dysphagia', *Nature Clinical Practice Gastroenterology & Hepatology* **5**, 393–403.

Cooper, M., Pettit, E. and Clibbens, J. 1998. 'Evaluation of a nursery based language intervention in a socially disadvantaged area', *International Journal of Language & Communication Disorders* **33**:(Suppl.), 526–31.

Correa, D. D., DeAngelis, L. M., Shi, W., Thaler, H., Glass, A. and Abrey, L. E. 2004. 'Cognitive functions in survivors of primary central nervous system lymphoma', *Neurology* **62**:4, 548–55.

Cosyns, M., Van Borsel, J., Wierckx, K., Dedecker, D., Van de Peer, F., Daelman, T., Laenen, S. and T'Sjoen, G. 2014. 'Voice in female-to-male transsexual persons after long-term androgen therapy', *Laryngoscope* **124**:6, 1409–14.

Council of Academic Programs in Communication Sciences and Disorders & American Speech-Language-Hearing Association 2016. *Communication sciences and disorders (CSD) education survey national aggregate data report: 2014–2015 academic year*. Available online: www.asha.org/uploadedFiles/2014–2015-CSD-Education-Survey-National-Aggregate-Data-Report.pdf. Accessed 5 September 2016.

Covington, M. A., He, C., Brown, C., Naçi, L., McClain, J. T., Fjordbak, B. S., Semple, J. and Brown, J. 2005. 'Schizophrenia and the structure of language: the linguist's view', *Schizophrenia Research* **77**:1, 85–98.

Cowan, N. 2008. 'What are the differences between long-term, short-term, and working memory?', *Progress in Brain Research* **169**, 323–38.

Cowley, J. and Glasgow, C. 1994. *The Renfrew bus story*, Centreville, DE: The Centreville School.

Craig, A., Hancock, K., Tran, Y., Craig, M. and Peters, K. 2002. 'Epidemiology of stuttering in the community across the entire life span', *Journal of Speech, Language, and Hearing Research* **45**:6, 1097–105.

Croft, S., Marshall, J., Pring, T. and Hardwick, M. 2011. 'Therapy for naming difficulties in bilingual aphasia: which language benefits?', *International Journal of Language & Communication Disorders* **46**:1, 48–62.

Crosbie, S., Holm, A. and Dodd, B. 2005. 'Intervention for children with severe speech disorder: a comparison of two approaches', *International Journal of Language & Communication Disorders* **40**:4, 467–91.

Crosson, B., Ford, A., McGregor, K. M., Meinzer, M., Cheshkov, S., Li, X., Walker-Batson, D. and Briggs, R. W. 2010. 'Functional imaging and related techniques: an introduction for rehabilitation researchers', *Journal of Rehabilitation Research and Development* **47**:2, vii–xxxiv.

Cruice, M., Worrall, L., Hickson, L. and Murison, R. 2003. 'Finding a focus for quality of life with aphasia: social and emotional health, and psychological well-being', *Aphasiology* **17**:4, 333–53.

Crystal, D. 1986. *Listen to your child: a parent's guide to children's language*, Harmondsworth: Penguin.

2003. *English as a global language*, 2nd edn, New York: Cambridge University Press.

Crystal, D. and Varley, R. 1998. *Introduction to language pathology*, 4th edn, London: Whurr.

Cummings, L. 2005. *Pragmatics: a multidisciplinary perspective*, Edinburgh: Edinburgh University Press.

2008. *Clinical linguistics*, Edinburgh: Edinburgh University Press.

2009. *Clinical pragmatics*, Cambridge: Cambridge University Press.

2010. 'Neuropragmatics', in L. Cummings (ed.), *The Routledge pragmatics encyclopedia*, London and New York: Routledge, 292–4.

2012. 'Establishing diagnostic criteria: the role of clinical pragmatics', *Lodz Papers in Pragmatics* **8**:1, 61–84.

2013. 'Clinical pragmatics and theory of mind', in A. Capone, F. Lo Piparo and M. Carapezza (eds.), *Perspectives on linguistic pragmatics*, Perspectives in Pragmatics, Philosophy & Psychology, Vol. 2, Dordrecht: Springer, 23–56.

2014a. *Pragmatic disorders*, Dordrecht: Springer.

2014b. 'Pragmatic disorders and theory of mind', in L. Cummings (ed.), *Cambridge handbook of communication disorders*, Cambridge: Cambridge University Press, 559–77.

2014c. *Communication disorders*, Basingstoke: Palgrave Macmillan.

2015. 'Pragmatic disorders and social functioning: a lifespan perspective', in A. Capone and J. L. Mey (eds.), *Interdisciplinary studies in pragmatics, culture and society*, Perspectives in Pragmatics, Philosophy & Psychology, Vol. 4, Dordrecht: Springer, 179–208.

Cureoglu, S., Schachern, P. A., Ferlito, A., Rinaldo, A., Tsuprun, V. and Paparella, M. M. 2006. 'Otosclerosis: etiopathogenesis and histopathology', *American Journal of Otolaryngology* **27**:5, 334–40.

D'haeseleer, E., Depypere, H. and Van Lierde, K. 2013. 'Comparison of speaking fundamental frequency between premenopausal women and postmenopausal women with and without hormone therapy', *Folia Phoniatrica et Logopaedica* **65**:2, 78–83.

Dabul, B. L. 2000. *Apraxia battery for adults – Second edition*, Austin, TX: Pro-Ed Inc.

Daly, D. A. 2006. *Predictive cluttering inventory*. Available online: www.mnsu.edu/comdis/isad10/papers/daly10/dalycluttering2006R.pdf. Accessed 13 May 2016.

Davies, D. G. and Jahn, A. F. 2004. *Care of the professional voice: a guide to voice management for singers, actors and professional voice users*, New York: Routledge.

Davis, L. A. 2007. 'Quality of life issues related to dysphagia', *Topics in Geriatric Rehabilitation* **23**:4, 352–65.

Daya, H., Hosni, A., Bejar-Solar, I., Evans, J. N. G. and Bailey, C. M. 2000. 'Pediatric vocal fold paralysis: a long-term retrospective study', *Archives of Otolaryngology – Head & Neck Surgery* **126**:1, 21–5.

De Sonneville-Koedoot, C., Stolk, E., Rietveld, T. and Franken, M.-C. 2015. 'Direct versus indirect treatment for preschool children who stutter: the RESTART randomized trial', *PLoS ONE* **10**:7, e0133758. doi: 10.1371/journal.pone.0133758.

Dean, E., Howell, J., Hill, A. and Waters, D. 1990. *Metaphon resource pack*, Windsor, Berks: NFER-Nelson.

Dean, E., Howell, J., Waters, D. and Reid, J. 1995. 'Metaphon: a metalinguistic approach to the treatment of phonological disorder in children', *Clinical Linguistics & Phonetics* **9**:1, 1–19.

Delis, D. C., Kaplan, E. and Kramer, J. 2001. *Delis-Kaplan executive function scale*, San Antonio, TX: The Psychological Corporation.

Department for Children, Schools and Families 2008. *Every child a talker: guidance for early language lead practitioners*, London: Author.

Dickson, K., Marshall, M., Boyle, J., McCartney, E., O'Hare, A. and Forbes, J. 2009. 'Cost analysis of direct versus indirect and individual versus group modes of manual-based speech-and-language therapy for primary school-age children with primary language impairment', *International Journal of Language & Communication Disorders* **44**:3, 369–81.

Dietrich, M., Verdolini Abbott, K., Gartner-Schmidt, J. and Rosen, C. A. 2008. 'The frequency of perceived stress, anxiety, and depression in patients with common pathologies affecting voice', *Journal of Voice* **22**:4, 472–88.

DiGiovanni, J. J. and McCarthy, J. W. 2016. 'IPE 102: innovative interprofessional education that includes audiology and speech-language pathology', in A. Johnson (ed.), *Interprofessional education and interprofessional practice in communication sciences and disorders: an introduction and case-based examples of implementation in education and health care settings*, Rockville, MD: American Speech-Language-Hearing Association, 29–55.

Dion, S., Duivestein, J. A., St Pierre, A. and Harris, S. R. 2015. 'Use of thickened liquids to manage feeding difficulties in infants: a pilot survey of practice patterns in Canadian pediatric centers', *Dysphagia* **30**:4, 457–72.

Dockrell, J., Stuart, M. and King, D. 2006. 'Implementing effective oral language interventions in pre-school settings: no simple solutions', in J. Clegg and J. Ginsborg (eds.), *Language and social disadvantage: theory into practice*, Wiley: Chichester, 177–87.

2010. 'Supporting early oral language skills for English language learners in inner city preschool provision', *British Journal of Educational Psychology* **80**:4, 497–515.

Dodd, B., Crosbie, S., McIntosh, B., Holm, A., Harvey, C., Liddy, M., Fontyne, K., Pinchin, B. and Rigby, H. 2008. 'The impact of selecting different contrasts in phonological therapy', *International Journal of Speech-Language Pathology* **10**:5, 334–45.

Dodd, B., Hua, Z., Crosbie, S., Holm, A. and Ozanne, A. 2006. *Diagnostic evaluation of articulation and phonology (DEAP)*, San Antonio, TX: Pearson.

Dondorf, K., Fabus, R. and Ghassemi, A. E. 2016. 'The interprofessional collaboration between nurses and speech-language pathologists working with patients diagnosed with dysphagia in skilled nursing facilities', *Journal of Nursing Education and Practice* **6**:4, 17–20.

Downey, L. E., Mahoney, C. J., Buckley, A. H., Golden, H. L., Henley, S. M., Schmitz, N., Schott, J. M., Simpson, I. J., Ourselin, S., Fox, N. C., Crutch, S. J. and Warren, J. D. 2015. 'White matter tract signatures of impaired social cognition in frontotemporal lobar degeneration', *NeuroImage: Clinical* **8**, 640–51.

Drummond, S. 1993. *Dysarthria examination battery*, Tucson, AZ: Communication Skill Builders.

Duchan, J. F. 2011. A history of speech-language pathology: overview. Available online: www.acsu.buffalo.edu/~duchan/new_history/overview.html. Accessed 1 February 2017.

Duchan, J. F. and Erickson, J. G. 1976. 'Normal and retarded children's understanding of semantic relations in different verbal contexts', *Journal of Speech and Hearing Research* **19**:4, 767–76.

Dufresne, D., Dagenais, L., Shevell, M. I. and REPACQ Consortium 2014. 'Epidemiology of severe hearing impairment in a population-based cerebral palsy cohort', *Pediatric Neurology* **51**:5, 641–4.

Dumer, A. I., Oster, H., McCabe, D., Rabin, L. A., Spielman, J. L., Ramig, L. O. and Borod, J. C. 2014. 'Effects of the Lee Silverman Voice Treatment (LSVT LOUD) on hypomimia in Parkinson's disease', *Journal of the International Neuropsychological Society* **20**:3, 302–12.

Dumontheil, I., Apperly, I. A. and Blakemore, S.-J. 2010. 'Online usage of theory of mind continues to develop in late adolescence', *Developmental Science* **13**:2, 331–8.

Duncan, A. F., Watterberg, K. L., Nolen, T. L., Vohr, B. R., Adams-Chapman, I., Das, A., Lowe, J. and Eunice Kennedy Shriver National Institute of Child Health and Human Development Neonatal Research Network 2012. 'Effect of ethnicity and race on cognitive and language testing at age 18–22 months in extremely preterm infants', *Journal of Pediatrics* **160**:6, 966–71.

Dunn, L. M. and Dunn, D. M. 2007. *Peabody picture vocabulary test – Fourth edition (PPVT-4)*, San Antonio, TX: Pearson Assessment.

Dunsby, A. M. and Davison, A. M. 2011. 'Causes of laryngeal cartilage and hyoid bone fractures found at postmortem', *Medicine, Science, and the Law* **51**:2, 109–13.

Dunsmuir, S., Clifford, V. and Took, S. 2006. 'Collaboration between educational psychologists and speech and language therapists: barriers and opportunities', *Educational Psychology in Practice* **22**:2, 125–40.

Eadie, P., Morgan, A., Ukoumunne, O. C., Ttofari Eecen, K., Wake, M. and Reilly, S. 2015. 'Speech sound disorder at 4 years: prevalence, comorbidities, and predictors in a community cohort of children', *Developmental Medicine and Child Neurology* **57**:6, 578–84.

Ebbels, S. H., Marić, N., Murphy, A. and Turner, G. 2014. 'Improving comprehension in adolescents with severe receptive language impairments: a randomized control trial of intervention for coordinating conjunctions', *International Journal of Language & Communication Disorders* **49**:1, 30–48.

Edwards, C. M., Newell, J. M., Rich, D. W. and Hitchcock, L. I. 2015. 'Teaching interprofessional practice: an exploratory course assignment in social work and speech language pathology', *Journal of Teaching in Social Work* **35**:5, 529–43.

Eigentler, A., Rhomberg, J., Nachbauer, W., Ritzer, I., Poewe, W. and Boesch, S. 2012. 'The scale for the assessment and rating of ataxia correlates with dysarthria assessment in Friedreich's ataxia', *Journal of Neurology* **259**:3, 420–6.

Elliott, R. 2003. 'Executive functions and their disorders', *British Medical Bulletin* **65**:1, 49–59.

Ellis Weismer, S. 2014. 'Specific language impairment', in L. Cummings (ed.), *Cambridge handbook of communication disorders*, Cambridge: Cambridge University Press, 73–87.

Enderby, P. and Palmer, R. 2008. *Frenchay dysarthria assessment – Second edition (FDA-2)*, Austin, TX: Pro-Ed.

Eriksson, K., Hartelius, L. and Saldert, C. 2016. 'On the diverse outcome of communication partner training of significant others of people with aphasia: an experimental study of six cases', *International Journal of Language & Communication Disorders* **51**:4, 402–14.

Feng, Y. M., Wu, Y. Q., Wang, J. and Yin, S. K. 2012. 'Cochlear implantation in a patient with severe cochlear hypoplasia', *Journal of Laryngology & Otology* **126**:11, 1172–5.

Fergadiotis, G., Wright, H. H. and West, T. M. 2013. 'Measuring lexical diversity in narrative discourse of people with aphasia', *American Journal of Speech-Language Pathology* **22**:2, S397-S408.

Field, J. 2015. 'Psycholinguistics', in N. Braber, L. Cummings and L. Morrish (eds.), *Exploring language and linguistics*, Cambridge: Cambridge University Press, 324–52.

Fodor, J. A. 1983. *The modularity of mind: an essay on faculty psychology*, Cambridge, MA: The MIT Press.

Food and Drug Administration 2015. *Premarket to postmarket shift in clinical data requirements for cochlear implant device approvals in pediatric patients*. Report prepared for the 1 May 2015 meeting of the Ear, Nose, and Throat Devices Panel of the Medical Devices Advisory Committee. Available online: www.fda.gov/downloads/AdvisoryCo mmittees/CommitteesMeetingMaterials/MedicalDevices/MedicalDe vicesAdvisoryCommittee/EarNoseandThroatDevicesPanel/UCM44 3996.pdf. Accessed 2 January 2016.

Franzen, M. D. 2002. *Reliability and validity in neuropsychological assessment*, 2nd edn, New York: Springer Science + Business Media, LLC.

Frattali, C. M., Thompson, C. K., Holland, A. L., Wohl, C. B. and Ferketic, M. M. 1995. *Functional assessment of communication skills for adults (ASHA FACS)*, Rockville, MD: American Speech-Language-Hearing Association.

Freeman, M. and Fawcus, M. 2000. *Voice disorders and their management*, London: Whurr Publishers.

Frost, L. A. and Bondy, A. 1994. *PECS: the picture exchange communication system*, Cherry Hill, NJ: Pyramid Educational Consultants.

Gale, N., Gnepp, D. R., Poljak, M., Strojan, P., Cardesa, A., Helliwell, T., Šifrer, R., Volavšek, M., Sandison, A. and Zidar, N. 2016. 'Laryngeal squamous intraepithelial lesions: an updated review on etiology, classification, molecular changes, and treatment', *Advances in Anatomic Pathology* **23**:2, 84–91.

Gardner, H. 2014. 'Collaborative working between pediatric speech and language therapy and ENT colleagues: what is good practice?', *Current Opinion in Otolaryngology & Head and Neck Surgery* **22**:3, 167–71.

Gartner-Schmidt, J. L., Roth, D. F., Zullo, T. G. and Rosen, C. A. 2013. 'Quantifying component parts of indirect and direct voice therapy related to different voice disorders', *Journal of Voice* **27**:2, 210–6.

George, M. and Monnier, P. 2010. 'Long-term voice outcome following partial cricotracheal resection in children for severe subglottic stenosis', *International Journal of Pediatric Otorhinolaryngology* **74**:2, 154–60.

Geurts, H. M., Verté, S., Oosterlaan, J., Roeyers, H., Hartman, C. A., Mulder, E. J., Berckelaer-Onnes, I. A. and Sergeant, J. A. 2004. 'Can the children's communication checklist differentiate between children with autism, children with ADHD, and normal controls?', *Journal of Child Psychology and Psychiatry* **45**:8, 1437–53.

Gierut, J. 1992. 'The conditions and course of clinically induced phonological change', *Journal of Speech and Hearing Research* **35**:5, 1049–63.

2001. 'Complexity in phonological treatment: clinical factors', *Language, Speech, and Hearing Services in Schools* **32**:4, 229–41.

Gierut, J., Elbert, M. and Dinnsen, D. 1987. 'A functional analysis of phonological knowledge and generalisation learning in misarticulating children', *Journal of Speech and Hearing Research* **30**:4, 462–79.

Gillam, R. B. and Pearson, N. 2004. *Test of narrative language*, Austin, TX: Pro-Ed.

Gillam, R. B., Logan, K. J. and Pearson, N. 2009. *Test of childhood stuttering*, Austin, TX: Pro-Ed.

Gillon, G. T. 2000. 'The efficacy of phonological awareness intervention for children with spoken language impairment', *Language, Speech, and Hearing Services in Schools* **31**:2, 126–41.

2004. *Phonological awareness: from research to practice*, New York: The Guilford Press.

Golden, C. J. 1978. *The Stroop color and word test: a manual for clinical and experimental uses*, Chicago, IL: Stoelting.

Goldman, R. and Fristoe, M. 2015. *Goldman-Fristoe test of articulation – Third edition (GFTA-3)*, Bloomington, MN: NCS Pearson, Inc.

Golub, J. S., Chen, P. H., Otto, K. J., Hapner, E. and Johns, M. M. 2006. 'Prevalence of perceived dysphonia in a geriatric population', *Journal of the American Geriatrics Society* **54**:11, 1736–9.

Goodglass, H., Kaplan, E. and Barresi, B. 2001. *Boston diagnostic aphasia examination – Third edition (BDAE-3)*, Baltimore, MD: Lippincott Williams & Wilkins.

Govil, N., Stapleton, A. L., Georg, M. W. and Yellon, R. F. 2015. 'The role of tympanostomy tubes in surgery for acquired retraction pocket cholesteatoma', *International Journal of Pediatric Otorhinolaryngology* **79**:12, 2015–19.

Gramuglia, A. C. J., Tavares, E. L. M., Rodrigues, S. A. and Martins, R. H. G. 2014. 'Perceptual and acoustic parameters of vocal nodules in children', *International Journal of Pediatric Otorhinolaryngology* **78**:2, 312–16.

Greenwood, N., Wright, J. A. and Bithell, C. 2006. 'Perceptions of speech and language therapy amongst UK school and college students: implications for recruitment', *International Journal of Language & Communication Disorders* **41**:1, 83–94.

Grice, H. P. 1975. 'Logic and conversation', in P. Cole and J. Morgan (eds.), *Syntax and semantics*, Vol. III, New York: Academic Press, 41–58.

Grisel, J. J. and Samy, R. N. 2010. 'Cochlear implant', in M. L. Pensak (ed.), *Otolaryngology cases*, New York: Thieme, 54–6.

Grogan-Johnson, S., Gabel, R. M., Taylor, J., Rowan, L. E., Alvares, R. and Schenker, J. 2011. 'A pilot exploration of speech sound disorder intervention delivered by telehealth to school-age children', *International Journal of Telerehabilitation* **3**:1, 31–42.

Grosjean, F. 2012. *Bilinguals in the United States: who are the millions of bilinguals in the US?* Available online: www.psychologytoday.com/blog/life-bilingual/201205/bilinguals-in-the-united-states. Accessed 5 August 2016.

Gualtieri, C. T. and Johnson, L. G. 2005. 'ADHD: is objective diagnosis possible?', *Psychiatry (Edgmont)* **2**:11, 44–53.

Gunn, A., Menzies, R. G., O'Brian, S., Onslow, M., Packman, A., Lowe, R., Iverach, L., Heard, R. and Block, S. 2014. 'Axis I anxiety and mental health disorders among stuttering adolescents', *Journal of Fluency Disorders* **40**, 58–68.

Harris, J. and Cottam, P. 1985. 'Phonetic features and phonological features in speech assessment', *British Journal of Disorders of Communication* **20**:1, 61–74.

Harrison, E. and Onslow, M. 1999. 'Early intervention for stuttering: the Lidcome Program', in R. F. Curlee (ed.), *Stuttering and related disorders of fluency*, New York: Thieme, 65–79.

Hartshorne, M. 2011. *Speech, language and communication in secondary aged pupils. I CAN Talk Series – Issue 10*. London: I CAN.

Hayden, D. A. 2006. 'The PROMPT model: use and application for children with mixed phonological-motor impairment', *International Journal of Speech-Language Pathology* **8**:3, 265–81.

  2008. *P.R.O.M.P.T. Prompts for restructuring oral muscular phonetic targets. Introduction to technique: a manual*, 2nd edn, Santa Fe, NM: The PROMPT Institute.

Healey, K. T., Nelson, S. and Scaler Scott, K. 2015. 'A case study of cluttering treatment outcomes in a teen', *Procedia – Social and Behavioral Sciences* **193**, 141–6.

Health & Care Professions Council (HCPC) 2013. *Standards of proficiency: speech and language therapists*, London: Health & Care Professions Council.

Health and Social Care Information Centre 2014. *NHS hospital and community health service (HCHS) workforce statistics in England, non-medical staff – 2003–2013, as at 30 September*. Available online: www.hscic.gov.uk/catalogue/PUB13741. Accessed 5 September 2016.

Health Workforce Australia 2014. *Australia's health workforce series: speech pathologists in focus*, Canberra: Health Workforce Division.

Hegde, M. N. and Freed, D. 2011. *Assessment of communication disorders in adults*, San Diego, Oxford and Brisbane: Plural Publishing.

Henry, A. 1992. 'Infinitives in a *for-to* dialect', *Natural Language and Linguistic Theory* **10**:2, 279–301.

Heuer, R. J., Hawkshaw, M. J. and Sataloff, R. T. 2006. 'The clinical voice laboratory', in R. T. Sataloff (ed.), *Vocal health and pedagogy, Vol. I: Science and assessment*, San Diego and Oxford: Plural Publishing, Inc., 159–98.

Heuer, R. J., Rulnick, R. K., Horman, M., Perez, K. S., Emerich, K. A. and Sataloff, R. T. 2006. 'Voice therapy', in R. T. Sataloff (ed.), *Vocal health and pedagogy, Vol. II: Advanced assessment and practice*, San Diego and Oxford: Plural Publishing, 227–52.

Higdon, C. W. and Vaughan, L. 2011. 'The role of speech-language pathology in life care planning', in S. Riddick-Grisham and L. M. Deming (eds.), *Pediatric life care planning and case management*, 2nd edn, Boca Raton, FL, London and New York: CRC Press, 189–274.

Hinton, R., Budimirovic, D. B., Marschik, P. B., Talisa, V. B., Einspieler, C., Gipson, T. and Johnston, M. V. 2013. 'Parental reports on early language and motor milestones in fragile X syndrome with and without autism spectrum disorders', *Developmental Neurorehabilitation* **16**:1, 58–66.

Hirano, M. 1981. *Clinical examination of voice*, New York: Springer Verlag.

Hodge, M. 2014. 'Developmental dysarthria', in L. Cummings (ed.), *Cambridge handbook of communication disorders*, Cambridge: Cambridge University Press, 26–48.

Hodson, B. W. and Paden, E. P. 1991. *Targeting intelligible speech: a phonological approach to remediation*, 2nd edn, Austin, TX: Pro-Ed.

Hoey, M. 1991. *Patterns of lexis in texts*, Oxford: Oxford University Press.

Hoffman, H. J., Ko, C.-W., Themann, C. L., Dillon, C. F. and Franks, J. R. 2006. 'Reducing noise-induced hearing loss (NIHL) to achieve US healthy people 2010 goals', *American Journal of Epidemiology* **163**:(Suppl. 11), S122.

Hogikyan, N. D. and Sethuraman, G. 1999. 'Validation of an instrument to measure voice-related quality of life (V-RQOL)', *Journal of Voice* **13**:4, 557–69.

Homack, S. and Riccio, C. A. 2004. 'A meta-analysis of the sensitivity and specificity of the Stroop Color and Word Test with children', *Archives of Clinical Neuropsychology* **19**:6, 725–43.

Hövels-Gürich, H. H., Bauer, S. B., Schnitker, R., Willmes-von Hinckeldey, K., Messmer, B. J., Seghaye, M.-C. and Huber, W. 2008. 'Long-term outcome of speech and language in children after corrective surgery for cyanotic or acyanotic cardiac defects in infancy', *European Journal of Paediatric Neurology* **12**:5, 378–86.

Howard, D. and Patterson, K. 1992. *Pyramids and palm trees test: a test of semantic access from pictures and words*, Bury St. Edmunds: Thames Valley Test Company.

Hsu, A. K., Rosow, D. E., Wallerstein, R. J. and April, M. M. 2015. 'Familial congenital bilateral vocal fold paralysis: a novel gene translocation', *International Journal of Pediatric Otorhinolaryngology* **79**:3, 323–7.

Hsu, H. J. and Bishop, D. V. 2014. 'Training understanding of reversible sentences: a study comparing language-impaired children with age-matched and grammar-matched controls', *PeerJ* **2**, e656.

Huber, J. E. 2008. 'Effects of utterance length and vocal loudness on speech breathing in older adults', *Respiratory Physiology & Neurobiology* **164**:3, 323–30.

IPDTOC Working Group 2011. 'Prevalence at birth of cleft lip with or without cleft palate: data from the International Perinatal Database of Typical Oral Clefts (IPDTOC)', *Cleft Palate-Craniofacial Journal* **48**:1, 66–81.

Iverach, L. and Rapee, R. M. 2014. 'Social anxiety disorder and stuttering: current status and future directions', *Journal of Fluency Disorders* **40**, 69–82.

Iverson, J. M. 2010. 'Developing language in a developing body: the relationship between motor development and language development', *Journal of Child Language* **37**:2, 229–61.

Jacobson, B. H., Johnson, A., Grywalski, C., Silbergleit, A., Jacobson, G., Benninger, M. S. and Newman, C. W. 1997. 'The voice handicap index (VHI): development and validation', *American Journal of Speech-Language Pathology* **6**:3, 66–70.

Janssens, L., Drooghmans, S. and Schaeken, W. 2015. 'But: do age and working memory influence conventional implicature processing?', *Journal of Child Language* **42**:3, 695–708.

Jarvis, E. J. and Rogers, L. E. 2008. 'A baseline survey looking at adult patients who no longer require percutaneous endoscopic gastrostomy (PEG) following joint intervention by a dietician and a speech and language therapist (SLT)', *Proceedings of the Nutrition Society*, **67**: (OCE), E138.

Jensen, D. R., Grames, L. M. and Lieu, J. E. C. 2013. 'Effects of aural atresia on speech development and learning: retrospective analysis from a multidisciplinary craniofacial clinic', *JAMA Otolaryngology – Head & Neck Surgery* **139**:8, 797–802.

Jokel, R., Kielar, A., Anderson, N. D., Black, S. E., Rochon, E., Graham, S., Freedman, M. and Tang-Wai, D. F. 2016. 'Behavioural and neuroimaging changes after naming therapy for semantic variant primary progressive aphasia', *Neuropsychologia* **89**, 191–216.

Jones, S. M., Carding, P. N. and Drinnan, M. J. 2006. 'Exploring the relationship between severity of dysphonia and voice-related quality of life', *Clinical Otolaryngology* **31**:5, 411–17.

Kahrilas, P. J. and Gupta, R. R. 1990. 'Mechanisms of acid reflux associated with cigarette smoking', *Gut* **31**:1, 4–10.

Kambanaros, M. and Grohmann, K. K. 2011. 'Profiling performance in L1 and L2 observed in Greek-English bilingual aphasia using the Bilingual Aphasia Test: a case study from Cyprus', *Clinical Linguistics & Phonetics* **25**:6–7, 513–29.

Karnell, M. P., Melton, S. D., Childes, J. M., Coleman, T. C., Dailey, S. A. and Hoffman, H. T. 2007. 'Reliability of clinician-based (GRBAS and CAPE-V) and patient-based (V-RQOL and IPVI) documentation of voice disorders', *Journal of Voice* **21**:5, 576–90.

Kaufman, N. R. 1995. *Kaufman speech praxis test*, Detroit: Wayne State University Press.

Kay Elemetrics 1993. *Multi-dimensional voice program (MDVP): computer program*, Pine Brook, NJ: Author.

Kay, J., Lesser, R. and Coltheart, M. 1992. *Psycholinguistic assessments of language processing in aphasia (PALPA): An introduction*, Hove, UK: Lawrence Erlbaum Associates.

1996. 'Psycholinguistic assessments of language processing in aphasia (PALPA): an introduction', *Aphasiology* **10**:2, 159–80.

Keck, C. S. and Doarn, C. R. 2014. 'Telehealth technology applications in speech-language pathology', *Telemedicine Journal and E-Health* **20**:7, 653–9.

Kell, C. A., Neumann, K., Behrens, M., von Gudenberg, A. W. and Giraud, A. L. 2017. 'Speaking-related changes in cortical functional connectivity associated with assisted and spontaneous recovery from developmental stuttering', *Journal of Fluency Disorders*, to appear.

Kell, C. A., Neumann, K., von Kriegstein, K., Posenenske, C., von Gudenberg, A. W., Euler, H. and Giraud, A. L. 2009. 'How the brain repairs stuttering', *Brain* **132**:10, 2747–60.

Kertesz, A. 2006. *Western aphasia battery-revised*, San Antonio, TX: Pearson.

Kessler, R. C., Aguilar-Gaxiola, S., Alonso, J., Chatterji, S., Lee, S., Ormel, J., Ustün, T. B. and Wang, P. S. 2009. 'The global burden of mental disorders: an update from the WHO World Mental Health (WMH) surveys', *Epidemiologia e Psichiatria Sociale* **18**:1, 23–33.

Khan, L. M. L. and Lewis, N. P. 2015. *Khan-Lewis phonological analysis – Third edition (KLPA-3)*, Bloomington, MN: Psychological Corporation.

Knowles, W. and Masidlover, M. 1982. *The Derbyshire language scheme*, Derbyshire County Council.

Kobayashi, Y., Tamiya, N., Moriyama, Y. and Nishi, A. 2015. 'Triple difficulties in Japanese women with hearing loss: marriage, smoking, and mental health issues', *PLoS ONE* **10**:2, e0116648.

Kojima, H., Tanaka, Y., Shiwa, M., Sakurai, Y. and Moriyama, H. 2006. 'Congenital cholesteatoma clinical features and surgical results', *American Journal of Otolaryngology* **27**:5, 299–305.

Korzeniewski, S. J., Birbeck, G., DeLano, M. C., Potchen, M. J. and Paneth, N. 2008. 'A systematic review of neuroimaging for cerebral palsy', *Journal of Child Neurology* **23**:2, 216–27.

Kosaka, B. 2006. 'Neuropsychological assessment in mild traumatic brain injury: a clinical overview', *BC Medical Journal* **48**:9, 447–52.

Kraft, S. J. and Yairi, E. 2012. 'Genetic bases of stuttering: the state of the art, 2011', *Folia Phoniatrica et Logopaedica* **64**:1, 34–47.

Kreher, D. A., Holcomb, P. J., Goff, D. and Kuperberg, G. R. 2008. 'Neural evidence for faster and further automatic spreading activation in schizophrenic thought disorder', *Schizophrenia Bulletin* **34**:3, 473–82.

Kuo, C.-L., Liao, W.-H. and Shiao, A.-S. 2015. 'A review of current progress in acquired cholesteatoma management', *European Archives of Otorhinolaryngology* **272**:12, 3601–9.

Labov, W. 1972. *Sociolinguistic patterns*, Philadelphia: University of Pennsylvania Press.

Lai, M. C., Lombardo, M. V., Auyeung, B., Chakrabarti, B. and Baron-Cohen, S. 2015. 'Sex/gender differences and autism: setting the scene for future research', *Journal of the American Academy of Child & Adolescent Psychiatry* **54**:1, 11–24.

Laiho, A. and Klippi, A. 2007. 'Long- and short-term results of children's and adolescents' therapy courses for stuttering', *International Journal of Language & Communication Disorders* **42**:3, 367–82.

Law, J., Lee, W., Roulstone, S., Wren, Y., Zeng, B. and Lindsay, G. 2012. *'What works': interventions for children and young people with speech, language and communication needs*, London: Department for Education.

Law, J., Reilly, S. and Snow, P. C. 2013. 'Child speech, language and communication need re-examined in a public health context: a new direction for the speech and language profession', *International Journal of Language & Communication Disorders* **48**:5, 486–96.

Law, J., Rush, R., Schoon, I. and Parsons, S. 2009. 'Modeling developmental language difficulties from school entry into adulthood: literacy, mental health, and employment outcomes', *Journal of Speech, Language, and Hearing Research* **52**:6, 1401–16.

Lee, A. S.-Y. and Gibbon, F. E. 2015. 'Non-speech oral motor treatment for children with developmental speech sound disorders', *Cochrane Database of Systematic Reviews*, Issue 3. Art. No.: CD009383. doi: 10.1002/14651858.CD009383.pub2.

Lee, S. J., Cho, Y., Song, J. Y., Lee, D., Kim, Y. and Kim, H. 2016. 'Aging effect on Korean female voice: acoustic and perceptual examinations of breathiness', *Folia Phoniatrica et Logopaedica* **67**:6, 300–7.

Letts, C., Edwards, S., Sinka, I., Schaefer, B. and Gibbons, W. 2013. 'Socioeconomic status and language acquisition: children's performance on the new Reynell Developmental Language Scales', *International Journal of Language & Communication Disorders* **48**:2, 131–43.

Levy, E. S. 2014. 'Implementing two treatment approaches to childhood dysarthria', *International Journal of Speech-Language Pathology* **16**:4, 344–54.

Litosseliti, L. and Leadbeater, C. 2013. 'Speech and language therapy/pathology: perspectives on a gendered profession', *International Journal of Language & Communication Disorders* **48**:1, 90–101.

Littlefield Cook, J. and Cook, G. 2005. *Child development: principles & perspectives*, Boston, MA: Allyn & Bacon.

Liu, T. 2012. 'Motor milestone development in young children with autism spectrum disorders: an exploratory study', *Educational Psychology in Practice* **28**:3, 315–26.

Lock, S., Wilkinson, R. and Bryan, K. 2001. *SPPARC: supporting partners of people with aphasia in relationships and conversations*, Bicester, Oxon: Winslow Press.

Lof, G. L. and Watson, M. M. 2008. 'A nationwide survey of nonspeech oral motor exercise use: implications for evidence-based practice', *Language, Speech, and Hearing Services in Schools* **39**:3, 392–407.

Logemann, J. A. 1991. 'Approaches to management of disordered swallowing', *Baillière's Clinical Gastroenterology* **5**:2, 269–80.

2006. 'Medical and rehabilitative therapy of oral, pharyngeal motor disorders', *GI Motility Online*. doi:10.1038/gimo50.

Lord, C., Rutter, M., DiLavore, P. C., Risi, S., Gotham, K., Bishop, S. L., Luyster, R. J. and Guthrie, W. 2012. *Autism diagnostic observation schedule – Second edition (ADOS-2)*, Torrance, CA: Western Psychological Services.

Loret, C. 2015. 'Using sensory properties of food to trigger swallowing: a review', *Critical Reviews in Food Science and Nutrition* **55**:1, 140–5.

Loukusa, S., Leinonen, E., Jussila, K., Mattila, M.-L., Ryder, N., Ebeling, H. and Moilanen, I. 2007. 'Answering contextually demanding questions: pragmatic errors produced by children with Asperger syndrome or high-functioning autism', *Journal of Communication Disorders* **40**:5, 357–81.

Lubinski, R. and Hudson, M. W. 2013. *Professional issues in speech-language pathology and audiology*, 4th edn, Clifton Park, NY: Delmar.

Maddy, K. M., Capilouto, G. J. and McComas, K. L. 2014. 'The effectiveness of semantic feature analysis: an evidence-based systematic review', *Annals of Physical and Rehabilitation Medicine* **57**:4, 254–67.

Maggio, V., Grañana, N. E., Richaudeau, A., Torres, S., Giannotti, A. and Suburo, A. M. 2014. 'Behavior problems in children with specific language impairment', *Journal of Child Neurology* **29**:2, 194–202.

Mahler, L. A., Ramig, L. O. and Fox, C. 2015. 'Evidence-based treatment of voice and speech disorders in Parkinson disease', *Current Opinion in Otolaryngology & Head and Neck Surgery* **23**:3, 209–15.

Marsh, K., Bertranou, E., Suominen, H. and Venkatachalam, M. 2010. *An economic evaluation of speech and language therapy*, London: Matrix Evidence.

Martinez, C. C. and Cassol, M. 2015. 'Measurement of voice quality, anxiety and depression symptoms after speech therapy', *Journal of Voice* **29**:4, 446–9.

Martins, R. H., do Amaral, H. A., Tavares, E. L., Martins, M. G., Gonçalves, T. M. and Dias, N. H. 2016. 'Voice disorders: etiology and diagnosis', *Journal of Voice* **30**:6, 761.e1–761.e9.

Marulis, L. M. and Neuman, S. B. 2010. 'The effects of vocabulary intervention on young children's word learning: a meta-analysis', *Review of Educational Research* **80**:3, 300–35.

Masuda, S., Usui, S. and Matsunaga, T. 2013. 'High prevalence of inner-ear and/or internal auditory canal malformations in children with sensorineural hearing loss', *International Journal of Pediatric Otorhinolaryngology* **77**:2, 228–32.

Matthews, J. L., Oddone-Paolucci, E. and Harrop, R. A. 2015. 'The epidemiology of cleft lip and palate in Canada, 1998 to 2007', *Cleft Palate-Craniofacial Journal* **52**:4, 417–24.

Maylor, E. A., Moulson, J. M., Muncer, A.-M. and Taylor, L. A. 2002. 'Does performance on theory of mind tasks decline in old age?', *British Journal of Psychology* **93**:4, 465–85.

McAllister, J. and Miller, J. 2013. *Introductory linguistics for speech and language therapy practice*, Chichester, West Sussex: Wiley-Blackwell.

McAllister, J., Collier, J. and Shepstone, L. 2012. 'The impact of adolescent stuttering on educational and employment outcomes: evidence from a birth cohort study', *Journal of Fluency Disorders* **37**:2, 106–21.

McCabe, D., Ashford, J., Wheeler-Hegland, K., Frymark, T., Mullen, R., Musson, N., Hammond, C. S. and Schooling, T. 2009. 'Evidence-based systematic review: oropharyngeal dysphagia behavioral treatments. Part IV – Impact of dysphagia treatment on individuals' postcancer treatments', *Journal of Rehabilitation Research and Development* **46**:2, 205–14.

McCabe, P. J., Sheard, C. and Code, C. 2008. 'Communication impairment in the AIDS dementia complex (ADC): a case report', *Journal of Communication Disorders* **41**:3, 203–22.

McCartney, E. 2007. *Language therapy manual*, Glasgow: University of Strathclyde.

McLeod, S. and McKinnon, D. H. 2007. 'Prevalence of communication disorders compared with other learning needs in 14,500 primary and secondary school students', *International Journal of Language & Communication Disorders* **42**:(Suppl. 1), 37–59.

McTear, M. F. 1985. 'Pragmatic disorders: a case study of conversational disability', *British Journal of Disorders of Communication* **20**:2, 129–42.

Mennen, I. and Stansfield, J. 2006. 'Speech and language therapy service delivery for bilingual children: a survey of three cities in Great Britain', *International Journal of Language & Communication Disorders* **41**:6, 635–52.

Menzies, R. G., Onslow, M., Packman, A. and O'Brian, S. 2009. 'Cognitive behavior therapy for adults who stutter: a tutorial for speech-language pathologists', *Journal of Fluency Disorders* **34**:3, 187–200.

Merrill, R. M., Anderson, Λ. E. and Sloan, A. 2011. 'Quality of life indicators according to voice disorders and voice-related conditions', *Laryngoscope* **121**:9, 2004–10.

Meurer, E. M., Fontoura, G. V., Corleta, H. V. and Capp, E. 2015. 'Speech articulation of low-dose oral contraceptive users', *Journal of Voice* **29**:6, 743–50.

Miccio, A. W. and Elbert, M. 1996. 'Enhancing stimulability: a treatment program', *Journal of Communication Disorders* **29**:4, 335–51.

Michael, S. E., Ratner, N. B. and Newman, R. 2012. 'Verb comprehension and use in children and adults with Down syndrome', *Journal of Speech, Language, and Hearing Research* **55**:6, 1736–49.

Mikulec, A. A. 2009. 'Congenital hearing loss (sensorineural and conductive)', in R. B. Mitchell and K. D. Pereira (eds.), *Pediatric otolaryngology for the clinician*, New York: Humana Press, 75–9.

Mildinhall, S. 2012. 'Speech and language in the patient with cleft palate', in M. T. Cobourne (ed.), *Cleft lip and palate: epidemiology, aetiology and treatment*, Basel: Karger, 137–46.

Miller, T., Deary, V. and Patterson, J. 2014. 'Improving access to psychological therapies in voice disorders: a cognitive behavioural therapy model', *Current Opinion in Otolaryngology & Head and Neck Surgery* **22**:3, 201–5.

Milman, L. H., Faroqi-Shah, Y. and Corcoran, C. D. 2014. 'Normative data for the WAB-R: a comparison of monolingual English speakers, Asian Indian-English bilinguals, and Spanish-English bilinguals,' Clinical Aphasiology Conference, 27 May-1 June 2014, St. Simons Island, GA.

Moore, D. R. 2002. 'Auditory development and the role of experience', *British Medical Bulletin* **63**:1, 171–81.

Moore, M. E. 2001. 'Third person pronoun errors by children with and without language impairment', *Journal of Communication Disorders* **34**:3, 207–28.

Moradi, N., Pourshahbaz, A., Soltani, M., Javadipour, S., Hashemi, H. and Soltaninejad, N. 2013. 'Cross-cultural equivalence and evaluation of psychometric properties of voice handicap index into Persian', *Journal of Voice* **27**:2, 258.e15–258.e22.

Moseley, D., Clark, J., Baumfield, V., Hall, E., Hall, I., Miller, J., Blench, G., Gregson, M. and Spedding, T. 2006. *Developing oral communication and productive thinking skills in HM Prisons*, London: Learning & Skills Research Centre.

Murray, E., McCabe, P. and Ballard, K. J. 2015. 'A randomized controlled trial for children with childhood apraxia of speech comparing rapid syllable transition treatment and the Nuffield Dyspraxia Programme – third edition', *Journal of Speech, Language, and Hearing Research* **58**:3, 669–86.

Myers, P. S. 1979. 'Profiles of communication deficits in patients with right cerebral hemisphere damage: implications for diagnosis and treatment', in *Clinical aphasiology conference*, Phoenix, AZ: BRK Publishers, 38–46.

Myers, B. R. and Finnegan, E. M. 2015. 'The effects of articulation on the perceived loudness of the projected voice', *Journal of Voice* **29**:3, 390.e9–390.e15.

Nascimento, W. V., Cassiani, R. A., Santos, C. M. and Dantas, R. O. 2015. 'Effect of bolus volume and consistency on swallowing events duration in healthy subjects', *Journal of Neurogastroenterology and Motility* **21**:1, 78–82.

National Academy of Neuropsychology 2001. *Nan definition of a clinical neuropsychologist*. Available online: www.nanonline.org/docs/PAIC/PDFs/NANPositionDefNeuro.pdf. Accessed 30 March 2016.

Nelson, A. P. and O'Connor, M. G. 2008. 'Mild cognitive impairment: a neuropsychological perspective', *CNS Spectrums* **13**:1, 56–64.

Nemr, K., Simões-Zenari, M., Cordeiro, G. F., Tsuji, D., Ogawa, A. I., Ubriq, M. T. and Menezes, M. H. 2012. 'GRBAS and Cape-V scales: high reliability and consensus when applied at different times', *Journal of Voice* **26**:6, e17–22.

Netten, A. P., Rieffe, C., Theunissen, S. C., Soede, W., Dirks, E., Korver, A. M., Konings, S., Oudesluys-Murphy, A. M., Dekker, F. W., Frijns, J. H. and the DECIBEL Collaborative Study Group 2015. 'Early identification: language skills and social functioning in deaf and hard of hearing preschool children', *International Journal of Pediatric Otorhinolaryngology* **79**:12, 2221–6.

Newman, R. D. 2012. 'Introduction to the videofluoroscopic swallowing study', in R. D. Newman and J. M. Nightingale (eds.), *Videofluoroscopy: a multidisciplinary team approach*, San Diego, Oxford and Melbourne: Plural Publishing, 3–18.

Nicholas, L. E. and Brookshire, R. H. 1992. 'A system for scoring main concepts in the discourse of non-brain-damaged and aphasic speakers', *Clinical Aphasiology* **21**, 87–99.

Niedermeyer, H. P., Häusler, R., Schwub, D., Neuner, N. T., Busch, R. and Arnold, W. 2007. 'Evidence of increased average age of patients with otosclerosis', in W. Arnold and R. Häusler (eds.), *Otosclerosis and stapes surgery: advances in oto-rhino-laryngology*, Vol. 65, 17–24.

Nishimura, Y. and Kumoi, T. 1992. 'The embryologic development of the human external auditory meatus: preliminary report', *Acta Oto-Laryngologica* **112**:3, 496–503.

Northern, J. L. and Downs, M. P. 2002. *Hearing in children*, 5th edn, Baltimore, MD: Lippincott Williams & Wilkins.

O'Daniel, M. and Rosenstein, A. H. 2008. 'Professional communication and team collaboration', in R. G. Hughes (ed.), *Patient safety and quality: an evidence-based handbook for nurses*, Rockville, MD: Agency for Healthcare Research and Quality (US), 271–84.

Obert, A., Gierski, F., Calmus, A., Portefaix, C., Declercq, C., Pierot, L. and Caillies, S. 2014. 'Differential bilateral involvement of the parietal gyrus during predicative metaphor processing: an auditory fMRI study', *Brain and Language* **137**, 112–19.

Olszewska, E., Wagner, M., Bernal-Sprekelsen, M., Ebmeyer, J., Dazert, S., Hildmann, H. and Sudhoff, H. 2004. 'Etiopathogenesis of cholesteatoma', *European Archives of Otorhinolaryngology* **261**:1, 6–24.

Onslow, M., Packman, A. and Harrison, E. (eds.) 2003. *The Lidcombe program of early stuttering intervention: a clinician's guide*, Austin, TX: Pro-Ed.

Onyett, S., Standen, R. and Peck, E. 1997. 'The challenge of managing community mental health teams', *Health and Social Care in the Community* **5**:1, 40–7.

Paluska, S. A. and Lansford, C. D. 2008. 'Laryngeal trauma in sport', *Current Sports Medicine Reports* **7**:1, 16–21.

Paneth, N., Hong, T. and Korzeniewski, S. 2006. 'The descriptive epidemiology of cerebral palsy', *Clinics in Perinatology* **33**:2, 251–67.

Papafragou, A. and Musolino, J. 2003. 'Scalar implicatures: experiments at the semantic-pragmatic interface', *Cognition* **86**:3, 253–82.

Papagno, C., Capasso, R. and Miceli, G. 2009. 'Reversed concreteness effect for nouns in a subject with semantic dementia', *Neuropsychologia* **47**:4, 1138–48.

Pardini, M. and Nichelli, P. F. 2009. 'Age-related decline in mentalizing skills across adult life span', *Experimental Aging Research* **35**:1, 98–106.

Passenger, T. 2014. 'Introduction to educational psychology practice', in A. J. Holliman (ed.), *The Routledge international companion to educational psychology*, London and New York: Routledge, 21–30.

Paul, R. and Norbury, C. F. 2012. *Language disorders from infancy through adolescence: listening, speaking, reading, writing, and communicating*, 4th edn, St Louis, MI: Elsevier Mosby.

Peccei, J. S. 1999. *Child language*, 2nd edn, London and New York: Routledge.

Peets, K. F. 2009. 'Profiles of dysfluency and errors in classroom discourse among children with language impairment', *Journal of Communication Disorders* **42**:2, 136–54.

Phelps-Terasaki, D. and Phelps-Gunn, T. 2007. *Test of pragmatic language – Second edition (TOPL-2)*, Austin, TX: Pro-Ed.

Pilleri, M. and Antonini, A. 2015. 'Therapeutic strategies to prevent and manage dyskinesias in Parkinson's disease', *Expert Opinion on Drug Safety* **14**:2, 281–94.

Plante, T. G. 2011. *Contemporary clinical psychology*, 3rd edn, Hoboken, NJ: John Wiley & Sons.

Pollock, K. E. and Hall, P. K. 1991. 'An analysis of the vowel misarticulations of five children with developmental apraxia of speech', *Clinical Linguistics & Phonetics* **5**:3, 207–24.

Pomerantz, A. M. 2014. *Clinical psychology: science, practice, and culture*, 3rd edn, Thousand Oaks, CA: Sage Publications, Inc.

Ponton, C. W., Eggermont, J. J., Kwong, B. and Don, M. 2000. 'Maturation of human central auditory system activity: evidence from multi-channel evoked potentials', *Clinical Neurophysiology* **111**:2, 220–36.

Porter, E. 1831. *Analysis of the principles of rhetorical delivery as applied in reading and speaking*, 4th edn, New York: J. Leavitt.

Preston, J. L., McAllister Byun, T., Boyce, S. E., Hamilton, S., Tiede, M., Phillips, E., Rivera-Campos, A. and Whalen, D. H. 2017. 'Ultrasound images of the tongue: a tutorial for assessment and remediation of speech sound errors', *Journal of Visualized Experiments* **119**, e55123, doi: 10.3791/55123.

PROMPT Institute 2016. *What is PROMPT?* Available online: www.promptinstitute.com/?page=FamiliesWIP. Accessed 21 June 2016.

Provencio-Arambula, M. H., Provencio, D. and Hegde, M. N. 2007. *Treatment of dysphagia in adults: resources and protocols in English and Spanish*, San Diego, CA: Plural Publishing.

Prutting, C. A. and Kirchner, D. M. 1987. 'A clinical appraisal of the pragmatic aspects of language', *Journal of Speech and Hearing Disorders* **52**:2, 105–19.

Quality Assurance Agency for Higher Education (QAA) 2001. *Benchmark statement: health care programmes – speech and language therapy*, Gloucester: Quality Assurance Agency.

Quesnel, A. M. and Cohen, M. S. 2015. 'Otologic considerations in microtia and atresia', in M. L. Cheney and T. A. Hadlock (eds.), *Facial surgery: plastic and reconstructive*, Boca Raton, FL: CRC Press, 537–48.

Raine, C. 2013. 'Cochlear implants in the United Kingdom: awareness and utilization', *Cochlear Implants International* **14**:S1, S32-S37.

Raine, R., Wallace, I., a' Bháird, C. N., Xanthopoulou, P., Lanceley, A., Clarke, A., Prentice, A., Ardron, D., Harris, M., Gibbs, J. S. R., Ferlie, E., King, M., Blazeby, J. M., Michie, S., Livingston, G. and Barber, J. 2014. 'Improving the effectiveness of multidisciplinary team meetings for patients with chronic diseases: a prospective observational study', *Health Services and Delivery Research* **2**:37.

Ramig, L., Pawlas, A. and Countryman, S. 1995. *Lee Silverman voice treatment: a practical guide to treating the voice and speech disorders in Parkinson disease*, Iowa City, IA: National Center for Voice and Speech.

Randolph, C. 2012. *Repeatable battery for the assessment of neuropsychological status update (RBANS Update)*, San Antonio, TX: Pearson.

Rautakoski, P. 2011. 'Training total communication', *Aphasiology* **25**:3, 344–65.

Reitan, R. M. and Wolfson, D. 1993. *The Halstead-Reitan neuropsychological test battery: theory and clinical interpretation*, 2nd edn, South Tucson, AZ: Neuropsychology Press.

Riley, G. D. 2009. *Stuttering severity instrument – Fourth edition (SSI-4)*, Austin, TX: Pro-Ed.

Rodney, J. P. and Sataloff, R. T. 2016. 'The effects of hormonal contraception on the voice: history of its evolution in the literature', *Journal of Voice* **30**:6, 726–30.

Roe, J. 2012. 'Alternative investigations', in R. D. Newman and J. M. Nightingale (eds.), *Videofluoroscopy: a multidisciplinary team approach*, San Diego, Oxford and Melbourne: Plural Publishing, 19–34.

Rohrer, J., Maturo, S., Hill, C., Bunting, G., Ballif, C. and Hartnick, C. 2014. 'Pediatric voice analysis: comparison of 2 computerized analysis systems', *JAMA Otolaryngology – Head & Neck Surgery* **140**:8, 742–45.

Rohrer, J. D., Rossor, M. N. and Warren, J. D. 2010. 'Apraxia in progressive nonfluent aphasia', *Journal of Neurology* **257**:4, 569–74.

Roid, G. H. 2003. *Stanford-Binet intelligence scales – Fifth edition (SB-5)*, Itasca, IL: Riverside Publishing.

Roland, P. S. and Marple, B. F. 1997. 'Disorders of the external auditory canal', *Journal of the American Academy of Audiology* **8**:6, 367–78.

Roth, T. N. 2015. 'Aging of the auditory system', in G. G. Celesia and G. Hickok (eds.), *Handbook of clinical neurology, Vol. 129, The human auditory system*, Elsevier, 357–73.

Roth, T. N., Hanebuth, D. and Probst, R. 2011. 'Prevalence of age-related hearing loss in Europe: a review', *European Archives of Oto-Rhino-Laryngology* **268**:8, 1101–7.

Roulstone, S. E., Marshall, J. E., Powell, G. G., Goldbart, J., Wren, Y. E., Coad, J., Daykin, N., Powell, J. E., Lascelles, L., Hollingworth, W., Emond, A., Peters, T. J., Pollock, J. I., Fernandes, C., Moultrie, J., Harding, S. A., Morgan, L., Hambly, H. F., Parker, N. K. and Coad, R. A. 2015. 'Evidence-based intervention for preschool children with primary speech and language impairments: Child Talk – an exploratory mixed-methods study', *Programme Grants for Applied Research* **3**:5. doi: 10.3310/pgfar03050.

Royal College of Speech and Language Therapists (RCSLT) 1998. *Good practice guidelines for speech and language therapists working with clients from linguistic minorities*, London: Royal College of Speech and Language Therapists.

2005. *Clinical guidelines*, Bicester, Oxon: Speechmark Publishing Ltd.

2010. *Guidelines for pre-registration speech and language therapy courses in the UK*, London: Royal College of Speech and Language Therapists.

2014. *Dysphagia training & competency framework: recommendations for knowledge, skills and competency development across the speech and language therapy profession*, London: RCSLT.

2017. *Young offenders and criminal justice*. Available online: www.rcslt.org/about/young_offenders_and_criminal_justice/intro. Accessed 26 March 2017.

RTI International and CDC 2004. 'Economic costs associated with mental retardation, cerebral palsy, hearing loss, and vision impairment: United States, 2003', *Morbidity and Mortality Weekly Report* **53**:3, 57–9.

Ruben, R. J. 2000. 'Redefining the survival of the fittest: communication disorders in the 21st century', *Laryngoscope* **110**:2 (Pt 1), 241–5.

Ruotsalainen, J. H., Sellman, J., Lehto, L., Isotalo, L. K. and Verbeek, J. H. 2007. 'Interventions for preventing voice disorders in adults', *Cochrane database of systematic reviews*, Issue 4. Art. No.: CD006372. doi: 10.1002/14651858.CD006372.pub2.

Ruscello, D. M. 2008. 'Nonspeech oral motor treatment issues related to children with developmental speech sound disorders', *Language, Speech, and Hearing Services in Schools* **39**:3, 380–91.

Rvachew, S. and Nowak, M. 2001. 'The effect of target-selection strategy on phonological learning', *Journal of Speech, Language, and Hearing Research* **44**:3, 610–23.

Saad, A. N., Parina, R. P., Tokin, C., Chang, D. C. and Gosman, A. 2014. 'Incidence of oral clefts among different ethnicities in the state of California', *Annals of Plastic Surgery* **72**:(Suppl. 1), S81-S83.

Sackett, D. L., Rosenberg, W. M. C., Gray, J. A. M., Haynes, R. B. and Richardson, W. S. 1996. 'Evidence based medicine: what it is and what it isn't', *British Medical Journal* **312**, 71.

Sacks, J. M. and Levy, S. 1959. 'The sentence completion test', in L. E. Abt and L. Bellak (eds.), *Projective psychology: clinical approaches to the total personality*, New York: Grove Press, 357–402.

Saeed, J. I. 2015. 'Semantics', in N. Braber, L. Cummings and L. Morrish (eds.), *Exploring language and linguistics*, Cambridge: Cambridge University Press, 168–93.

2016. *Semantics*, 4th edn, Chichester: Wiley Blackwell.

Sahlén, B. and Nettelbladt, U. 1993. 'Context and comprehension: a neurolinguistic and interactional approach to the understanding of semantic-pragmatic disorder', *European Journal of Disorders of Communication* **28**:2, 117–40.

Sandberg, C. and Kiran, S. 2014. 'Analysis of abstract and concrete word processing in persons with aphasia and age-matched neurologically healthy adults using fMRI', *Neurocase* **20**:4, 361–88.

Sato, Y., Kosugi, S. I., Aizawa, N., Ishikawa, T., Kano, Y., Ichikawa, H., Hanyu, T., Hirashima, K., Bamba, T. and Wakai, T. 2016. 'Risk factors and clinical outcomes of recurrent laryngeal nerve paralysis after esophagectomy for thoracic esophageal carcinoma', *World Journal of Surgery* **40**:1, 129–36.

Saunders, A. Z., Stein, A. V. and Shuster, N. L. 1990. 'Audiometry', in H. K. Walker, W. D. Hall and J. W. Hurst (eds.), *Clinical methods: the history, physical, and laboratory examinations*, 3rd edn, Boston: Butterworths, 628–30.

Saur, D., Lange, R., Baumgaertner, A., Schraknepper, V., Willmes, K., Rijntjes, M. and Weiller, C. 2006. 'Dynamics of language reorganization after stroke', *Brain* **129**:6, 1371–84.

Scaler Scott, K. 2017. 'Stuttering and cluttering', in L. Cummings (ed.), *Research in clinical pragmatics*, Cham, Switzerland: Springer, 471–90

Schilling-Estes, N. 2006. 'Dialect variation', in R. W. Fasold and J. Connor-Linton (eds.), *An introduction to language and linguistics*, New York: Cambridge University Press, 311–42.

Schmid, H.-J. 2015. 'Morphology', in N. Braber, L. Cummings and L. Morrish (eds.), *Exploring language and linguistics*, Cambridge: Cambridge University Press, 77–110.

Schöttke, H. and Giabbiconi, C. M. 2015. 'Post-stroke depression and post-stroke anxiety: prevalence and predictors', *International Psychogeriatrics* **27**:11, 1805–12.

Schrauwen, I. and Van Camp, G. 2010. 'The etiology of otosclerosis: a combination of genes and environment', *Laryngoscope* **120**:6, 1195–202.

Schuele, C. M. and Dykes, J. C. 2005. 'Complex syntax acquisition: a longitudinal case study of a child with specific language impairment', *Clinical Linguistics & Phonetics* **19**:4, 295–318.

Scientific Learning Corporation 2016. *Fast ForWord*. Available online: www.scilearn.com/products/fast-forword. Accessed 28 June 2016.

Scott, D. A. and Carey, J. C. 2006. 'Inner ear', in R. E. Stevenson and J. G. Hall (eds.), *Human malformations and related anomalies*, 2nd edn, New York: Oxford University Press, 366–72.

Scripture, E. W. 1912. *Stuttering and lisping*, New York: The Macmillan Company.

 1923. *Stuttering, lisping and correction of the speech of the deaf*, New York: The Macmillan Company.

Sell, D., Harding, A. and Grunwell, P. 1994. 'A screening assessment of cleft palate speech (Great Ormond Street Speech Assessment)', *European Journal of Disorders of Communication* **29**:1, 1–15.

 1999. 'GOS.SP.ASS.'98: An assessment for speech disorders associated with cleft palate and/or velopharyngeal dysfunction (revised)', *International Journal of Language & Communication Disorders* **34**:1, 17–33.

Sellars, C., Hughes, T. and Langhorne, P. 2005. 'Speech and language therapy for dysarthria due to non-progressive brain damage', *Cochrane database of systematic reviews*, Issue 3. Art. No.: CD002088. doi: 10.1002/14651858. CD002088.pub2.

Semel, E., Wiig, E. H. and Secord, W. A. 2003. *Clinical evaluation of language fundamentals*, 4th edn, Australia: Psychological Corporation.

Shah, R. K., Woodnorth, G. H., Glynn, A. and Nuss, R. C. 2005. 'Pediatric vocal nodules: correlation with perceptual voice analysis', *International Journal of Pediatric Otorhinolaryngology* **69**:7, 903–9.

Shanks, B. 2001. *Speaking and listening through narrative*, Keighley, UK: Black Sheep Press.

Sharland, M., Burch, M., McKenna, W. M. and Paton, M. A. 1992. 'A clinical study of Noonan syndrome', *Archives of Disease in Childhood* **67**:2, 178–83.

Sharma, G. and Goodwin, J. 2006. 'Effects of aging on respiratory system physiology and immunology', *Clinical Interventions in Aging* **1**:3, 253–60.

Shehata, G. A., El Mistikawi, T., Risha, A. S. and Hassan, H. S. 2015. 'The effect of aphasia upon personality traits, depression and anxiety among stroke patients', *Journal of Affective Disorders* **172**, 312–14.

Shipley, K. G. and McAfee, J. G. 2009. *Assessment in speech-language pathology: a resource manual*, 4th edn, Clifton Park, NY: Delmar Cengage Learning.

Shipster, C., Hearst, D., Dockrell, J. E., Kilby, E. and Hayward, R. 2002. 'Speech and language skills and cognitive functioning in children with Apert syndrome: a pilot study', *International Journal of Language & Communication Disorders* **37**:3, 325–43.

Shriberg, L. D., Campbell, T. F., Karlsson, H. B., Brown, R. L., McSweeny, J. L. and Nadler, C. J. 2003. 'A diagnostic marker for childhood apraxia of speech: the lexical stress ratio', *Clinical Linguistics & Phonetics* **17**:7, 549–74.

Sibbald, B. and Roland, M. 1998. 'Understanding controlled trials: why are randomised controlled trials important?', *British Medical Journal* **316**, 201.

Sichel, J. Y., Dangoor, E., Eliashar, R. and Halperin, D. 2000. 'Management of congenital laryngeal malformations', *American Journal of Otolaryngology* **21**:1, 22–30.

Sidavi, A. and Fabus, R. 2010. 'A review of stuttering intervention approaches for preschool-age and elementary school-age children', *Contemporary Issues in Communication Science and Disorders* **37**, 14–26.

Sielska-Badurek, E., Rzepakowska, A., Sobol, M., Osuch-Wójcikiewicz, E. and Niemczyk, K. 2016. 'Adaptation and validation of the voice-related quality of life measure into Polish', *Journal of Voice* **30**:6, 773.e7–773.e12.

Skuse, D. H. 2000. 'Imprinting, the X-chromosome, and the male brain: explaining sex differences in the liability to autism', *Pediatric Research* **47**:1, 9–16.

Sliwinska-Kowalska, M. 2015. 'Hearing', in M. Lotti and M. L. Bleecker (eds.), *Occupational neurology*, Handbook of clinical neurology, Vol. 131. Elsevier, 341–63.

Smile Train 2015. *2015 annual report*, New York: Author.

Solazzo, A., Monaco, L., Del Vecchio, L., Tamburrini, S., Iacobellis, F., Berritto, D., Pizza, N. L., Reginelli, A., Di Martino, N. and Grassi, R. 2012. 'Investigation of compensatory postures with videofluoromanometry in dysphagia patients', *World Journal of Gastroenterology* **18**:2, 2973–8.

Special Eurobarometer 2012. *Europeans and their languages: report*, Brussels: European Commission.

St Louis, K. O., Myers, F. L., Cassidy, L. J., Michael, A. J., Penrod, S. M., Litton, B. A., Coutras, S. W., Olivera, J. L. R. and Brodsky, E. 1996. 'Efficacy of delayed auditory feedback for treating cluttering: two case studies', *Journal of Fluency Disorders* **21**:3–4, 305–14.

Steele, C. M., Alsanei, W. A., Ayanikalath, S., Barbon, C. E. A., Chen, J., Cichero, J. A. Y., Coutts, K., Dantas, R. O., Duivestein, J., Giosa, L., Hanson, B., Lam, P., Lecko, C., Leigh, C., Nagy, A., Namasivayam, A. M., Nascimento, W. V., Odendaal, I., Smith, C. H. and Wang, H. 2015. 'The influence of food texture and liquid consistency modification on swallowing physiology and function: a systematic review', *Dysphagia* **30**:1, 2–26.

Steele, S. C. and Mills, M. T. 2011. 'Vocabulary intervention for school-age children with language impairment: a review of evidence and good practice', *Child Language Teaching and Therapy* **27**:3, 354–70.

Stiles, J. and Jernigan, T. L. 2010. 'The basics of brain development', *Neuropsychology Review* **20**:4, 327–48.

Stow, C. and Dodd, B. 2003. 'Providing an equitable service to bilingual children in the UK: a review', *International Journal of Language & Communication Disorders* **38**:4, 351–77.

Stow, C. and Pert, S. 2015. *SLT assessment and intervention: best practice for children and young people in bilingual settings*, London: Royal College of Speech and Language Therapists.

Stroke Association 2014a. *Research spend in the UK: comparing Stroke, Cancer, Coronary Heart Disease and Dementia*, London: Author.

2014b. *Stroke association research strategy 2014–2019*, London: Author.

Strong, C. J. 1998. *The strong narrative assessment procedure*, Eau Claire, WI: Thinking Publications.

Stroop, J. R. 1935. 'Studies of interference in serial verbal reactions', *Journal of Experimental Psychology* **18**:6, 643–62.

Sudhir, P. M., Chandra, P. S., Shivashankar, N. and Yamini, B. K. 2009. 'Comprehensive management of psychogenic dysphonia: a case illustration', *Journal of Communication Disorders* **42**:5, 305–12.

Sullivan, S. and Ruffman, T. 2004. 'Social understanding: how does it fare with advancing years?', *British Journal of Psychology* **95**:1, 1–18.

Swigert, N. 2016. 'Successful collaboration on breathing and swallowing', *The ASHA Leader* **21**:1, 34–5.

Tatar, E. C., Sahin, M., Demiral, D., Bayir, O., Saylam, G., Ozdek, A. and Korkmaz, M. H. 2016. 'Normative values of voice analysis parameters with respect to menstrual cycle in healthy adult Turkish women', *Journal of Voice* **30**:3, 322–8.

Taylor, B., Jick, H. and MacLaughlin, D. 2013. 'Prevalence and incidence rates of autism in the UK: time trend from 2004–2010 in children aged 8 years', *BMJ Open* **3**, e003219.

Thevasagayam, M., Rodger, K., Cave, D., Witmans, M. and El-Hakim, H. 2010. 'Prevalence of laryngomalacia in children presenting with sleep-disordered breathing', *Laryngoscope* **120**:8, 1662–6.

Thomas, P. 1997. 'What can linguistics tell us about thought disorder?', in J. France and N. Muir (eds.), *Communication and the mentally ill patient: developmental and linguistic approaches to schizophrenia*, London: Jessica Kingsley Publishers, 30–42.

Thompson, C. K., Riley, E. A., den Ouden, D.-B., Meltzer-Asscher, A. and Lukic, S. 2013. 'Training verb argument structure production in agrammatic aphasia: behavioral and neural recovery patterns', *Cortex* **49**:9, 2358–76.

Thordardottir, E. 2015. 'The relationship between bilingual exposure and morphosyntactic development', *International Journal of Speech-Language Pathology* **17**:2, 97–114.

Thorne, M. C. and Garetz, S. L. 2016. 'Laryngomalacia: review and summary of current clinical practice in 2015', *Paediatric Respiratory Reviews* **17**, 3–8.

Titone, D. and Levy, D. L. 2004. 'Lexical competition and spoken word identification in schizophrenia', *Schizophrenia Research* **68**:1, 75–85.

Tomblin, J. B., Records, N. L., Buckwalter, P., Zhang, X., Smith, E. and O'Brien, M. 1997. 'Prevalence of specific language impairment in kindergarten children', *Journal of Speech, Language, and Hearing Research* **40**:6, 1245–60.

Towey, M. 2013. 'Speech therapy telepractice', in S. Kumar and E. R. Cohn (eds.), *Telerehabilitation*, London: Springer, 101–24.

Trupe, L. A., Varma, D. D., Gomez, Y., Race, D., Leigh, R., Hillis, A. E. and Gottesman, R. F. 2013. 'Chronic apraxia of speech and "Broca's area"', *Stroke* **44**:3, 740–4.

Turkstra, L. S., Coelho, C. and Ylvisaker, M. 2005. 'The use of standardized tests for individuals with cognitive-communication disorders', *Seminars in Speech and Language* **26**:4, 215–22.

Tyler, A. A. and Macrae, T. 2010. 'Stimulability: relationships to other characteristics of children's phonological systems', *Clinical Linguistics & Phonetics* **24**:4–5, 300–10.

Tyrrell, J., White, M. P., Barrett, G., Ronan, N., Phoenix, C., Whinney, D. J. and Osborne, N. J. 2015. 'Mental health and subjective well-being of individuals with Ménière's: cross-sectional analysis in the UK Biobank', *Otology & Neurotology* **36**:5, 854–61.

Ullrich, D., Ullrich, K. and Marten, M. 2014. 'A longitudinal assessment of early childhood education with integrated speech therapy for children with significant language impairment in Germany', *International Journal of Language & Communication Disorders* **49**:5, 558–66.

Van Borsel, J. and Tetnowski, J. A. 2007. 'Fluency disorders in genetic syndromes', *Journal of Fluency Disorders* **32**:4, 279–96.

Van Borsel, J., Reunes, G. and van den Bergh, N. 2003. 'Delayed auditory feedback in the treatment of stuttering: clients as consumers', *International Journal of Language & Communication Disorders* **38**:2, 119–29.

Van der Lely, H. K. J. and Battell, J. 2003. 'Wh-movement in children with grammatical SLI: a test of the RDDR hypothesis', *Language* **79**:1, 153–81.

Van Zaalen, Y. and Reichel, I. K. 2015. *Cluttering: current views on its nature, diagnosis, and treatment*, Bloomington, IN: iUniverse.

Vandenborre, D., van Dun, K. and Mariën, P. 2015. 'Apraxic agraphia following bithalamic damage', *Brain and Cognition* **95**, 35–43.

Vannson, N., James, C., Fraysse, B., Strelnikov, K., Barone, P., Deguine, O. and Marx, M. 2015. 'Quality of life and auditory performance in adults with asymmetric hearing loss', *Audiology & Neuro-otology* **20**:(Suppl. 1), 38–43.

Vanryckeghem, M. and Brutten, G. J. 2007. *KiddyCAT: communication attitude test for preschool and kindergarten children who stutter*, San Diego, CA: Plural Publishing.

Velleman, S. L. 2004. 'Speech disorders in children: descriptive linguistic approaches', in R. D. Kent (ed.), *The MIT encyclopedia of communication disorders*, Cambridge, MA: MIT Press, 198–9.

Verbuk, A. and Shultz, T. 2010. 'Acquisition of relevance implicatures: a case against a rationality-based account of conversational implicatures', *Journal of Pragmatics* **42**:8, 2297–313.

Verdolini, K. 2004. 'Voice therapy for adults', in R. D. Kent (ed.), *The MIT encyclopedia of communication disorders*, Cambridge, MA: The MIT Press, 88–91.

Vos, R. C., Dallmeijer, A. J., Verhoef, M., Van Schie, P. E., Voorman, J. M., Wiegerink, D. J., Geytenbeek, J. J., Roebroeck, M. E., Becher, J. G. and PERRIN + Study Group 2014. 'Developmental trajectories of receptive and expressive communication in children and young adults with cerebral palsy', *Developmental Medicine and Child Neurology* **56**:10, 951–9.

Vose, A., Nonnenmacher, J., Singer, M. L. and González-Fernández, M. 2014. 'Dysphagia management in acute and sub-acute stroke', *Current Physical Medicine and Rehabilitation Reports* **2**:4, 197–206.

Wake, M., Levickis, P., Tobin, S., Zens, N., Law, J., Gold, L., Ukoumunne, O. C., Goldfeld, S., Le, H. N. D., Skeat, J. and Reilly, S. 2012. 'Improving outcomes of preschool language delay in the community: protocol for the *Language for Learning* randomised controlled trial', *BMC Pediatrics* **12**, 96.

Wales, C. J., Corsar, K. and Devlin, M. F. 2009. 'Submucous cleft palate', *British Dental Journal* **207**, 254. doi: 10.1038/sj.bdj.2009.822.

Wall, L. R., Ward, E. C., Cartmill, B., Hill, A. J. and Porceddu, S. V. 2017. 'Examining user perceptions of SwallowIT: a pilot study of a new telepractice application for delivering intensive swallowing therapy to head and neck cancer patients', *Journal of Telemedicine and Telecare* **23**:1, 53–9.

Ward, D. 2006. *Stuttering and cluttering: frameworks for understanding and treatment*, New York: Psychology Press.

Watts, C. R., Diviney, S. S., Hamilton, A., Toles, L., Childs, L. and Mau, T. 2015. 'The effect of stretch-and-flow voice therapy on measures of vocal function and handicap', *Journal of Voice* **29**:2, 191–9.

Wechsler, D. 2008. *Wechsler adult intelligence scale – Fourth edition (WAIS-IV)*, San Antonio, TX: Psychological Corporation.

2014. *Wechsler intelligence scale for children – Fifth edition (WISC-V)*, San Antonio, TX: Pearson.

Weiss, L. G., Saklofske, D. H., Holdnack, J. A. and Prifitera, A. 2015. 'WISC-V: advances in the assessment of intelligence', in L. G. Weiss, D. H. Saklofske, J. A. Holdnack and A. Prifitera (eds.), *WISC-V assessment and interpretation: scientist-practitioner perspectives*, New York: Elsevier, 3–23.

Weissman, A. N. and Beck, A. T. 1978. 'Development and validation of the dysfunctional attitudes scale: a preliminary investigation', paper presented at the 62nd Annual Meeting of the American Educational Research Association, Ontario, Canada, March 1978.

Wellman, H. M. and Lagattuta, K. H. 2000. 'Developing understandings of mind', in S. Baron-Cohen, H. Tager-Flusberg and D. J. Cohen (eds.), *Understanding other minds: perspectives from developmental cognitive neuroscience*, New York: Oxford University Press, 21–49.

Whitehouse, A. J., Watt, H. J., Line, E. A. and Bishop, D. V. 2009. 'Adult psychosocial outcomes of children with specific language impairment, pragmatic language impairment and autism', *International Journal of Language & Communication Disorders* **44**:4, 511–28.

Whitworth, A., Perkins, L. and Lesser, R. 1997. *Conversation analysis profile for people with aphasia (CAPPA)*, London: Whurr Publishers.

Whitworth, A., Webster, J. and Howard, D. 2005. *A cognitive neuropsychological approach to assessment and intervention in aphasia*, Hove, UK: Psychology Press.

(eds.) 2014. *A cognitive neuropsychological approach to assessment and intervention in aphasia: a clinician's guide*, Hove, UK, and New York: Psychology Press.

Whitworth, A., Webster, J. and Morris, J. 2014. 'Acquired aphasia', in L. Cummings (ed.), *Cambridge handbook of communication disorders*, Cambridge: Cambridge University Press, 436–56.

WHO Multicentre Growth Reference Study Group 2006. 'WHO motor development study: windows of achievement for six gross motor development milestones', *Acta Paediatrica* **450**:(Suppl.), 86–95.

Wight, S. and Miller, N. 2015. 'Lee Silverman voice treatment for people with Parkinson's: audit of outcomes in a routine clinic', *International Journal of Language & Communication Disorders* **50**:2, 215–25.

Wiig, E. H., Semel, E. and Secord, W. A. 2013. *Clinical evaluation of language fundamentals-Fifth Edition*, San Antonio, TX: Pearson.

Williams, A. L. 2000. 'Multiple oppositions: case studies of variables in phonological intervention', *American Journal of Speech-Language Pathology* **9**:4, 289–99.

2005. 'Assessment, target selection and intervention: dynamic interactions within a systemic perspective', *Topics in Language Disorders* **25**:3, 231–42.

Williams, P. and Stephens, H. (eds.) 2004. *Nuffield Centre dyspraxia programme – Third edition*, Windsor, UK: The Miracle Factory.

Wilson, S. M., Galantucci, S., Tartaglia, M. C., Rising, K., Patterson, D. K., Henry, M. L., Ogar, J. M., DeLeon, J., Miller, B. L. and Gorno-Tempini, M. L. 2011. 'Syntactic processing depends on dorsal language tracts', *Neuron* **72**:2, 397–403.

Wingate, M. E. 2002. *Foundations of stuttering*, San Diego, CA: Academic Press.

World Gastroenterology Organisation 2014. *Dysphagia: global guidelines & cascades*, Milwaukee, MI: Author.

World Health Organization (WHO) 1997. *WHOQOL: measuring quality of life*, Geneva: World Health Organization.

2001. *International classification of functioning, disability and health*, Geneva: World Health Organization.

2010. *Framework for action on interprofessional education & collaborative practice*, Geneva: World Health Organization.

2018. *International classification of diseases – Eleventh edition*, Geneva: World Health Organization.

Wright, T. 2015. 'Ménière's disease', Systematic Review 505, 5 November. *BMJ Clinical Evidence*. Available online: http://clinicalevidence.bmj.com/x/systematic-review/0505/overview.html. Accessed 17 August 2017.

Yaruss, J. S. 2014. 'Disorders of fluency', in L. Cummings (ed.), *Cambridge handbook of communication disorders*, Cambridge: Cambridge University Press, 484–98.

Yaruss, J. S. and Quesal, R. 2010. *Overall assessment of the speaker's experience of stuttering (OASES)*, Bloomington, MN: Pearson Assessments.

Yavaş, M. 1998. *Phonology: development and disorders*, San Diego, CA: Singular Publishing Group, Inc.

Young, E. C., Diehl, J. J., Morris, D., Hyman, S. L. and Bennetto, L. 2005. 'The use of two language tests to identify pragmatic language problems in children with autism spectrum disorders', *Language, Speech, and Hearing Services in Schools* **36**:1, 62–72.

Zarchi, O., Avni, C., Attias, J., Frisch, A., Carmel, M., Michaelovsky, E., Green, T., Weizman, A. and Gothelf, D. 2015. 'Hyperactive auditory processing in Williams syndrome: evidence from auditory evoked potentials', *Psychophysiology* **52**:6, 782–9.

Zur, K. B., Cotton, S., Kelchner, L., Baker, S., Weinrich, B. and Lee, L. 2007. 'Pediatric voice handicap index (pVHI): a new tool for evaluating pediatric dysphonia', *International Journal of Pediatric Otorhinolaryngology* **71**:1, 77–82.

Index

abduction, 36, 122, 126, 203, 318
academic
    achievement, 12, 211–12, 222, 263, 279, 365–6
    impact, 12–14, 305, 318
    underachievement, 12–14, 165, 318, 344, 375
acalculia, 185, 318, *See* dyscalculia
accent, 3, 10–11, 65–6, 68, 250, 318, 347
accommodation, 135, 140
accreditation, 285, 289, 301, 316, 318
achalasia, 121, 318, 348
acid laryngitis, 122, 318
acoustic neuroma, 113, 318, 371
acoustic reflex test, 111, 310, 318
acquired communication disorder, 18–19, 22, 32, 265, 267, 318
active articulator, 36, 318, *See* passive articulator
adduction, 36, 122, 202–3, 250–1, 254, 319, 341
advocacy, 1, 5, 269, 287–9, 294–5, 298, 301, 304, 316, 319
aetiology, 15–16, 88–91, 95, 100, 106, 121–2, 124–5, 198, 201, 207, 209, 231, 236, 308, 319, 321, 326, 334, 339, 351
affective
    flattening, 363
    state, 56–7, 137, 140, 165, 370
affix, 47, 319
aging, 89, 95, 108, 121, 123, 132, 204, 332, 339, 359
agrammatism, 15, 32, 50, 319
AIDS dementia complex, 63, 319
alcohol, 144, 251, 354, 374
alcohol-related dementia, 331
allophone, 42, 45, 319, 328
alogia, 118–19, 158–9, 162, 213, 319, 352, 359, *See* poverty of speech
Alport syndrome, 101, 319
Alzheimer's dementia, 20, 23, 33, 131, 165, 226, 237, 319
Alzheimer's disease, 125, 151, 237, 319, 331, 338, 348, 360
ambiguity, 58, 365
American Psychiatric Association, 4, 118, 167, 211, 331
American Speech-Language-Hearing Association, 1, 7–8, 225, 268, 274, 276, 280, 287, 336

amplification, 16, 113, 116–17, 320, 340
amyotrophic lateral sclerosis, 320, 350, *See* motor neurone disease
anaphoric reference, 62, 118, 320, 328
anatomy, 16–17, 35, 87–8, 92, 94–6, 101, 106, 121, 124–5, 176–7, 182, 250, 253, 309, 320, 332, 349, 352, 358
androgen therapy, 88, 93, 123, 250, 320
anomia, 243, 266, 274, 294–5, 320, *See* word-finding difficulty
anxiety, 12, 14, 122, 159–60, 162, 201, 247, 253, 259, 290, 310, 313, 320, 324, 361
anxiety disorder, 320
Apert syndrome, 178, 320
aphasia
    agrammatic, 54, 319, 360
    anomic, 219, 320
    battery, 173, 323
    Broca's, 219, 320
    conduction, 320
    global, 320
    non-fluent, 180, 295, 319–20, 360
    transcortical motor, 320
    Wernicke's, 52, 320, 375
aphasiology, 148, 398
aphonia, 105, 159–61, 213, 320, 341
apraxia of speech, 83, 97, 177–8, 180, 183, 210, 234, 236, 306, 311, 320, 332, 343, 350, 352, 354
apraxic agraphia, 76, 321
argument structure, 53–5, 84, 321, 365
Arnold-Chiari malformation, 105, 321
articulation, 10, 17, 36, 42, 67, 72, 85, 124, 168–9, 172, 176, 178–83, 198, 217, 234, 248–9, 266, 318, 330, 333, 341, 349, 374
articulation disorder, 8–9, 83, 321, 367
articulatory groping, 321
artificial larynx, 255, 335, *See* electrolarynx
Asperger's syndrome, 56–7, 321
aspiration, 105, 173, 207–8, 219–20, 257, 259, 267, 272, 294, 311, 314, 321, 325, 353, 365, 373, *See* silent aspiration
aspiration pneumonia, 256, 260, 301, 321
atherosclerosis, 93, 321
atresia, 96, 101, 106, 108, 116, 125–6, 321, 325, 329, 340, 373

411

atrophy, 98, 251, 321, 341, 350, 356, 367
attention, 17, 67–8, 99, 129, 131–3, 146, 151–2, 154, 156, 158, 174, 187–8, 236, 238, 247–8, 322, 348, 364, 369, *See* selective attention
attention deficit hyperactivity disorder (ADHD), 6, 62, 119, 131–2, 156–7, 170, 211, 215, 223, 322, 341–2, 352
audiogram, 103–4, 108–9, 127, 322, 353, 361
audiology, 16, 88, 107, 117, 124, 276, 285, 288, 322
audiometry, 109, 112, 127, 170, 322
auditory brainstem response audiometry, 117, 318, 322
augmentative and alternative communication (AAC), 5, 9, 24, 26, 216, 228, 235–7, 266, 301, 322, 338
aural atresia, 102
aural rehabilitation, 88, 102, 113, 117, 322
Austin, J. L., 55, 367
autism spectrum disorder (ASD), 6, 9, 33, 56, 92, 131, 170, 185, 211, 214, 216, 222, 232, 271, 287, 321–2, 325, 332, 336, 343, 352, 366, 370
auxiliary verb, 49, 237, 323, 344
avoidance behaviour, 200, 218, 247, 323, *See* stuttering
avolition, 212, 352, 363

Babinski reflex, 98, 100, 323
backing, 44, 182, 306
basal ganglia, 341
basilar membrane, 108, 323
Beckwith-Wiedemann syndrome, 94, 323, 347
bedside assessment, 2, 172, 209, 272, 323
behavioural impact, 12–14, 305, 323
bifid uvula, 177, 324
bilingual aphasia, 67, 324
bilingualism, 65, 67–9, 280–1, 324, 351
bipolar disorder, 88, 117–18, 158, 324
blending, 46–7, 230, 233, 324, 376
block, 247, 324, *See* stuttering
bolus, 206–8, 252, 256–7, 260, 314, 324, 354, 374
bowing, 202, 251, 324
brain tumour, 90, 99, 255, 324, 360
brainstem, 40, 93, 322, 324, 330, 341, 347, 372
breathiness, 105, 168, 203–4, 206, 324
breathing, 104, 169, 318, 363, 373
Broca's area, 93, 325

cancer, 25, 106, 258, 260, 291, 324, 326, 330, 340, 347, 354, 356–7, 362, 368, *See* carcinoma
candida albicans, 207, 325, 354
canonical babbling, 134, 325
capillary ectasias, 374, *See* varices
carcinoma, 106, 122, 124, 127, 251, 345, *See* cancer
carryover, 248, 253, 325, *See* generalization

case history, 64, 134, 171, 198–200, 207, 218, 270, 325, 350
cell biology, 92, 320, 325
central auditory processing, 107, 109, 325
central nervous system, 16, 93, 98–100, 103, 105, 152, 325, 330, 332, 351–3, 357
cerebellum, 76–7, 321, 324, 338
cerebral palsy, 31, 36, 92, 97, 100, 126, 134, 164, 206, 219, 231–2, 235, 251, 255, 266, 283, 286, 292, 309, 325, 332–3, 340–1, 363, 367
cerebrovascular accident, 19, 50, 52, 90–1, 93, 125–6, 207, 294, 309, 321, 324–5, 352, 356, 365, 368, *See* stroke
CHARGE syndrome, 101, 326
chemotherapy, 99–100, 249, 254, 324, 326, 345, 354
child language acquisition, 35, 47, 78, 80–1, 326, 366
childhood apraxia of speech, 9, 19, 32, 178, 210, 226, 232, 290, 296, 326, 331–2, 367, *See* developmental verbal dyspraxia
cholesteatoma, 103, 106, 108, 126, 326, 348
choral speech, 248–9, 326, 338, *See* stuttering
circumlocution, 243, 266, 323, 326, 347
cleft lip and palate, 15, 94, 96, 165, 291, 293–4, 326, 369, *See* submucous cleft palate
clinical education, 55, 87, 92, 119, 123, 129, 133, 144, 166, 184, 268, 274, 285
clinical neuropsychology, 132–3, 152, 326, 353
clinical pragmatics, 55, 326
clinical psychology, 18, 129, 132–3, 157, 160, 162, 327
clipping, 46–7, 327, 376
cluttering, 8, 195, 198, 200, 210, 213, 218, 245, 248–9, 327, 337
cochlea, 39, 41, 73, 92, 102–3, 106, 108, 114, 126, 327, 342–3, 349, 353, 355, 359, 363, 368, 373
cochlear
 aplasia, 102, 106, 327
 hypoplasia, 102, 106, 109, 126, 327, 371
 implant, 102, 107, 113–14, 229, 320, 327, 340
 implantation, 102, 114, 117, 327
cochleostomy, 114, 327
cognition, 100, 129, 131, 137, 161–2, 197–8, 319, 328
cognitive behavioural therapy, 119, 132, 160–2, 165, 247, 249, 327
cognitive development, 130, 135–7, 139–40, 327, 358
cognitive module, 147, 327, 343, *See* modularity
cognitive neuropsychology, 130–2, 328
cognitive psychology, 16, 18, 129, 131–3, 146–7, 151, 162, 327
cognitive-communication disorder, 8–9, 12, 20, 63, 152, 164, 174, 328
coherence, 63–4, 192, 194, 328
cohesion, 16, 20, 62, 64, 85, 118, 162, 165, 212, 320, 328, 335, 346, 369

cohesive device, 62
collaborative working, 159, 162, 268, 270, 273–5, 328
communication disorder, 1–3, 5–6, 8, 10–15, 18–24, 27–30, 32, 64, 66, 77, 88–91, 97, 125, 152, 158–9, 162, 166, 200, 210–11, 213–16, 221–3, 226, 250, 265, 269, 272, 280, 285, 288–90, 294, 296, 298, 300–1, 304–5, 315–16, 318–20, 323, 328, 330, 333, 338, 340, 364, 371, 375
communicative
　intention, 57–8, 71, 74, 138, 328, 336, 345
　partner, 24, 235
complementary distribution, 42, 328
componential analysis, 52, 55, 328, 364
compounding, 46–7, 329
comprehensibility, 62, 235, 266, 329
comprehension, 2, 18, 20, 22, 27, 35, 50, 53, 56, 65, 69–72, 74, 77, 80, 84, 89, 142–3, 159, 172–3, 184–6, 188, 190, 195, 209–10, 238, 240–1, 274, 278, 295, 312, 320, 325, 342, 345, 364, 371, 375–6
computerized axial tomography, 329
conductive hearing loss, 8, 16, 88, 95, 101, 103, 106–9, 116–17, 125, 127, 309, 320, 329, 340, 355, 372
confrontation naming, 46, 185, 329
congenital heart disease, 93
consonant cluster reduction, 15, 43, 45, 79, 82, 306, 311, 329, 358
constancy under negation, 60–1, 329
contact ulcer, 335, *See* granuloma
context, 20, 23, 30, 40, 55, 59, 61–2, 64, 66, 68, 73–4, 76, 83, 133, 141, 143, 147, 161, 167, 175–6, 179, 191–4, 197, 200, 210–12, 218, 234, 242, 244, 261, 267–8, 270, 275–6, 279, 281, 283, 287, 311, 313, 320, 329–31, 339, 344, 359, 362–3
continuing professional development (CPD), 34, 269, 285, 289, 301, 316, 329
contrastive function, 41, 45, 329
conversation analysis, 24, 166, 168, 171, 174, 176, 184, 329
conversational
　discourse, 63
　exchange, 85, 191, 195
　partner, 22, 24, 27, 226–7, 235, 244, 266, 304
　repair, 192, 330
conversion aphonia, 127, 320, 361
cooperative principle, 57–8, 61, 330, 348
coordinating conjunction, 278, 330
correct information unit, 174, 194, 330
coughing, 201, 207, 259, 267, 314
cranial
　nerve, 32, 40, 88, 93, 98, 100, 126, 177, 324, 330, 336, 341, 360, 373
　radiotherapy, 99–100, 330
craniofacial syndrome, 371

cricothyroid approximation, 250, 330
cricothyroid joint, 105, 330
cueing, 33, 168, 236, 243, 330
cytomegalovirus, 19, 97, 109, 125, 330

deixis, 59–61, 331, 359
delayed auditory feedback, 248–9, 331, 338
delusion, 32, 118, 212, 224, 331, 358, 363, *See* schizophrenia
dementia, 8, 14, 20, 53, 55, 89, 98, 121, 124, 128, 132, 149, 151, 153, 156, 216, 223, 258, 286, 319, 323, 331, 338, 349, 351, 360, 364, 371
demyelination, 351, *See* multiple sclerosis
depression, 12, 14, 25, 33, 158–62, 201, 214, 219, 225, 228, 253, 263, 304, 311, 314, 324, 331, 361, 366
derailment, 118, 331, 370
derivational morphology, 46–7, 331
developmental apraxia of speech, 36, 127, 331
developmental language disorder, 265, 305, 367
developmental period, 18–19, 22, 98, 159, 211–12, 254, 323, 325–6, 331, 365
developmental phonological disorder, 331, 357, *See* speech sound disorder
developmental psychology, 16, 18, 129–30, 133–4, 137, 139–40, 305, 332
developmental verbal dyspraxia, 164, 229, 332, 334, *See* childhood apraxia of speech
diadochokinetic (DDK) rate, 178, 332
Diagnostic and Statistical Manual of Mental Disorders (DSM), 118, 332
dialect, 40, 42, 65–6, 68, 85, 181, 332, 351
diaphragm, 72, 93, 332, 358
dietician, 33, 257, 271–2, 275, 314, 332
diffusion tensor imaging (DTI), 332
diphthong, 36, 83, 332
diplegia, 97, 332
discourse, 15–17, 20, 34–5, 57, 59, 61, 63–5, 83, 85, 152–3, 157, 159, 171, 175–6, 184, 191, 193–5, 198, 210, 311, 328, 330–3, 343–4, 351, 363, 371–2
discourse analysis, 62, 168, 176, 184, 333
disorganized speech, 118–19, 212, 333, 358, 370, *See* formal thought disorder
distal aetiology, 90–1, 333, 361, *See* proximal aetiology
distinctive feature, 43, 233–4, 333
dopamine, 346, 356, *See* Parkinson's disease
Down syndrome, 22, 80, 83–4, 90, 94, 134, 139, 195, 225, 237, 245, 306, 333, 337, 339, 343, 347, 372, *See* trisomy 21
Duchenne muscular dystrophy, 98, 100, 126, 231, 309, 333
dysarthria, 16, 18–19, 26, 31–2, 36, 39, 83, 88–9, 92, 97–8, 120, 126–7, 172–3, 177–8, 180, 183, 210, 214, 219, 228–9, 231–2, 234–6, 251, 276, 286–7, 293–4, 301, 306, 311, 333, 337–8, 341, 343, 350–2, 356

dyscalculia, 131, 133, 146, 318, 333, *See* acalculia
dysfluency, 24, 91, 196–200, 245, 331, 333, 352, 361
dyskinesia, 97, 99, 333, 346
dyslexia, 16, 32, 89, 131, 133, 144, 146, 334
dysphagia, 2, 9, 19, 22, 33, 97, 121, 124, 126, 152, 168, 170, 206–10, 216, 220, 256–60, 262, 265, 267, 271–6, 281, 286–7, 293–4, 300–1, 311, 314, 321, 332–4, 339, 351, 374
dysphonia, 4, 15, 31, 37, 88, 90–1, 105, 121–4, 126–7, 159–60, 162–3, 165, 201–2, 204–6, 213, 221, 250, 252, 267, 270, 274, 310, 334, 353, 362
dyspraxia, 131, 134, 146, 229–30, 232, 236, 334

ear canal, 39, 41, 96, 101, 108, 111, 113, 125, 329, 334, 349, 361
early corrective heart surgery, 93
ecological validity, 171, 175, 191, 194, 334
education, 1, 4, 12–13, 34–5, 40, 87, 89, 122, 131, 141, 157, 163, 166, 175, 243, 245, 252, 267–8, 274–5, 279–80, 282–9, 300, 304, 316, 318, 358, 366
educational psychologist, 16, 64, 131, 133, 141, 144–6, 163–4, 171, 271, 310, 334
educational psychology, 16, 18, 129, 131, 133, 140, 145–6, 305, 334
egocentric discourse, 165
electroencephalography (EEG), 99, 334
electroglottography (EGG), 203, 206, 335
electrolarynx, 236, 250, 253–5, 266, 335, 345, 354, *See* artificial larynx
electropalatography (EPG), 17, 169, 182–3, 229, 278, 335
ellipsis, 62, 64, 307, 328, 335
embryology, 94, 105, 335
emotion, 320, 327, 360, 363
emotional and behavioural disorder, 132, 361
emotional state, 57
encephalitis, 340, *See* herpes simplex encephalitis
endocrinology, 88, 120, 123–4, 127, 310, 335
endotracheal intubation, 105, 335
ENT medicine, 16–17, 88, 100, 106, 335, 355, *See* otolaryngology, otorhinolaryngology
entailment, 60–1, 329, 335
epidemiology, 15–16, 28, 88–91, 106, 305, 308, 335
epiglottis, 257, 336, 345, 373
Estuary English, 66, 336
euphoria, 324
Eustachian tube, 95, 103, 111, 336, 349, 352, 355
euthymia, 324
evidence-based practice, 232, 260–2, 264–5, 267, 287, 336
executive dysfunction, 336, 360
executive function, 17, 20, 152, 154–7, 163, 300, 315, 319, 322, 336, 360

external auditory meatus, 39, 101, 106, 334, 336
eye
    contact, 64, 189
    gaze, 57, 81, 189, 281

facial expression, 93, 186, 235, 281, 336, 341
facial nerve, 93, 98, 177, 336, 355
false belief test, 138–40, 336
fasciculation, 98, 177, 336, 341
fibreoptic endoscopic evaluation of swallowing (FEES), 169, 207, 287, 337
fibreoptic laryngoscopy, 202, 337, 346
figurative language, 16, 159, 337
final consonant deletion, 43, 233, 306, 311, 337
finger agnosia, 185, 337
fistula, 125, 177, 182–3, 337, 351, 373
flaccid dysarthria, 97, 337, 358, *See* dysarthria
fluency, 4, 24, 77, 166, 170, 195, 197, 199–200, 213, 216, 218, 220, 226, 245–7, 249, 265, 286, 326, 328, 331, 337–8, 347, 360
fluency disorder, 8–9, 21, 170, 195–6, 200, 213, 216, 245, 327, 337, 369
fluent aphasia, 59, 127, 320, 338
foetal alcohol spectrum disorder, 164
forensic impact, 12–14, 305, 338
formal thought disorder, 118, 212, 338, 370, *See* disorganized speech
fragile X syndrome, 32, 92, 125, 134, 245, 338–9, 360
frequency altered feedback, 248, 338
Friedreich's ataxia, 178, 338
friendship, 12–14, 200, 222, 263, 366
frontal lobe, 152, 157, 172, 336
frontotemporal dementia, 32, 77, 338, 360, 364
frontotemporal lobar degeneration, 180, 338
functional communication, 174, 189, 198, 244, 251, 338
functional dysphonia, 122, 160, 201, 338, *See* functional voice disorder
functional magnetic resonance imaging (fMRI), 76, 99, 338
functional voice disorder, 91, 201, 205, 338, *See* organic voice disorder
fundamental frequency, 94, 123, 179, 202, 338, 344, 350, 358, 375, *See* pitch

gag reflex, 177, 337–8, 346
gastroenterologist, 121, 123, 208–9, 268, 270–1, 275, 315, 339
gastroenterology, 16, 88, 120–4, 127, 257, 308, 310, 339
gastroesophageal reflux disease (GERD), 88, 122, 124, 201, 208, 270, 345, 354
gender dysphoria, 127, 339
gender reassignment, 133, 250, 339

general practitioner, 122, 288, 290, 298, 339
generalization, 43, 67, 233, 243–4, 266, 325, 339, *See* carryover
genetic syndrome, 81, 90, 92, 134, 245, 339, 360
genetics, 92, 125, 339
geriatrics, 89, 120, 123, 125, 127, 310, 339
gerontology, 120, 124, 310, 339
gesture, 2, 57–8, 94, 185–6, 195, 235–6, 330, 338–9, 341, 371
glossectomy, 25, 96, 106, 121, 125–6, 176, 206, 339, 347, 354
Goldenhar syndrome, 101, 339
grammar, 29, 48, 50, 59, 175, 184–5, 211–12, 238, 240, 329, 347, 356, 366, 372, *See* syntax
granuloma, 335, *See* contact ulcer
greeting, 74, 165, 189, 212
Grice, H.P., 57–8, 330, 342, 348
grimace, 178, 197, 218, 340
group therapy, 2–3, 17, 225, 227, 245, 263, 266, 313

hallucination, 32, 118, 158, 162, 212, 224, 340, 358, 363
hard palate, 83, 177, 182, 306, 324, 326, 337, 354, 366, *See* soft palate
head and neck cancer, 133, 225, 270–1, 273, 286, 340, 348
head injury, 2, 25, 91, 126, 165, 266, 270–1, 274, 309, 315, 371, *See* traumatic brain injury
hearing
 aid, 107, 113, 117, 124, 214, 235, 248, 320
 impairmant, 229, 278, 340
hearing loss
 conductive, 16, 88, 95, 101, 103, 106–9, 116–17, 125, 127, 309, 320, 329, 340, 355, 371
 sensorineural, 16, 19, 102–3, 106–8, 110, 117, 126, 327, 331, 340, 348, 353, 359, 365
hemiparesis, 340
hemiplegia, 97, 340
herpes simplex encephalitis, 90, 127, 340, *See* encephalitis
histology, 92, 320, 340, 344
HIV infection, 331
hoarseness, 19, 32, 105, 122, 125, 161, 168, 202–4, 270, 340
homonymy, 52, 55, 365
humour, 20, 212, 340, *See* joke
Huntington's disease, 127
hyoid bone, 105, 340, 370
hyperactivity, 119, 223, 322, 341
hyperadduction, 19, 267, 341, 374
hyperfunctional voice disorder, 201, 205, 341, 351
hypernasal resonance, 182, 341, 352
hypernasality, 95, 213, 341, 351
hyperreflexia, 98, 341, 367
hypertonia, 177, 341
hypoglossal nerve, 98, 177, 341

hypokinetic dysarthria, 90, 92, 341, 349
hypomimia, 251, 341
hyponasality, 213, *See* hypernasality
hypophonia, 251, 342

idiom, 16, 20, 32, 57, 159, 193, 212, 315, 337, 342
illocutionary force, 356
immittance audiometry, 111, 322, 342
impedance audiometry, 111, 117, 342
implicature, 57–9, 61, 77, 81–2, 85, 307, 330, 342, 348, 359
impulsivity, 119, 223, 322, 342
inattention, 119, 223, 322, 342
incidence, 16, 33, 89, 91, 95, 103–4, 125, 198, 259, 308, 323, 333, 336, 342, 373
incomplete partition dysplasia, 102, 342
incus, 39, 103, 342, 349, 355
indirect speech act, 20, 57, 342
inference, 60–1, 81, 137, 153, 187–8, 193, 212, 241, 343, 364
inferencing, 238, 240, 242, 343
inflectional morphology, 45–7, 343
inflectional suffix, 46–7, 66, 78, 82, 237, 307, 343
information management, 174, 343
informational encapsulation, 147, 151, 343, 349
inner ear, 73, 102, 106, 108–9, 327, 340, 343, 348–9, 355, 363, 365, 373
intellectual disability, 5, 90, 97, 139, 185, 211–12, 237, 245, 271, 320, 331–3, 338, 343, 346, 353, 360, 363, 365–7, 376, *See* learning disability
intelligence quotient (IQ), 343
intelligibility, 41, 44–5, 72, 83, 92, 167, 172, 176, 178, 181, 198, 213–14, 221, 223, 263, 273, 320, 329, 339, 343
intercostal muscle, 93, 344
intercostal nerve, 93, 344
International Classification of Functioning, Disability and Health (ICF), 167, 197, 214–15, 344
intonation, 80, 360
intubation, 335, 369
inversion, 49, 56, 80, 344
irony, 58–9, 77–8, 344, 353, 363, *See* sarcasm
iteration, 195, 200, 333, 369, *See* stuttering

jargon, 295, 338, 375
jitter, 123, 202, 204, 206, 344, *See* shimmer
joke, 193, 279, *See* humour

lamina propria, 92, 344
Landau-Kleffner syndrome, 235, 351, 356
language
 acquisition, 65, 75, 78, 81–2, 86, 140, 325–6, 331, 366
 battery, 168, 184–5, 194
 decoding, 22, 73–4, 76, 344

language (cont.)
  delay, 13, 33, 89, 168, 239, 243, 262, 266, 278, 344
  development, 19, 33, 47–8, 67, 69, 78, 80–2, 84, 86, 116–17, 134, 146, 199, 240, 243, 271, 344, 351, 357, 364
  encoding, 22, 71–2, 76, 345
  expressive, 19, 31, 56, 65, 80, 116, 165, 168, 170–3, 184–5, 194, 240, 244, 266, 344, 349, 375
  pathology, 205
  receptive, 19, 28, 65, 116, 165, 167–8, 170–3, 184–5, 194, 244, 266, 344, 349
  signed, 320
  spoken, 18, 26, 66, 69, 71–2, 76, 233, 235, 237, 239, 266, 271, 280, 320, 333, 347, 364
  written, 18, 69, 71–2, 76, 165, 216, 320, 333, 355, 364
language disorder
  expressive, 13, 15, 18–22, 32, 336, 345
  receptive, 13, 18–19, 21–2, 32, 278, 305, 345
laryngeal apraxia, 236, 335, 345
laryngeal cancer, 16, 88, 106, 121, 126, 204, 206, 249, 251, 266, 335, 345, 355, *See* cancer
laryngectomy, 25, 106, 121, 126, 207, 249, 253, 266, 287, 291, 309, 335, 339, 345, 352, 354, 357, 369
laryngology, 287, 345
laryngomalacia, 104, 106, 126, 345, 369
laryngopharyngeal reflux, 252, 345
laryngoscopy, 19, 202, 206, 270, 345
larynx, 35, 72, 88, 94, 100, 104–6, 126–7, 169, 178, 201–2, 205–6, 209, 250, 252, 320, 330, 335, 337–8, 340, 345, 355, 357, 362, 370, 375
learning disability, 158, 287, 292, 343, 346, *See* intellectual disability
left hemisphere, 32, 77, 88, 209, 346, *See* right hemisphere
left-hemisphere damage, 363, *See* right-hemisphere damage
lesion, 19, 88, 90, 97–8, 100, 110, 122, 149, 202, 250, 321, 337, 341, 346, 363, 373
levator veli palatini, 93, 95–6, 346
levodopa, 99, 333, 346
Lewy body dementia, 360
lexical
  diversity, 192, 194, 346
  reiteration, 62, 64, 328, 346
  relation, 16, 51, 55, 70–1, 346
  retrieval, 168, 326, 329, 337, 346, 376, *See* word retrieval
  semantics, 51, 55, 191, 194, 347, 365
  stress, 210, 347
limb apraxia, 180, 347
linguistic competence, 48, 347
linguistics, 15–16, 34–5, 48, 51, 54–5, 59, 61–2, 64, 68, 77–8, 82, 87, 371, 374

literacy, 9, 28, 31, 144, 229, 231, 233, 236, 263, 287, 347
lower motor neuron, 98, 337, 341, 347, 350, 361, 372, *See* upper motor neuron

macroglossia, 94, 177, 323, 347
magnetoencephalography (MEG), 99, 347
Makaton, 5, 22, 24, 235, 347
mandible, 94, 106, 177, 347, 349, 355, 358, 371
mandibulectomy, 106, 126, 347
mania, 342, 370
manner of articulation, 36, 40, 83, 233, 347, *See* place of articulation
manometry, 208–9, 347
mastication, 124, 207, 348
mastoid bone, 103, 109, 348
mastoidectomy, 103, 348
maxillofacial surgery, 100, 120, 123, 127, 310, 348
maxim, 58, 61, 81, 159, 348
mean length of utterance (MLU), 348
memory
  autobiographical, 348
  episodic, 131, 165, 319, 348
  long-term, 348
  semantic, 53, 55, 348, 364
  short-term, 187, 274, 348
  working, 17, 142–4, 152, 187, 348, 376
Ménière's disease, 109–10, 309, 348, 362, 371
meningitis, 19, 92, 97, 103, 126, 309, 348, 365
mental
  flexibility, 152, 336
  health, 2, 28, 88, 116–17, 119–20, 133, 158–9, 162, 275, 286–7, 305, 361, 371
  representation, 70, 136, 147, 328
  state, 56–7, 130, 137–8, 140, 164, 328, 370
  status, 98, 349
metaphor, 16, 20, 32, 57–8, 77–8, 147, 159, 193, 212, 315, 349, 353
micrognathia, 94, 96, 128, 176–7, 349, 358, 371
microtia, 101, 106, 321, 340, 349
middle ear, 39, 95, 101, 103, 106, 109, 111, 124, 127, 321–2, 326, 329, 336, 340, 342, 348–9, 355, 368, 372
middle ear cleft, 103, 349
mild cognitive impairment, 132, 156, 349
minimal pair, 41, 230, 233–4, 329, 349
Möbius syndrome, 126, 309
modularity, 131, 147, 151, 349, *See* cognitive module
monoloudness, 178, 349
monophthong, 36, 41, 85, 307, 349
monopitch, 178, 350, 358
morpheme, 45, 47–8, 80, 82, 190, 218, 319, 343, 348, 350, 359, 369, 376
morphology, 9, 15, 17, 34–5, 45–8, 65, 78, 82–3, 149, 183, 186–7, 193, 306, 326, 343, 350
morphosyntax, 237, 350
motor development, 64, 134–5, 332, 350

motor execution, 72, 76, 177, 350
motor milestone, 134, 140, 163, 171–2, 198, 350
motor neurone disease, 23, 25, 31, 98, 125, 127, 219, 221, 228, 235, 255, 265, 273, 320, 337–8, 350, 356, 363, *See* amyotrophic lateral sclerosis
motor programming, 177, 230–2, 320, 345, 350, 354
motor speech disorder, 2, 8, 15–16, 39, 98, 178, 180, 183, 216, 232, 234, 236, 265, 301, 320, 350
motor speech execution, 22, 266, 313, 350
motor speech programming, 22, 266, 313, 350
multidisciplinary team, 100, 133, 146, 157, 163–4, 268–75, 300, 326, 350
multilingualism, 34, 67, 69, 351
multiple negation, 66, 351
multiple sclerosis (MS), 98
muscle tension dysphonia, 253, 267, 341, 351
mutism, 18, 26, 351

naming, 52–3, 67, 77, 139, 149, 154, 190, 197, 210, 243, 266
narrative
  coherence, 16, 20, 63–4, 220
  discourse, 174–5, 192, 351
  oral, 187
  production, 62, 64, 164, 168, 172, 174, 194
nasal
  emission, 178, 266, 351
  polyp, 125
  turbulence, 178, 351
nasogastric tube, 169, 258, 260, 272, 351
nasometer, 17, 169, 182, 351
nasometry, 169, 182–3, 352
nasopharynx, 93, 336, 349, 352, 357, 366
nativism, 78, 82, 326, 352
near infrared spectroscopy (NIRS), 99, 352
neck stoma, 254, 352
negative symptom, 118, 158, 212, 352, 358, 363, *See* positive symptom, schizophrenia
neoplasm, 324, 345, 354, 357
neurodegenerative
  disease, 25, 98, 235, 273, 319, 324, 337–8, 350, 363
  disorder, 100, 180, 221, 270
neurodevelopment, 97
neurodevelopmental disorder, 81, 119, 134, 157, 211, 213, 215, 271, 321–2, 325, 338, 341, 352
neurogenic communication disorder, 88, 91, 352
neurogenic dysphagia, 207, 257–8, 334, 352, *See* dysphagia
neurogenic stuttering, 91, 195, 200, 357, *See* psychogenic stuttering
neurologist, 2, 98–100, 167, 172, 209, 268, 271–2, 275, 300, 314, 352

neurology, 15–17, 35, 88, 96, 99, 305, 308, 352, 359
neuropragmatics, 77–8, 353
neuropsychologist, 17, 132, 152, 154, 157, 163, 174, 268, 275, 310, 315, 326, 353
neuropsychology, 17–18, 129–30, 132–3, 151, 157, 326, 353
neurosurgery, 18, 99–100, 353
noise-induced hearing loss, 103, 109, 126, 309, 353, 371, *See* hearing loss
noise-to-harmonics ratio, 204, 353
non-literal language, 58, 193, 337
non-oral feeding, 2, 19, 121, 260, 334, 353, 355
non-verbal communication, 130, 328, 336, 365
Noonan syndrome, 134, 353
norm-referenced test, 174, 176, 180, 183, 191, 194, 353
nosology, 119, 166, 215, 353

occupational
  functioning, 116–17, 160, 220, 222, 244, 375
  therapist, 268, 271, 283, 315, 353
oesophageal
  dysphagia, 121, 208–9, 318, 334, 348, 354, *See* dysphagia
  speech, 250, 253–4, 266, 354
  voice, 254, 370
oesophagectomy, 105, 121, 354
oesophagitis, 207, 354
oesophagoscopy, 208, 354
oesophagus, 106, 121, 206, 208, 219, 254, 318, 325, 339, 345, 353–4, 362, 369, 373
olfaction, 93, 354
oncologist, 271, 354
oncology, 120, 123, 125, 127, 310, 354, 359
oral
  apraxia, 178, 180, 183, 321, 354
  cancer, 96, 106, 121, 126, 339, 354
  cavity, 40, 42, 94, 100, 106, 202, 206, 208–9, 250, 253, 257, 314, 335, 340, 354, 356–7
  feeding, 33, 168, 258, 272, 315, 353, 355
orbicularis oris, 93, 336, 355
organ of Corti, 39, 103, 327, 355
organic voice disorder, 90, 201, 205, 355, *See* functional voice disorder
oropharyngeal dysphagia, 208–9, 257, 314, 334, 355, *See* dysphagia
orthodontics, 120, 123, 127, 310, 337, 355
orthography, 149, 355
ossicle, 39, 101, 103, 108, 111, 126, 326, 342, 348–9, 355, 368, 372
otitis media, 88, 95, 108, 111, 125, 329, 348, 355, 372
otolaryngologist, 103–6, 122–3, 127, 160, 201–2, 208, 268, 270, 274, 355, 368
otolaryngology, 15, 88, 122, 126, 308, 355

otorhinolaryngology, 16–17, 88, 100, 305, 335, 345, 355, *See* ENT medicine
otosclerosis, 95, 329, 355, 368

paediatrician, 163, 167, 171–2, 271, 356
paediatrics, 120, 123, 127, 310, 355
palatal lift, 234, 356
palate
  artificial, 183, 335
  hard, 83, 177, 182, 306, 324, 326, 337, 354, 366
  soft, 36, 72, 83, 95, 177, 182, 202, 207, 209, 266, 306, 324, 326, 337, 346, 356, 366, 373
palliative care, 120, 123, 127, 310, 356
paralysis, 96, 105, 201, 251, 340–1, 366, 373
paresis, 96, 251, 366, 374
Parkinson's disease, 90, 92, 98–9, 126, 202, 205, 219, 234, 251, 258–9, 267, 292, 301, 324, 333, 341, 346, 349, 356
partial cricotracheal resection, 105, 356
particularization, 48–9, 356, 372
passive articulator, 36, 318, 347, 356, *See* active articulator
pathogenesis, 122, 251, 356
pause, 118–19, 158, 193, 195, 248, 254, 323
perception, 6, 10, 25, 35, 37, 39–41, 65, 69, 73–4, 76, 86, 104, 129, 131, 145–6, 151, 168, 182, 198, 204, 248, 251, 269, 280–1, 285, 288, 315–16, 328, 340, 343, 349, 352, 356–8, 361–2
percutaneous endoscopic gastrostomy, 258, 260, 353, 356
performative verb, 56, 356
peripheral nervous system, 16, 88, 93, 333, 353, 357
perseveration, 195, 200, 295, 333, 369
pharyngectomy, 106, 357
pharynx, 105–6, 126, 202, 206, 209, 219, 252, 257, 335, 338, 340, 345, 352, 356–7, 373, 375
phenotype, 92, 357
phonation, 93, 96, 106, 124, 126, 161, 177, 179, 202, 205–6, 250, 254, 267, 310, 320, 333, 341, 345, 357
phonemic cue, 210, 311, 330
phonetics, 15, 17, 34–7, 39–41, 83, 305, 357
phonological
  awareness, 229, 231, 233, 236, 238, 240–1, 357
  development, 29, 78–9, 344, 357
  disorder, 9, 15, 33, 42–3, 79, 82, 223, 237, 357, 367
  feature, 42, 45, 52, 357
  process, 43–5, 79, 82–3, 181, 183, 217, 332, 358
phonology, 15, 17, 34–5, 41–2, 45, 78–9, 82–3, 149, 172, 175–6, 183, 193, 230, 240–1, 326, 347, 358
phrenic nerve, 93, 358
physiology, 16–17, 35, 87–8, 92–6, 101, 106, 121, 124–5, 177, 250, 253, 256–7, 260, 305, 309, 337, 358

physiotherapist, 268, 283, 315–16, 358
Piaget, J., 358
Pierre Robin syndrome, 94, 101, 128, 349, 358
pitch, 37, 88, 94, 123, 178, 202, 204–5, 248, 250, 272, 322, 330, 338, 349, 358, 368, *See* fundamental frequency
place of articulation, 36, 41, 43, 83, 233, 358, *See* manner of articulation
planning, 7, 16, 29, 72, 76, 86, 152, 220, 230–3, 236, 245, 266, 284–5, 313, 315, 336, 347, 350
pointing, 50, 56, 81
politeness, 342
positive symptom, 32, 213, 331, 352, 358, 363, 370, *See* negative symptom, schizophrenia
positron emission tomography (PET), 99, 359
posterior fossa tumour, 351, *See* brain tumour
post-natal period, 325
poverty of speech, 118, 158, 162, 213, 319, 352, 359, 363, *See* alogia
Prader-Willi syndrome, 164, 337
pragmatic development, 78, 81–2, 345, 359
pragmatic language impairment, 20, 192, 222, 359, 366
pragmatics, 9, 15–17, 34–5, 55, 57, 61, 63, 78, 82–3, 153, 171, 175–6, 184, 189, 191–2, 195, 198, 248–9, 305, 312, 326, 359, 363
prefixation, 46–7, 359, 376
pre-natal period, 96–7
presbycusis, 107, 109, 117, 309, 359, 362, 371
presbylarynx, 202, 324
presupposition, 60–1, 85, 184, 307, 329, 359
prevalence, 16, 28, 32, 89, 91, 94, 97, 103–4, 108, 117, 120–1, 125, 245, 308, 324, 335, 351, 359
primary CNS lymphoma, 360
primary motor cortex, 93, 325, 360–1
primary progressive aphasia, 77, 360, *See* dementia
prison, 28–9, 133, 275
problem-solving, 15, 17–18, 132, 146, 151–2, 360–1
procedural discourse, 64, 194
professional voice user, 90, 125, 253, 360, 375
prognosis, 88, 360
progressive non-fluent aphasia, 235, 338, *See* dementia
progressive supranuclear palsy, 338, 356, *See* Parkinson's disease
prolongation, 195, 247, 360, 369, *See* stuttering
prolonged speech, 247, 249, 313, 360
prosody, 178–9, 198, 234, 333, 341, 358, 360, 363
protraction, 369, *See* stuttering
proximal aetiology, 90–1, 360, *See* distal aetiology
psychiatrist, 118–20, 127, 211, 271, 275, 361
psychiatry, 15, 17, 88, 117, 119–20, 127, 305, 308, 361
psychogenic dysphonia, 120, 132, 159–60, 162, 165, 201, 270, 310, 319, 361

psychogenic stuttering, 91, 195, 200, 357, *See* neurogenic stuttering
psychological impact, 12–14, 305, 361
psychologist, 13, 17, 84, 132–3, 135, 138–41, 143, 146–7, 158–9, 161–3, 165, 175, 211, 270, 310, 327, 332, 358, 361
psychology, 17, 121, 129–33, 146, 151, 157, 163, 262, 282, 327, 332, 334, 349
psychometric test, 131, 141, 143–4, 146, 164, 361
psychopathology, 157–9, 162, 361
psychotherapy, 119–20, 327, 361
puberphonia, 8, 361
pure tone audiometry, 16, 107, 109–10, 117, 124, 310, 361, 367
pyramidal system, 98, 361
pyriform sinus, 258–9, 357, 361, 373

quality of life, 33, 116–17, 162, 197–8, 200, 204–6, 218, 221, 225, 244, 253, 255, 293, 322, 358, 362, 366

radiotherapy, 99, 249, 253–4, 324, 330, 345, 362
randomized controlled trial, 261–2, 264, 267, 362
reading, 9, 13–14, 31, 35, 40, 76, 143, 148–9, 171, 184–5, 187–8, 190, 229, 233, 238, 240–1, 251, 295, 312, 334, 364
reasoning, 81, 131–2, 137–8, 142–4, 146, 151, 238, 242, 263, 327, 338, 361–2
recruitment, 11, 98, 103, 106, 362
recurrent laryngeal nerve, 105, 362, 370
reference, 34, 51, 54, 63–4, 94, 150, 213, 268, 320, 347, 362, 371
referent, 27, 60, 62–3, 74, 193, 362
reflux laryngitis, 88, 318, 362
register, 65–6, 68, 362
rehabilitation, 2–3, 25–7, 102, 113, 132–3, 152, 154, 163, 243, 268, 270–1, 273, 275–6, 284, 295, 300, 322, 326, 353, 370
reliability, 174–5, 198, 363
repair, 27, 195, 218, 293, 330, *See* trouble source
repetition, 27, 56, 149, 178, 190, 197, 213, 236, 241–2, 247, 304, 332, 346, 363, 369, *See* stuttering
repetitive language, 32
reported speech, 168
request for clarification, 330
resonance, 9, 95, 99, 178, 250–1, 341, 351
resonation, 124, 177, 179, 333
respiration, 92, 106, 124, 177–8, 333, 345, 355, 363, 371
respiratory therapist, 273, 363
response inhibition, 132, 363
Rett syndrome, 214, 363
right hemisphere, 98, 363, *See* left hemisphere
right-hemisphere damage, 16, 20, 32, 153, 328, 363, *See* left-hemisphere damage
right-hemisphere language disorder, 31, 363

Royal College of Speech and Language Therapists, 1, 14, 34, 68, 87, 129, 166, 268, 272, 294, 336

sarcasm, 57, 77, 137, 139, 193, 363, *See* irony
scala tympani, 114, 323, 327, 363
schema, 147, *See* script
schizophrenia, 15, 32, 46, 58–9, 66, 71, 86, 88, 117–20, 157–9, 162, 211–13, 215, 224, 331–2, 340, 352, 358, 363, 366, 370–1
script, 190, *See* schema
Searle, J. R., 367
seizure, 235, 274, 315, 363
selective attention, 154, 157, 322, 364, *See* attention
selective mutism, 9, 320
self-esteem, 12–14, 31, 122, 219, 221–2, 253, 279, 361, 364
semantic
  component, 52–3, 55, 328, 364
  cue, 311, 330
  dementia, 53, 334, 338, 364, *See* primary progressive aphasia
  development, 80–2, 364
  field, 16
  impairment, 127, 150
  knowledge, 52, 65, 364
  network, 71, 76, 86, 243, 364
  paraphasia, 52, 71, 347, 364
  relation, 51, 70–1, 73, 80, 82, 86, 185, 188, 312, 321, 335, 346, 364–5
  role, 53–5, 84, 365, 370
  system, 147, 149–50
semantics, 9, 15, 17, 34–5, 51–5, 76, 78, 82–3, 149–50, 159, 162, 168, 183–4, 191–2, 194, 237–8, 244, 305, 326, 328, 347, 364–5
semicircular canal, 102, 327, 343, 365, 373
sense, 51, 54, 63, 69, 147, 262, 291, 328, 343, 354, 365, 374
sensorineural hearing loss, 16, 19, 102–3, 106–8, 110, 117, 126, 327, 331, 340, 348, 353, 359, 365
sexual dimorphism, 94, 365
shimmer, 202, 204, 206, 365, *See* jitter
silence, 281
silent aspiration, 168, 172, 219, 321, 365, *See* aspiration
single-photon emission computed tomography (SPECT), 76, 365
social
  communication, 56, 192, 211–13, 321–2, 365
  context, 35, 191, 212
  functioning, 116, 263, 366
  impact, 12–14, 301, 304, 366
  integration, 263, 366
  interaction, 13, 19, 56, 64, 189, 192, 281, 322, 330, 366
  interactionism, 78, 82, 326, 366
  isolation, 14, 22, 304

social (cont.)
    relationship, 57, 59, 61, 159, 211–12, 362, 365
    withdrawal, 12, 122, 217, 363, 366
    worker, 271, 274–5, 366
social (pragmatic) communication disorder, 4, 211, 214, 359, 365
social communication skill, 3, 171–2, 211, 279, 366
socioeconomic status, 28, 89, 91, 191, 366
soft palate, 36, 72, 83, 95, 177, 182, 202, 207, 209, 266, 306, 324, 326, 337, 346, 350, 356, 373, *See* hard palate
spasmodic dysphonia, 122–3, 351
spastic dysarthria, 97, 126, 177, 366, *See* dysarthria
spasticity, 97, 274, 367
specific language impairment (SLI), 46, 222, 237
speech act, 55–6, 61, 74, 171, 174, 184, 191–2, 342, 359, 367
speech and language therapist, 1, 4, 10, 94, 116, 129, 131–2, 160, 167, 192–3, 218, 281–2, 295, 314, 350, 367
speech and language therapy, 1–3, 10–11, 14, 30–1, 34, 87, 129, 133–4, 152, 243, 259–61, 263, 268, 271–3, 276, 282, 299–301, 367
speech audiometry, 110, 117, 124, 310, 322, 367
Speech Pathology Australia, 5, 268, 284, 286–8
speech production, 35, 65, 69, 77, 92–5, 97, 99, 120, 125–6, 134, 140, 172, 177–83, 195, 203, 209, 219, 228–36, 245–6, 249, 254, 266–7, 274, 278, 320–1, 325–6, 334, 337, 339, 341, 345–6, 349–50, 354, 357, 363, 367, 373
speech sound disorder, 8, 14, 23, 31, 42–5, 66, 83, 85, 219, 221, 225–6, 231–2, 234, 236, 262–3, 329, 358, 367, *See* developmental phonological disorder
Speech-Language and Audiology Canada, 286, 288–9
speech-language pathologist, 1, 3, 7–9, 124–5, 214, 225, 232, 282, 299, 328, 367, 373
speech-language pathology, 214, 216, 259, 265, 276, 285, 288, 320, 367
spinal nerve, 93, 344, 367
spirometer, 179, 367
stammering, 10, 213, 216, 246, 291, 293, 298, 337, 368–9, *See* stuttering
standardized test, 166, 173
stapedectomy, 96, 355, 368
stapedius muscle, 111, 127, 368
stenosis, 101, 369
stimulability, 181, 231, 234, 237, 368
stoma, 352, 369
stopping, 15, 44, 79, 82, 182, 306, 312, 332, 358, 368
story
    generation, 194
    grammar, 192, 194–5, 238, 266, 368
    telling, 175, 212, 240

stress, 72, 161, 164, 195, 250, 347, 360
stria vascularis, 108, 368
stridor, 104, 126, 345, 368
stroboscopy, 202–3, 206, 368
strobovideolaryngoscopy, 202, 368
stroke, 4, 12, 19, 21, 25, 31–3, 50, 52, 76–7, 93, 96–7, 100, 125, 132, 148–9, 156–7, 165, 180, 191, 206, 209, 214, 219–20, 225, 234, 237, 255, 258, 260, 265–6, 271, 276, 293, 295, 298, 320, 325, 334, 340–1, 346, 355, 363–4, 367–8, 373, *See* cerebrovascular accident
struggle behaviour, 247, 369, *See* stuttering
stuttering, *See* stammering
    developmental, 5, 77, 89–90, 125, 127, 164, 199, 331
    neurogenic, 91, 195, 200, 352
    psychogenic, 91, 195, 200, 361
style, 26, 65, 67–8, 141, 175, 245, 283, 369
subdural haematoma, 18, 273, 369
subglottic stenosis, 104–6, 356, 369
submucous cleft palate, 177, 324, 369, *See* cleft lip and palate
substance use disorder, 162
substantia nigra, 356, *See* Parkinson's disease
substitution, 43–5, 62, 64, 232, 266, 321, 328, 368–9
suck reflex, 177, 369
suffixation, 46–7, 369, 376
sulcus vocalis, 251, 369
supraglottic laryngectomy, 206, 345, 369, *See* laryngectomy
supraglottoplasty, 105, 369
surgical voice reconstruction, 254
surgical voice restoration, 253–4, 369
swallowing, 1–2, 4, 8, 11–12, 14–22, 25, 27, 29–31, 33, 87, 90–1, 93, 96–7, 99–100, 106, 121, 126–7, 132–3, 152, 166–70, 172, 182, 206–10, 213, 215, 219–20, 225, 254, 256–60, 267–73, 275–6, 281–2, 284–91, 294–6, 298, 301, 314, 319, 321, 323–4, 330, 334, 336, 348, 350, 352, 361, 366–7, 372–5
syntactic development, 29, 79, 82, 370, 372
syntax, *See* grammar
    expressive, 50, 65
    receptive, 84, 168, 171, 185, 195, 263, 362, 370
systematic review, 25, 31, 232, 235–6, 258, 262–4, 267, 370

tangentiality, 118
teasing, 193
telerehabilitation, 223, 225, 227, 370
thematic role, 54–5, 370
theory of mind, 57, 121, 130, 137, 140, 336, 364, 370
thought disorder, 71, 333, 338, 358, 363, 370, *See* schizophrenia
thyroid cartilage, 203, 330, 340, 370

thyroidectomy, 105, 126, 370
tic disorder, 213, 370
tinnitus, 104, 106, 109, 318, 348, 371
tongue cancer, 206, *See* cancer
top-down processing, 40, 74, 76, 371
topic
   development, 371
   digression, 328
   management, 174, 184, 192, 195, 217, 371
   termination, 371
total communication, 244, 266, 371
Tourette's syndrome, 144
tracheostomy, 169, 287, 349, 371
tracheotomy, 105, 126, 371, 374
transcranial magnetic stimulation, 99, 371
traumatic brain injury, 9, 12, 16, 25, 149, 151–3, 194, 216, 231, 293, 309, 323, 328, 336, 351, 366, 369, 371, *See* head injury
Treacher Collins syndrome, 94, 101, 106, 371
trisomy 21, 90, 333, 339, 372, *See* Down syndrome
trouble source, 330, *See* repair
T-unit, 194, 372
turn-taking, 167, 174, 192, 195, 372
tympanic membrane, 39, 103, 111, 334, 349, 372
tympanometry, 111, 310, 342, 372

ultrasound, 182, 278, 372
universal grammar, 48–9, 356, 372
upper motor neuron, 98, 341, 361, 366, 372, *See* lower motor neuron
upper oesophageal sphincter, 207, 251, 254, 257, 354, 373
utterance interpretation, 74, 76, 328

VACTERL/VATER association, 101, 373
vagus nerve, 93, 346, 362, 373
validity, 170, 174, 198, 247, 373
vallecula, 257–9, 373
varices, 374, *See* capillary ectasias
vascular dementia, 338, 360, *See* dementia
velopharyngeal
   closure, 126, 234
   incompetence, 95–6, 125, 214, 219, 234, 340–1, 346, 356, 373
   insufficiency, 182, 352, 373
   port, 16, 35, 95, 182, 228, 351, 356, 373
velum, 32, 36, 93, 95–6, 182, 373
vernacular, 67, 85, 351, 373
vestibule, 102, 314, 327, 342, 373
vestibulocochlear nerve, 40, 327, 355, 373

videoendoscopy, 207, 209, 374
videofluoroscopy, 4, 168, 182–3, 207–9, 257, 273, 275, 287, 301, 311, 374
vision, 93
visual
   agnosia, 150, 374
   field, 235
vocabulary
   expressive, 374
   receptive, 143, 362
vocal
   abuse and misuse, 90, 250, 374–5
   fold paralysis, 104–6, 123, 126, 202, 321, 355, 374
   hygiene, 122, 161, 252–4, 270, 274, 374–5
   intensity, 202, 253, 349, 356, 374
   nodule, 19, 88, 90, 105–6, 125–7, 201–2, 205, 250, 267, 309, 360, 374
   polyp, 32, 205, 375
   tract, 42, 229, 250, 358, 375
vocal fold haemorrhage, 252, 374
vocational impact, 12, 14, 305, 375
voice
   mutation, 94, 361, 375
   onset time, 40, 375
   prosthesis, 250, 253–5, 369, 375
   quality, 160, 178, 204, 254, 351, 365, 375
   therapy, 160–1, 249–50, 253–4, 267, 311, 339, 375
   transsexual, 124
voice disorder
   functional, 91, 201, 205, 338
   hyperfunctional, 201, 205, 341, 351
   neurogenic, 374
   organic, 90, 201, 205, 355
   psychogenic, 91, 133, 160, 205
voicing, 36, 40–2, 44, 79, 82–3, 161, 180–2, 204, 233, 306, 311, 375

Wernicke's area, 93, 375
Williams syndrome, 90, 107, 125, 144, 339, 376
word retrieval, 243, 376, *See* lexical retrieval
word-finding difficulty, 220, 320, 376, *See* anomia
word-formation, 45, 47, 324, 327, 329, 331, 359, 369, 376
World Health Organization, 167, 174, 197, 211, 214–15, 243, 274, 344, 362
world knowledge, 74, 76
writing, 9, 66, 76, 78, 140, 184–5, 189–90, 194, 198, 234, 273, 321, 346, 350, 355, 371

Printed in Great Britain
by Amazon